FAMILY CARE OF OLDER PEOPLE IN EUROPE

Biomedical and Health Research

Volume 46

Earlier published in this series

Vol. 15. N. Katunuma, H. Kido, H. Fritz and J. Travis (Eds.), Medical Aspects of Proteases and Protease Inhibitors
Vol. 16. P.I. Haris and D. Chapman (Eds.), New Biomedical Materials
Vol. 17. J.J.F. Schroots, R. Fernandez-Ballesteros and G. Rudinger (Eds.), Aging in Europe
Vol. 18. R. Leidl (Ed.), Health Care and its Financing in the Single European Market
Vol. 19. P. Jenner and R. Demirdamar (Eds.), Dopamine Receptor Subtypes
Vol. 20. P.I. Haris and D. Chapman (Eds.), Biomembrane Structures
Vol. 21. N. Yoganandan, F.A. Pintar, S.J. Larson and A. Sances Jr. (Eds.), Frontiers in Head and Neck Trauma
Vol. 22. J. Matsoukas and T. Mavromoustakos (Eds.), Bioactive Peptides in Drug Discovery and Design: Medical Aspects
Vol. 23. M. Hallen (Ed.), Human Genome Analysis
Vol. 24. S.S. Baig (Ed.), Cancer Research Supported under BIOMED 1
Vol. 25. N.J. Gooderham (Ed.), Drug Metabolism: Towards the Next Millennium
Vol. 26. P. Jenner (Ed.), A Molecular Biology Approach to Parkinson's Disease
Vol. 27. P.A. Frey and D.B. Northrop (Eds.), Enzymatic Mechanisms
Vol. 28. A.M.N. Gardner and R. Fox, The Venous System in Health and Disase
Vol. 29. G. Pawelec (Ed.), EUCAMBIS: Immunology and Ageing in Europe
Vol. 30. J.F. Stoltz, M. Singh and P. Riha, Hemorheology in Practice
Vol. 31. B.J. Njio, A. Stenvik, R.S. Ireland and B. Prahl-Andersen (Eds.), EURO-QUAL
Vol. 32. In production
Vol. 33. H.H. Goebel, S.E. Mole and B.D. Lake (Eds.), The Neuronal Ceroid Lipofuscinoses (Batten Disease)
Vol. 34. G.J. Bellingan and G.J. Laurent (Eds.), Acute Lung Injury: From Inflammation to Repair
Vol. 35. M. Schlaud (Ed.), Comparison and Harmonisation of Denominator Data for Primary Health Care Research in Countries of the European Community
Vol. 36. F.F. Parl, Estrogens, Estrogen Receptor and Breast Cancer
Vol. 37. J.M. Ntambi (Ed.), Adipocyte Biology and Hormone Signaling
Vol. 38. N. Yoganandan and F.A. Pintar (Eds.), Frontiers in Whiplash Trauma
Vol. 39. J.-M. Graf von der Schulenburg (Ed.), The Influence of Economic Evaluation Studies on Health Care Decision-Making
Vol. 40. H. Leino-Kilpi, M. Välimäki, M. Arndt, T. Dassen, M. Gasull, C. Lemonidou, P.A. Scott, G. Bansemir, E. Cabrera, H. Papaevangelou and J. Mc Parland, Patient's Autonomy, Privacy and Informed Consent
Vol. 41. T.M. Gress (Ed.), Molecular Pathogenesis of Pancreatic Cancer
Vol. 42. J.-F. Stoltz (Ed.), Mechanobiology: Cartilage and Chondrocyte
Vol. 43. B. Shaw, G. Semb, P. Nelson, V. Brattström, K. Mølsted and B. Prahl-Andersen, The Eurocleft Project 1996-2000
Vol. 44. R. Coppo and L. Peruzzi (Eds.), Moderately Proteinuric IgA Nephropathy in the Young
Vol. 45. L. Turski, D.D. Schoepp and E.A. Cavalheiro (Eds.), Excitatory Amino Acids: Ten Years Later

ISSN: 0929-6743

Family Care of Older People in Europe

Edited by

Ian Philp

*Community Sciences Centre, Northern General Hospital,
Sheffield Institute for Studies on Ageing,
The University of Sheffield, Sheffield, United Kingdom*

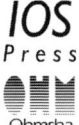

IOS Press

Ohmsha

Amsterdam • Berlin • Oxford • Tokyo • Washington, DC

© 2001, The authors mentioned in the Table of Contents

All rights reserved. No part of this book may be reproduced, stored in a retrieval system, or transmitted, in any form or by any means, without the prior written permission from the publisher.

ISBN 1 58603 153 8 (IOS Press)
ISBN 4 274 90449 0 C3047 (Ohmsha)
Library of Congress Catalog Card Number: 2001089336

Publisher
IOS Press
Nieuwe Hemweg 6B
1013 BG Amsterdam
The Netherlands
fax: +31 20 688 33 55
e-mail: order@iospress.nl

Distributor in the UK and Ireland
IOS Press/Lavis Marketing
73 Lime Walk
Headington
Oxford OX3 7AD
England
fax: +44 1865 75 0079

Distributor in the USA and Canada
IOS Press, Inc.
5795-G Burke Centre Parkway
Burke, VA 22015
USA
fax: +1 703 323 3668
e-mail: iosbooks@iospress.com

Distributor in Germany, Austria and Switzerland
IOS Press/LSL.de
Gerichtsweg 28
D-04103 Leipzig
Germany
fax: +49 341 995 4255

Distributor in Japan
Ohmsha, Ltd.
3-1 Kanda Nishiki-cho
Chiyoda-ku, Tokyo 101
Japan
fax: +81 3 3233 2426

LEGAL NOTICE
The publisher is not responsible for the use which might be made of the following information.

PRINTED IN THE NETHERLANDS

Preface

There is now universal recognition that populations are ageing. Initial concerns about economic and social burden are giving way to more positive views about the potential for older people to contribute to the welfare of their families, communities and societies.

Many older people remain fit, active and independent into old age, but most will experience a period of frailty prior to death. With the extension of healthy active life, frailty is commonly experienced in late old age. Frailty results from the interaction of multiple problems, including long-term (chronic) diseases, increased susceptibility to new (acute) illnesses, and decline in physiological control of balance, strength, bladder control, vision, hearing and cognitive (brain) function. This is exacerbated by environmental challenge, for example from social isolation, inadequate housing and poverty.

- An appropriate response to frailty is therefore complex. Its components include:
- Promoting health and well-being through multi-sectoral co-ordinated activity involving health, social care, housing, transport, education, crime and incomes policies.
- Responding rapidly to acute illness before a chain of events leads to irreversible decline.
- Active management of chronic diseases.
- Rehabilitation to maximise independent functioning.
- Environmental adjustment using assistive technology.
- The provision of personal care.

It should be noted that to maximise the independence and autonomy of frail older people, personal care should only be required when all possibilities for health promotion, medical treatment, rehabilitation and environmental adjustment have been pursued. Furthermore, personal care can be delivered in a variety of ways, involving formal services as well as informal care by families, friends, neighbours, and in a variety of settings, including institutional care.

Overly simplistic responses to individual and population ageing based on fear and ignorance lead to premature deployment of long-term care services and missed opportunities for restoring the independence of the older person. Also, a false dichotomy can develop between informal and formal care. Families can be expected to meet all the care needs of the older person, whose needs therefore remain hidden from service providers, until a catastrophe occurs, the exhausted carer withdraws, the potential for rehabilitation is lost and the older person is admitted to long-term institutional care, sometimes after a prolonged period of inappropriate hospital care.

Policy makers need to understand that care for older people must involve, from an early stage, a partnership between formal services and informal carers. Furthermore, informal carers have needs in their own right and many are themselves elderly.

In this book we review the literature on family caregiving for older people, focusing on the impact of caregiving on caregivers, and on evidence for effectiveness in supporting caregivers. We then describe the care systems for older people in ten European countries (France, Germany, Greece, Italy, Netherlands, Poland, Portugal, Spain, Sweden and the United Kingdom) the contributions of informal caregivers and formal services, and how the needs of informal caregivers are assessed and met. We illustrate these descriptions with nine fictional case scenarios using three levels of dependency in an older person, and three different social environments.

Contents

Preface	v
Chapter 1: Europe (April 1998)	1
Liesbeth Borgermans, Mike Nolan and Ian Philp	
Chapter 2: France (October 1998)	27
Judith Chwalow, Andrea Bagnall, Christine Baudoin and Fabienne Elgrably	
Chapter 3: Germany (November 2000)	49
Hanneli Döhner and Christopher Kofahl	
Chapter 4: Greece (September 1998)	75
Judith Triantifillou and Elizabeth Mestheneos	
Chapter 5: Italy	97
Giovanni Lamura, Maria Gabriella Melchiorre, Sabrina Quattrini, Massimo Mengani and Alberto Albertini	
Chapter 6: The Netherlands (February 2000)	135
Susan G.M. Adam and Jack B.F. Hutten	
Chapter 7: Poland (September 1998)	161
Barbara Bień, Beata Wojszel, Barbara Polityńska and Jolanta Wilmańska	
Chapter 8: Portugal (January 2000)	189
Daniela Figueiro and Liliana Sousa	
Chapter 9: Spain (December 1999)	211
Arantza Larizgoitia Jauregi	
Chapter 10: Sweden (August 1999)	237
Rolf Hässler	
Chapter 11: United Kingdom (December 1999)	255
Kate Lothian, Kevin McKee, Ian Philp and Mike Nolan	
Author Index	281

Chapter 1

Europe
(April 1998)

Liesbeth Borgermans
Arthur Andersen Business Consulting
Warandeberg No 4
B-1000
Brussels
Belgium

Mike Nolan
Professor of Gerontological Nursing
University of Sheffield
Samuel Fox House
Northern General Hospital
Herries Road
Sheffield S5 7AU
United Kingdom

Ian Philp
Professor of Health Care for Older People
University of Sheffield
Sheffield Institute for Studies on Ageing
Community Sciences Centre
Northern General Hospital
Herries Road
Sheffield S5 7AU
United Kingdom

Introduction

Caregivers in Europe

The terms "informal caregiver" or "family caregiver" have become part of the caregiving literature vocabulary. However, there is no consensus among researchers, policy makers, service-providers, caregivers or cared-for persons as to what constitutes an "informal caregiver". Definitions of an informal caregiver greatly vary. For example, researchers have defined informal caregivers according to the kind and amount of caregiving tasks they perform, the frequency of contact between caregiver and cared-for person and the type of relationship between them. Furthermore, the centrality of the caregiver in the caregiving system is often used for defining caregivers, e.g. primary caregivers having total responsibility for providing care, primary caregivers with informal help, primary caregivers with both informal and formal help, or secondary caregivers who are primarily responsible for the cared-for person.

For practical reasons, we will use the term "family caregiver" throughout this chapter because the majority of caregivers are family members. This does not mean we ignore the possible important contributions of neighbours and friends to the care of the older person. In fact, this chapter is dedicated to all informal caregivers of older persons in Europe.

A report on the assessment of family caregivers, must take into account varying aspects and concepts of family care for older persons in Europe. In previous chapters, current health policies and the cultural, social and economical-political background to family care in Europe were described. The trend toward increased longevity, increased chronic health conditions, containment of spiralling health care costs, and a decrease in the length of hospital stay, all place an increased emphasis on the family and informal caregiving system.

The aim of this chapter is the development of a *common approach* and related *framework* that will guide future *assessment* and *interventions* of *family caregivers* in Europe.

Assessment is the process of defining needs and determining eligibility for assistance against stated policy criteria [1]. Needs of the family caregiver are the requirements to enable them to achieve, maintain or restore an acceptable level of quality of life, primarily objectively defined by the family carer him/herself. A (family) caregiver is considered a person who has a significant responsibility and role in providing care for an older person.

In order to understand the conceptual pillars used in the development of both the common approach and the framework, different core components of family caregiving (assessment) will be described and discussed.

Two main perspectives towards family caregivers will be discussed in the context of this chapter, including an economical-political and a family oriented perspective. The economical-political perspective in which caregivers are perceived as resources often experiencing burden, has highly influenced the theoretical concepts of family caregiving and the interventions proposed in caregiving literature. As a result, the needs of the caregiver are poorly conceptualised and explained only through the negative consequences of caregiving.

The guiding premises and aims of family caregiver assessment are presented thereafter, as well as the eligibility criteria for the assessment of the family caregiver.

Different Perspectives on Family Caregiving

Assessment and outcome evaluation of family caregiving can be discussed from different perspectives, including an economical-political and more in particular, a family and patient-oriented perspective [2]. These perspectives are the first component taken into account in the development of a common approach and framework that guides the assessment of the family caregiver.

An economical-political perspective

The response of virtually all developed countries to their ageing population has been to institute a policy of community care in an effort to achieve more cost-effective use of scarce resources [3,4]. In achieving this aim, increasing emphasis has been placed on the role of the family (informal) system as the mainstay of care provision [5]. Informal support systems have been found to be an alternative to institutional care of the older person by providing concrete services and emotional support, financial assistance as well as by linking the older person to needed formal community resources [6,7]. In this context, the willingness and availability of families to deliver these services to the cared-for older person are easy to document [8-12].

On one hand, family caregivers are seen as resources who are able to substitute for formal service providers [13]. At present, this is seen to be the dominant view of caregivers; their value based on financial considerations. On the other hand, caregivers are often perceived as co-clients [13], who need care from formal service providers, which blurs the boundary between who is the user and who is the carer [14].

The lack of a coherent, integrated policy and relevant assessment and service interventions for family caregivers has been documented both in the U.K [13-15], and in the U.S [16]. There is little contemporary evidence for the effectiveness of supporting family caregivers in terms of health/economic benefits, although substantial evidence is available on the impact of caregiver burden in the decision to institutionalise the cared-for person [17-21]. Moreover, the family's sense of well-being or burden is an important factor in the use of community services as well [22]. In order to develop predictive models for service use, and to improve the effectiveness of the interventions offered, separate assessments of the needs of family caregivers have become a statutory right within some European countries. Despite the rhetoric, there are many complicated issues in the heart of the family caregiver assessment debate that threaten to limit effective implementation. In the context of the COPE project, we have identified the following issues as important to take into account before and during the development of the COPE trials.

These issues are (modified and adapted [1]):

- The different organisational and value frameworks among the different national and local health authorities in Europe.
    - How will the organisational and value framework concerning family caregivers influence the development of the trials?
    - Which are the current health policies and laws in the country concerning the rights of the family caregiver?
- The generally low priority and value ascribed to care of the family caregiver within society.
    - Which of the current policies/tendencies of the national and local governments recognise the role of the family caregiver?
- The difficulty of defining "informal care and caregiver".
    - How to define "informal care" and "carer" in the trial?
- The lack of appropriate and properly validated methods of assessing need of family carers.

— Which validated measurement instruments are available in each country for the assessment of the family caregiver (for use in daily practice or for research purposes)?
- The role of the general practitioner in the application of assessment methods and instruments.
  — What role will the general practitioner play in the development of each trial?
- The implications of assessment for the way in which professionals relate to each other.
  — What role will community services centres play in the development of each trial?
  — Who will provide the assessment of the family caregiver?
  — Which are the consequences of the assessment method in the way professionals will relate to each other?
- The need to develop a common professional language in the context of family care.
  — How will the trial facilitate the development of a common language concerning family care?

A family and patient-oriented perspective

At present, geriatric assessment programs provide detailed information on the older person's functional, medical, cognitive abilities in an effort to identify conditions amenable to treatment, and ultimately to delay or prevent institutional care. General agreement exists on the components of those assessment, and reasonable instruments to measure those domains [23,24]. In comparison, measurement of components of needs, burdens and satisfactions of family caregivers, is rarely a part of regular assessment of both the cared-for person and the family carer within countries of the European Union. Even if in some circumstances the social sphere is sometimes assessed, it is the domain least likely to be subjected to standardised indicators. Nevertheless, caregiver well-being or burden appears to be an important social indicator for the quality of life of the cared-for person. Therefore, separate measurement of components of the social domain is as important as measurements of health and physical functioning [25].

From a family and patient oriented perspective, we will try to establish a partnership approach between the formal service provider and the (family) caregiver. The partnership approach in the COPE project is defined as the interactive, personalised, contextual (cultural, political and socio-economical) determined helping relationship aimed at the provision of effective support of both the family carer and the care-for person, within the resources available to the state and the family carer. In the context of this partnership approach, carers are not viewed as resources [13], but their needs are given the same status as those of the cared-for person [26]. Their co-partnership and expertise is ought to be fully acknowledged in all circumstances.

Therefore, carers' opinions and expertise are actively incorporated into the assessment process. If the latter does not occur, services offered by formal caregivers might become rejected by family caregivers [27,28]. This partnership approach within the COPE project will build further on the existing carers' charter [29], in which caregivers are perceived to have the right to:

- acknowledge and address their own needs for personal fulfilment
- easy access to information and advice
- counselling made available to them at different stages of the caring process, including bereavement counselling
- practical help in carrying out the tasks of caregiving and financial support

- skills' training and development of their potential
- support services (e.g. public health nurses, day centres, ...)
- emotional and social support
- respite care both for short spells as in day hospitals and for longer periods to enable them to have time for themselves
- expect their families, public authorities and community members to provide a plan for services and support for caregivers
- involvement at all levels of policy planning, to participate and contribute to the planning of an integrated and co-ordinated service for carers

Theoretical Concepts in the Context of Family Care

Literature on caregiving has grown significantly in both volume and sophistication in the last ten years [30], focusing on almost all aspects of family caregiving for older persons. This review includes research literature of which two important critical remarks need to be made:

> *The literature is dominated by a burden perspective, seldom including the positive aspects of family caregiving.*
> *There is an apparent lack of practice literature, describing the dynamic nature and complexity of family caregiving.*

In the context of assessment, the assessor should have a basic knowledge of the most important concepts of family caregiving that are researched today, and their use in measurement instruments, in order to understand the complexity of caregiving. The burden perspective should be replaced by a broader view on family caregiving, including positive aspects of care as well. This broader perspective might have important implications for the training of the assessor.

The following is an attempt to clarify the meanings and use of terms, in order to enhance the understanding on the components of caregiver assessment. This review does not pretend to be exhaustive.

Caregiver burden

There has been no uniform definition of burden [31]. Caregiver burden is a multifaceted construct, referring to enduring problems in a caregiving situation. Sometimes burden is described as the load or responsibilities carried, or to the time and effort required for a person to attend to the needs of another [32]. Burden is also described as an outcome variable, including decreased feelings of well-being and increased health problems [33]. Some authors describe burden as stress, the latter operationalized as hassles, or minor irritations of daily living [34]. Hassles are both transient and chronic events that are appraised by an individual as threatening his or her well-being.

Some times a distinction is made between subjective burden and objective burden. Subjective burden is defined as the mediating emotional response of a subject to caregiving, whereas objective burden refers to the impact of caregiving in terms of the amount of care given and other variables [32-35].

The consequence of this conceptual diversity is that no unequivocal conclusions can be drawn with respect to the nature of burden on caregivers, and its relationship to the functioning of those receiving care and to other psychological characteristics of the carers themselves [36]. Moreover, some authors advocate the removal of the term burden from the health care lexicography because of its pejorative connotations [37].

Caregiver stress

Caregiver burden is related to, or used as a synonym for of stress. In some stress-models stress is seen as the simply result of some kind of antecedent stimulus or event. According to this stimulus-response model, disturbing behaviour for example of the cared-for person, causes feelings of stress within family caregivers. The implicit assumption here is that there is a linear relationship between a stimulus and the stress response [38].

A transactional model of stress [39,40] seems more appropriate to understand the complexity of caregiver reactions towards different stimuli [41-43]. Folkman & Lazarus [39] define stress as "a relationship between the person and the environment that is appraised by the person as relevant to his or her well-being and in which the person's resources are taxed or exceeded". Within this transactional model of stress the existence of events in a person's life is not automatically assumed to be stress-provoking. An event only becomes a stressor when the mind identifies it as such [44]. So it is the subjective interpretation of events and not their objective characteristics that best determine stress [16].

Thompson [45] describes two major perspectives applied to an understanding of stress and burden. They call these the stress perspective and the social context perspective. The focus of the first perspective is on the individual caregiver. In the second, a broader perspective is taken which includes the family unit which can mediate between stressors and their impact [38]. Stressors that are ambiguous [46] or unpredictable [47] seem to pose the most problems to caregivers.

Caregiver well-being & satisfaction

The measurement of well-being [48] is a non-specific-burden measure that can be applied to diverse groups of caregivers as well as to non-caregivers. Caregiver well-being and caregiver burden might be considered as opposite sides of the same coin [48]. An absence of satisfaction is likely to be associated with a poorer and fragile caring relationship. It may also serve as an indicator suggesting the need to look closely at the situation to determine if both the caregiver and the cared-for person are at risk. Helping caregivers to identify sources of satisfaction can result in an improved caring relationship [49].

Caregiver burnout

The term burnout is rarely used in the literature about informal caregiving, [50] in contrast to literature on professional caregivers [51,52]. Caregiver burnout emerges when a person reaches a state of physical, emotional and mental exhaustion due to strain, most often after a chronic day-to-day type [53,54].

Correlates of burden

In caregiving literature, there is conflicting evidence about the relationships between burden and particular characteristics of the cared-for person, the caregiver and the caregiving situation. In the context of assessment of the family caregiver, it remains important that the assessor has a basic knowledge of the variables that might contribute to subjective reported feelings of burden in family caregivers.

Correlates of burden may not be interpreted as directly *causing* feelings of burden within family caregivers. Especially in the light of the development of more dynamic models of burden and stress, caution is warranted. For example, deviant behaviours of the cared-for person are considered to be positively associated with feelings of burden. While some family caregivers may view deviant behaviours as extremely burdensome, other carers may not interpret these as burdens.

Patient related variables - Severity of the disease (dementia) in general

In only a few studies using multivariate measures of severity of dementia an association is found between the general severity of dementia and caregivers' psychological well-being or burden [55,56]. In one study, increasing severity of dementia was associated with an increase in caregiver's burden [57] and another found a linear relationship between severity of cognitive impairment and breakdown in care [58]. However, in most studies no association was found between the general severity of dementia and indicators of caregivers' burden or psychological well-being [48,59-62].

Cognitive impairment

Cognitive impairment of the cared-for person is positively associated with caregivers' psychological [36,63,64]. However, one must be critical of these findings. Incongruity in findings of the different studies can be explained by the various phases in patients' dementia. A study by Zarit [22] was conducted with severely demented people. Pruchno & Resch [63] showed that caregivers' levels of burden were elevated as the frequency of the cared-for person's forgetful behaviours increased. Other studies did not show an association between the cared-for person's cognitive impairment and caregivers' burden or psychological well-being [60,62,65,66]. On the whole, there seems to be no strong association between cognitive impairment of the cared-for person and burden of the family caregiver.

Functional status

Functional impairment, as measured by the impairment in the cared-for activities of daily living (e.g. washing and eating), is in most studies found not to be associated with caregivers' psychological distress or burden [55,60,65-68]. Only in a few studies did ADL-impairment appear to be significantly associated with burden [36,59]. ADL impairment does appear to be predictive of breakdown in care leading to institutionalisation [69].

IADL impairment, (e.g. impairment in shopping or cooking) has been associated with caregivers' scores for depression [36,65,66]. Functional impairment does not appear to be strongly related to caregivers' burden or psychological well-being, although IADL impairment seems to be more strongly associated with caregivers' outcomes than does ADL impairment.

Behavioural disturbances

In general, it is assumed that problems like aggressive behaviour and agitation are especially troublesome for caregivers. A positive association between the occurrence and or severity of behavioural problems in totality and caregivers' burden, psychological distress and breakdown of care has been found in many studies [59,63,64,68,70-76]. Only a few studies did not find an association between patients' behavioural problems and caregivers' burden or depressive symptomatology [22,66,67].

Perceived impact on caregivers feelings of well-being and burden

Significant correlations are reported between caregivers' appraisal of cognitive impairment, ADL and IADL dependency of the cared-for person as either hassles or uplifts and caregiver's depressive symptomatology, except for ADL hassles. The more hassles experienced by the caregivers, the higher their depressive symptomatology [26,76]. Haley [66] established that caregivers reported more depressive complaints as they appraised dependency in ADL and IADL and patients' behavioural problems as more stressful, and as they perceive themselves as less effective in coping with these dementia symptoms. Motenko [77] found that more frustration with ADL-impairment was associated with decreased well-being.

Caregivers' coping

Coping represents the behaviour and practices of individuals in response to stressful activities [33], or it refers to the things people do (acting or thinking) to increase a sense of well-being in their lives and to avoid being harmed by stressful events [78]. Patterson [79] believes that the word adaptation is to be preferred, whereas others opt for managing [41,46].

In Lazarus & Folkman's terms [40], coping is defined mainly in terms of problem-solving efforts that people employ when a perceived demand is seen to tax their adaptive resources. In this context a distinction must be made between coping strategies and coping resources [38]. Coping strategies or coping styles concern how people cope. These refer to problem-focused coping strategies such as reframing, and emotion-focused coping strategies such as grieving, wishful thinking and acceptance. Problem-solving coping if often held to be most effective [80-83], although emotion-focused strategies are considered to play an important role in the promotion of health. To determine its effectiveness, the coping strategy should be matched to the nature of the stressor. Individuals who have a range of coping strategies are likely to cope more effectively [38].

Five general points are important with regard to coping strategies:

1. Individuals usually access more than one coping strategy in their attempts to manage stressful situations [38].

2. The coping strategies applied can involve behavioural as well as cognitive approaches [38].

3. Very little is known about the economic and social costs and benefits to individuals of different coping strategies [38].

4. All coping strategies are potentially useful but must be matched with the nature of the stressor faced [82].

5. Effectiveness of the coping strategy should be considered with regard to the intended outcome [41,84].

Coping resources usually refer to the kinds of resources people might call upon. Internal resources refer to personal skills, relevant life experiences, psychological disposition and analytic ability. External resources refer to income, housing, socio-economic status, formal services and also social resources such as social networks, social support available through such networks. There is strong evidence to suggest that social resources are heavily implicated in mediating stress and coping [42,85-87].

One of caregivers' resources that may influence caregivers' psychological well-being of burden are their coping strategies. Lazarus & Folkman [40] distinguish between two different coping strategies: problem-focused and emotion-focused. Problem-focused coping aims at managing or altering the problem situation in order to diminish stress. Emotion-focused coping aims at regulating emotional reactions to the problem-situation. The relationship between caregivers' problem-focused coping and their burden or psychological well-being is still unclear. Pratt found that more confidence in problem-solving and more re-framing of problems were associated with less burden of caregivers, although the associations were weak [88]. Furthermore, Haley [66] found that more use of logical analysis or problem-solving was associated with less depression and more satisfaction with life. In most studies published later, a beneficial influence of problem-focused coping strategies was not found on caregivers' burden or psychological well-being [36,66,67,89].

Findings on some emotion-focused coping strategies showed even a detrimental influence of these strategies on caregivers' burden and psychological well-being. Passivity, escape, avoidance or evasive coping appeared to be negatively associated with psychological well-being and positively with burden [89]. Remarkably, emotion-focused coping strategies also had a beneficial influence. What these coping strategies seem to have in common is that they do not seek to ignore, minimise, nor work off emotional distress, but focus on the positive found that focusing on more on the positive ("rediscover what's important in life) was associated with better mental health [89,90]. Other emotion-focused coping strategies (blaming oneself, fantasising, wishful thinking) showed different or no influence on caregivers' well-being and burden [36,89].

Caregivers' neuroticism

There are a few studies on the association between caregivers' neuroticism and burden or psychological well-being. A higher level of neuroticism is associated with a higher level of burden or psychological distress [91]. Caregivers with a high level of neuroticism are more likely to perceive themselves as currently being under more stress, which in turn is associated with poor mental health ratings [91].

Social support

Burden is likely to vary according to categories of families. For example, when the family network is closed-knit and there is a strong cohesion and solidarity within the group, the caregivers' lot would be more bearable, even in the absence of practical assistance.

Networks, both formal and informal, which support the work of the family caregiver are considered as essential in continuing to look after the cared-for person, despite all difficulties. Networks can play a role in the prevention of the carer being immersed gradually in greater and greater isolation.

The coping strategy "seeking social support" may be both palliative and instrumental [36]. Although social support is a frequently used coping strategy among caregivers, in most studies no association is found between seeking social support and indicators of caregivers' burden of psychological well-being [36,66,67,89].

Interventions for the family caregiver

As the caregiving literature is dominated by the burden perspective, so are the interventions proposed to support the family caregiver. A critical analysis reveals:

- Most interventions focus on the reduction of stress resulting from caregiving activities.

- Very few interventions are designed to focus on the positive aspects of care.

- Interventions are seldom organised within a multidisciplinary context.

Comprehensive assessment of the family caregiver should lead to the planning and creation of individualised care packages. In this context, the recognition of caregiver expertise and how their knowledge can compliment that of professionals is considered extremely important [28,92]. This assumes the development of models that are sensitive to the stage of caregiving and assist carers to make various transitions [15,93].

A general intervention strategy: The concept of social support

While family caregivers are an important source of social support to older persons, caregivers experience a strong need for social support as well. There is a consistent finding that social support may help buffer or mitigate the negative effects of caregiving [17]. Family caregivers with low levels of social support have more negative mental and physical health outcomes than family caregivers who perceive high levels of social support.

Social support seems to be a multidimensional construct. The concept has been studied abundant in caregiving literature in relation to depression [17,48], stress [48,68], and burden [48,93,94]. Social support research has been obstructed by a lack of clarity in both terms of definitions and components. The terms social support, social integration and social network are often used interchangeably, leading to confusion over their difference and exact definitions. Researchers have developed a social support hierarchy including three levels of social relationships. These three levels mutually influence each other and both the network and functional properties are important. ssessment, as well as interventions for the family caregiver should include these three levels of social relationships.

Social integration; meaning the number, density and range of relationships.

Social network; which refers to the structure and sources of relationships surrounding the individual.

Social support; which explores the functionality of social relationships, and the resources that are provided by other persons.

Social support from the part of formal service providers can be assumed to represent:

A. Emotional support: which include listening, concern, trust, reassurance and professional intimacy, which all contribute to the feeling that one is cared about [95].

B. Informational support: which includes giving useful information, suggestions and advice which can help family caregivers solving their problems. Examples of informational support interventions are (a) enhancing the extent to which caregivers are prepared for their role and acquire the necessary skills, knowledge and expertise [95,96], and (b) help carers to develop new coping resources/responses. Supporting and enhancing caregivers' coping efforts is a major intention underlying professional [28].

C. Appraisal support: which is feedback that affirms self-worth. Examples of appraisal support are the achievement of autonomy and dealing with feelings of guilt and inadequacy.

D. Instrumental support: which refers to direct aid or services such as help with ADL and IADL activities solve a problem. Examples of instrumental support activities are home-based nursing and hygienic care, as well as help with household.

Consequences of external caregiving

Before accepting external help, the caregiver has to recognise the limits of his or her own resources, which is not always simple after years of devoted care. The arrival of external caregivers means that family carer has to give up some territory and accept the intrusion of strangers to his area, dispossessing them of the exclusive intimacy of the patient, part of the decisions, and also part of their power.

Needs of the family caregiver

The literature review on caregiver needs reveals the following conclusions:

- The needs of the family caregiver are extremely important in the context of assessment. It is found however, that caregivers' needs are poorly researched and conceptualised.
- Limited instruments are available to assess the needs of family caregiver. If the literature fails to reveal a suitable instrument, investigators create an assessment tool for their specific study, with often limited information on psychometric properties.
- Caregivers have generally a great need for support in the sense of emotional, social, practical and material support. The needs vary according to individual situations , the stage of caregiving and to a more general context.
- Only through identification and clarification of the needs of caregivers, health care providers will be able to focus their attention and shape treatments that contribute to the long-term success of home care.

Caregiver needs explained through the negative consequences of caregiving

A variety of physical and psychological health problems is reported within family caregivers [48], such as high blood pressure, backaches, headaches, insomnia, anxiety, depression and exhaustion [8,97-99]. Especially fatigue is reported in 75-85 percent of all family caregivers. Family caregivers report themselves to be in poorer health in comparison with other groups, and there is evidence suggesting that stress resulting form caregiving has a negative impact on the functioning of the immune system, which in turn may lead to increased mobility [100]. In this context, findings show caregivers to have more physician visits and to receive more prescription for medication as compared to non-caregivers [67]. Despite the physical, emotional, social and financial demands of caregiving, it is only recently that in some ways the needs of caregivers have been appreciated [17]. In a study, conducted to explore formal needs of caregivers of frail older persons, it was found that just under half of the caregivers were satisfied with the attention they received from the health care system [101]. The needs of caregivers are often overlooked when health care professionals focus their attention of the one receiving the more obvious care, being the cared-for person [102].

The question: "what do carers need in the different stages of caregiving" is most difficult to answer, as each caring situation has many facets, and it takes in almost all aspects of life. Moreover, caregivers find difficulties in formulating their needs. This is particularly true when they are unaware of what exists or could exist in terms of formal services [29].

Caregiver needs explained through the positive consequences of caregiving

Understanding Family Care" [38] describes the number of authors who have become critical of the predominant focus of stressors and burdens of care, and who have suggested that a true picture will not emerge until the potentially satisfying aspects of caregiving are not explored in greater detail [92].

A report on family caregiving in the United Kingdom [29] points out that the everyday needs of the carer is mostly a function of three criteria:

- the type and degree of dependence of the patient, and the needs for care deriving from this
- the extent of the personal involvement of the carer
- the type of household and the possible presence within the household of other people besides the carer and the cared-for person

Other criteria who seem most decisive in their effects on caregivers' needs are:

- siting, accessibility, capacity and professionalism of home-based services
- the caregivers' state of health, emotional strength and physical well-being
- the economical level
- social isolation
- participation (or non participation) in the labour market
- co-residence or not

Psycho-social needs

Psycho-social needs most often reported in literature are the need to talk about one's difficulties and satisfactions caused by the care situation, the need to be listened to, and to receive some sympathy [28,48,68,94,103]. Also the need for acknowledgement, even praise in turn for most efforts is reported [29]. The development of a warm, therapeutic relationship with formal service providers increases the caregiver's ability to cope effectively [9].

Attending a support group is very rarely mentioned as a need among carers, with the exception of those who belong to such groups. It is more the case that the positive results obtained by this type of assistance underline the needs at this level [9,104].

The need for information and learning

The lack of information on services, allowances and rights is felt particularly strongly in the early stage of the caregiving process, especially when dependency is caused by a sudden event. Complaints about information include for example the fragmented way in which some information is presented.

Family caregivers have identified information and education needs related to resources, community services, respite care, stress management, support groups and communication techniques [105]. Family caregivers need both practical teaching to build up skill, and acquisition of knowledge about the illnesses, dependency and its course [8]. The latter seems most pressing when the patient suffers from mental deterioration.

Financial needs

Financial needs exist on various levels such as the substitution on income, covering medical and paramedical expenses, hospitalisation, medicine and equipment costs [106], although in some communities financial impact of caregiving may be relatively low [58].

Need for practical assistance

Research demonstrate that caregivers, many of whom provide intensive home care, make little use of community services [32]. In case of dementia, a significantly greater use of services is noted in combination with a high level of unmet needs, mainly for mainstream medical services and help with the supervision of the older person [58]. These studies reflect the views of caregivers already in receipt of specialist services, whereas those using only primary care teams may be resistant to using secondary care services [70].

Need for respite care

Some studies suggest that family caregivers of demented older persons report services such as respite care and adult day care to be helpful *in order* to have some time for oneself and time to breathe [102,104]. The need for intermittent breaks covers a number of ranges: respites for a few hours, for a day or two and for several weeks in a row for holidays.

Need for technical equipment

Appropriate technical equipment such as the hospital bed, the commode, and a wheelchair, might considerably facilitates the carers work.

Premises and Aims of the Assessment of the Family Caregiver

A critical analysis of the literature on theoretical concepts of family care and interventions as well as the needs of the family caregiver reveal that the burden perspective is apparent, and that caregivers are primarily perceived as resources, rather than co-partners and experts. We propose the premises directing the assessment of the family caregiver primarily to be based on a family centred perspective, as described below.

The premises are based on a family and patient centred perspective, rather than a economical-political perspective. The latter need to be taken into account as well, because of current health policies and restricted financial resources within countries of the European Community which can not be ignored. Each COPE partner need to determine how they will operationalise the different premises in their country before the development of their trial(s).

Premises directing the assessment of the family caregiver

- The family caregiver and the cared- for person should have the same right of access to needs assessment [15].
- In any assessment, four perspectives need to be included: those of the carer, the client, the assessor and that of the agency [15].
- There has to be an individual assessment of caregiver need that moves beyond the instrumental, and takes a multidimensional and longitudinal [45,107-109].
- Both the carer and the cared-for person's interactions and the assessment process itself has to be considered within the context of a relationship [15].
- The relationship between carer and assessor should be based on a genuine partnership, rather than perceiving the carer as a resource [15].
- The carer should have the equal right to decide whether to continue or to abrogate existing responsibilities of caring [15].

Aims directing assessment of the family caregiver

The aims of assessment of the family caregiver will differ again, from the perspective one is holding. Each COPE partner needs to determine how the aims of assessment of the family caregiver will be operationalised before the development of their trial(s). It is important that the different COPE-partners try to find a balance between both the caregivers perceived as partners and resources in the development of their trials.

Caregivers as partners, clients or experts

Family caregivers are considered being partners, clients or experts, depending on their physical and mental abilities, expertise, willingness and possibilities to co-operate. If caregivers are viewed as partners, clients or experts, then the aim of assessment is primarily:
- to acknowledge the (unmet) needs of the family caregiver
- to identify and build on the strengths of the family carer, and their social and environmental support
- to plan individualised care packages
- to communicate more effectively with colleagues
- to provide appropriate services and interventions
- to allow a range of options for consumers
- to measure individual outcomes of care

Caregivers as resources

If caregivers are viewed as resources, then the aim of assessment is primarily:
- to determine if services are necessary
- to determine in what form services will be provided (which services are cost-effective, available and affordable)
- to intervene no more than is necessary to foster independence
- to concentrate on those with the greatest needs
- to understand population needs

- measuring case-mix and outcomes for service audit, for population health targets and for cross-national comparison

Eligibility criteria for the assessment of the family caregiver

In the development of a common approach and the framework the eligibility criteria for the assessment of the family caregiver need to be taken into account. Eligibility criteria have been developed for the assessment of the cared-for person and entry to care and case management programs. This means that the assessment of needs and the services that flow from it have to meet certain criteria. In some authorities these have been defined in terms of crisis management, such as avoiding imminent breakdown of care arrangements, risk of abuse and neglect, or requiring help and support with personal care. Other authorities have defined eligibility criteria more broadly to encompass psycho-social needs, e.g. living alone, presence of serious physical/mental illness/disability/degree of stress unacceptable to person, carer or community.

Eligibility criteria for the assessment of the family caregiver are difficult to establish. The presence of a family caregiver might already be enough reason to consider a first stage assessment of the perceived needs and difficulties. Each COPE partner needs to decide if eligibility criteria for both assessment and assistance of the family caregiver will be established.

If the family caregiver reports more difficulties than satisfactions resulting from the caregiving situation, this might be considered as a trigger towards a more in-depth and comprehensive assessment.

At present, most measurements target family carers taking care for demented older people [34,36,57,66,68,90,110,111]. The assessment in the context of research studies is highly dominated by a burden perspective often ignoring the possible satisfactions of caregiving.

A minority of measurements focus on family carers of frail older people [32,35], memory impaired adults [48], neurological impaired older people [112], and older people after a primary stroke [113], with hip surgery or heart disease [114], and with chronic degenerative disorders such as arthritis, cognitive impairment and incontinence.

Assessment instruments for the family caregiver

A detailed overview of measurement instruments for the family caregiver is presented below (Table 1). From a critical literature review on instruments of the family caregiver the following conclusions can be drawn:

- At present, despite the overwhelming volume of on caregiving literature, rather few instruments are available which account for the complexity of caregiving. This might be explained by the fact that family care is provided in diverse circumstances and cultural and social determined situations. As such, it is almost impossible to include all possible relevant factors within one set of indices.

- In contrast to the U.S and the U.K, few research studies are available on caregiver well-being in countries of the European Union, although cultural differences are important in the understanding of possible different perceptions and behaviours of family caregivers towards caregiving for their relatives.

- Carers' needs are likely to remain poorly addressed because of the scope of assessment [15,115]. Caregiving literature has been dominated by a focus on tasks and the physical aspects of caring as well as burdens or difficulties of caring, relatively neglecting the potential for satisfactions or uplifts. The concept most studied from different perspectives and with different instruments is burden [116], although the measurement of burden itself remains controversial. Many of these studies are heavily influenced by a psychosocial approach to caregiving which challenged the prevalent medical model of care [117]. In a medical model of care, caregiving is automatically perceived as a synonym of decrements in selected dimensions of well-being, such as physical health, mental health, social participation and financial resources.

- The different measurements are based on a rather quantitative approach of stress and burden. Although quantitative studies of stress and burden have some value, there is an increasing realisation that the search for powerful and enduring predictors of caregiver burden or stress are likely to prove fruitless, and that in turn emphasis should be placed how to achieve a comprehensive individualised assessment of carers' needs [118]. A re-emerge of qualitative studies is required [119,120], because of the uniqueness of each caregiving situation in which the subjective experiences of the caregiver play a major role.

- The predominant focus has been on the use of cross-sectional designs neglecting the dynamic nature of caregiving wherein positive and negative consequences of caregiving and the condition of the cared-for person s well, are often changing over time.

- Some investigators advocate the use of multidimensional measures that differentiate the task of caregiving from its effects [25,35]. Others measure only the current feelings of caregivers about this responsibility [22,60,68,88,93,121]. As a result, items of a scale are scored into different subscales (multidimensional), according to the dimension they represent, or scored upon the global scale (unidimensional). Unidimensional burden scales [68,90,112,114] produce an overall burden score, tapping similar effects of burden [48,57]. Multidimensional measurements [35,48] reveal scores distinguishing between various areas of caregiver's well-being and functioning. Items on the subscales represent the dimension of the concept they are referring to. Researchers acknowledge that multidimensional scaling of constructs for caregiver burden and strain is needed to accurately reflect the caregiving situation [57,122,123]. Such instruments should have good internal consistency, modest to moderate intercorrelation of subscales, and high factor loadings.

- The varied measures have sometimes limited psychometric justification. Many instruments now being used in research on caregiving lack for example sufficient face and content validity for their use in clinical practice with families [36,124,125]. In the development of valid and reliable instruments three problems are noticed [57]:
    - Research on measures, which is not theoretically grounded makes it difficult to understand the clinical perspective of the clinical researcher.
    - Ill-defined terms and overlapping definitions to represent caregiver burden and other aspects of the caregiving situation causes difficulty to distinguish the concepts from one another.
    - Global measures of caregiving make it difficult to interpret exactly what is being measured.

- With exception of the concept of well-being all measurements are tied to samples of caregivers, varying from spouses to adult children or other close relatives, being primary caregivers of the cared-for person. Sometimes these measurements differ in the way they are tied to informal caregiving as a family task [66] instead of being a more personified task of one of the family carers.

We might conclude that at present only one set of instruments developed by Nolan [38] is available in which difficulties, coping behaviours and satisfactions are measured. This instrument has potential for in-depth assessment of the caregiver in routine practice. No instrument is currently available which meets the needs to cover these domains at the stage of screening for caregiver needs.

Table 1: Overview of Measurement Instruments for the Family Caregiver

The symbol * refers to the establishment of the psychometric property, whether the symbol "?" refers to missing information on the establishment of the psychometric property.

Instrument	Psychometric properties	
Burden Interview [68]	Content validity: * Construct validity: * Convergent validity: *	Internal consistency: * Test-retest reliability:* Sensitivity: * Specificity: Establishment of cut-off-points: *
Caregiver Strain Instrument [114]	Content validity: * Construct validity: * Convergent validity:	Internal consistency: * Test-retest reliability: ? Sensitivity: ? Specificity: ? Establishment of cut-off-points: ?
Measuring Family Well-Being of Demented Elderly [48]	Content validity: ? Construct validity: ? Convergent validity: ?	Internal consistency: ? Test-retest reliability: ? Sensitivity: ? Specificity: ? Establishment of cut-off-points: ?
Model of Burden [35]	Content validity: ? Construct validity: * Convergent validity: ?	Internal consistency: ? Test-retest reliability: ? Sensitivity: ? Specificity: ? Establishment of cut-off-points: ?
Inventories [32]	Content validity: ? Construct validity: * Convergent validity: ?	Internal consistency: * Test-retest reliability: ? Sensitivity: ? Specificity: ? Cut-off-points: ?
Cost of Care Instrument [111]	Content validity: ? Construct validity: * Convergent validity: ?	Internal consistency: * Test-retest reliability: ? Sensitivity: ? Specificity: ? Cut-off-points: ?

Table 1 continued

Instrument	Psychometric properties
Caregiver Burden Inventory [57]	Content validity: * Internal consistency: * Construct validity: ? Test-retest reliability: ? Convergent validity: * Sensitivity: * Specificity: ? Cut-off-points: ?
Caregiver Appraisal Measure [74]	Content validity: ? Internal consistency: * Construct validity: * Test-retest reliability: ? Convergent validity: ? Sensitivity: ? Specificity: ? Cut-off-points: ?
Caregiver Hassles Scale [34]	Content validity: ? Internal consistency: * Construct validity: * Test-retest reliability: ? Convergent validity: ? Sensitivity: ? Specificity: * Cut-off-points: ?
Screen for Caregiver Burden [36]	Content validity Internal consistency: * Construct validity: * Test-retest reliability: * Convergent validity: * Sensitivity: * Specificity: ? Cut-off-points: ?
Family Caregiver Assessment Inventory and the Impact of Caregiving Inventory [66]	Content validity: ? Internal consistency: * Construct validity: ? Test-retest reliability: ? Convergent validity: * Sensitivity: * Specificity: * Cut-off-points: ?
Rasch Scale: Self-Perceived Pressure from Informal Care Scale [90]	Content validity: * Internal consistency: * Construct validity: * Test-retest reliability: * Convergent validity: ? Sensitivity: * Specificity: ? Cut-off-points: ?
A Novel Caregiver Burden Scale [113]	Content validity: * Internal consistency: * Construct validity: ? Test-retest reliability: * Convergent validity: ? Sensitivity: ? Specificity: ? Cut-off-points: ?
The Parent Caregiver Burden and Strain Scale [112]	Content validity: * Internal consistency: * Construct validity: * Test-retest reliability: * Convergent validity: ? Sensitivity: ? Specificity: ? Establishment of cut-off-points: ?
Caregiver's Assessment of Difficulties Scale, Caregiver's Assessment of Managing Scale, Caregiver's Assessment of Satisfaction Scale [15]	Content validity: Internal consistency: Construct validity: Test-retest reliability: Convergent validity: Sensitivity: Specificity: Establishment of cut-off-points:

Assessment Strategies

Every assessment strategy should include the type and timeframe of data gathering, who should do the assessment, ethical issues in assessment and a description and operationalisation of the principles of good assessment.

Type of data gathering

Measurement-data on caregiver burden, needs and satisfactions are at present obtained through self-report data [68,112], gathered by interview or in writing by a questionnaire with open-ended and/or fixed-choice questions [114], (which are self-administered or interviewer administered).

Authors elect a method or are using different ones, according to the way of conceptualising burden. As an example, objective burden has been be operationalized by prevalence of the number of behavioural problems [36] or by using a questionnaire with fixed-choice ('yes-no') questions [34,114]. Subjective burden, referring to the subjective view of the caregiver on a demand or situational aspect has been measured in different exploratory degrees. It has been rated on a Likert-scale, for example as distress [36], or satisfaction, in relation to each experience [74], or as the degree of a hassle [34].

Timeframe for data gathering

Assessment of family caregivers is comprehensive, complex and time consuming. It cannot be completed quickly, certainly not in one session, and requires that a relationship or trust exists between the assessor, carer and cared-for person. As a result, adequate assessment can only occur within the context of a continuing relationship [126].

Who should do the assessment?

Part of the debate about costs of assessment of the family caregiver, is the question who should do it. From a cost perspective, there is ambivalence amongst members of the primary care team about who should be responsible, and the implications on service delivery such as decision making, resource allocation, confidentiality and responsibility. From the clinical point of view it is clear that certain professionals, such as practice and district nurses, are in a good position to assess the family carer, because of their familiarity with the situation of each particular family member [127].

Ethical issues in assessment

An important ethical issue is "the right of family caregivers to refuse or to accept an assessment." Some family carers may feel with justification that a home visit and interview is an intrusion to their privacy. Formal caregivers should be aware of duplication of assessment between agencies, and possibly over-assessment too.

Principles of good assessment

Providing good assessment requires a specific training of the assessors. Clearly the training issues are related to the philosophy and approach to the assessment. Not only is a positive view of ageing required, but also sophisticated and sensitive interviewing and communication skills, as well as an in-depth knowledge about elderly and family care.

Nolan [15] brought together the conclusions of Write and Ellis [115,127] concerning the principles of good assessment, which are:

- empower people-inform fully, clarify users' and carers' understanding of the situation and the role of the assessor before going ahead
- shed their professional perspective-have an open mind, be prepared to learn
- start from where the user/carer is, establish their existing level of knowledge and what their hope and expectations are
- be interested in the carer as a person, not just a resource
- take time-build trust/rapport/overcome the brief visitor syndrome; this may take more than one visit
- be sensitive/imaginative/creative in responding-carers may not know what is possible, available
- avoid value judgements whenever possible-if such judgements are needed make them explicit
- offer honest, realistic options with an indication of any delay or limitations in service delivery
- listen to and value users' and carers' expertise/opinion, even if this runs counter to the assessor's values
- establish a suitable environment for the assessment, which ensures there is privacy, quiet and sufficient time
- involve rather than just inform the user and carer; make them feel they are a full participant in the assessment
- consider social, emotional, relationship needs, as well as practical needs; pay attention to the quality of the relationship between user and carer
- not make assessment a "battle" so people feel they have to fight for services
- balance all perspectives
- clarify understanding at the end of the process and agree the way forward

References

[1] F. Ross. Assessment in the Community. In: Assessing Elderly People I Philp (ed.), Farrand Press, London, 1994.

[2] I. Philp, An overview. In: Outcomes Assessment for Healthcare in Elderly People. In:. Philp (ed.), Farrand Press, London, 1997.

[3] G. Dooghe, Informal caregiving of elderly people: a European review. *Ageing and Society,* 12 (1992), 369-80.

[4] A. Walker *et al*, Older People in Europe: Social and Economic Policies: the 1993 Report of the European Observatory, Brussels: Commission of the European Communities, 1993.

[5] J. Alber, Health and social services. In A. Walker *et al* (eds). Older People in Europe: Social and Economic Policies: the 1993 Report of the European Observatory. Brussels: Commission of the European Communities, 1993.

[6] A. Horowitz, Predictors of caregiving involvement among adult children of the frail elderly. Paper presented ate the Annual Meeting of the Gerontological Society of America, Boston, MA, 1982.

[7] S.S. Tobin and R. Kulys, The family in the institutionalization of the elderly. *Journal of Social Issues,* 37 (1981) 145-157.

[8] P. Krach and J. Brooks, Identifying the responsabilities & needs of working adults who are primary caregivers. *Journal of Gerontological Nursing,* 21 (1995) 41-50.

[9] R. Davidhizar, Powerlessness of caregivers in home care. *Journal of Clinical Nursing,* 3 (1994) 155-158.

[10] E.M. Brody,. Prospects for family caregiving: response to change, continuity and diversity. In: R.A. Kane and J.D. Penrod (eds.), Family caregiving in an Aging Society. Sage, Thousand Oaks,

California, 1995.
[11] A. Monk, Family supports in old age. *Home Health Services Quaterly* 3 (1983) 101-111.
[12] R. Moroney, Families, care of the handicapped and public policy. *Home Health Care Services Quaterly* 3 (1983) 188-213.
[13] J. Twigg and K. Atkin, Carers perceived: Policy and Practice in informal Care, Open University Press, Buckinghamshire, 1994.
[14] M.R. Nolan, Carers. In I.Philp (ed.), Outcomes Assessment for Healthcare in Elderly People, Farrand Press, London, 1997.
[15] M. Nolan *et al*, A framework for assessing the needs of family carers: a multidisciplinary guide, Base Publications, Stroke-on-Trent, Shafffordshire, 1994.
[16] R.A. Kane and J.D. Penrod, Family Caregiving in an Aging Society, Sage, Thousand Oaks, California, 1995.
[17] J.J. Gallo, The effect of social support on depression in caregivers of the elderly. *The Journal of Family Practice* 30 (1990) 430-440.
[18] R. Montgomery and S. Kokoski, A longitudinal analysis of nursing home placement for dependent elders cared for by spouses vs.adult children. *Journal of Gerontology* 49 (1994) 862-869.
[19] S. McFaul and B.H. Miller, Caregiver burden and nursing home admission of frail elderly persons. *Journal of Gerontology* 47 (1992) 73-79.
[20] B. Chenoweth and B. Spencer, Dementia: The experience of family caregivers. *The Gerontologist* 26 (1986) 267-272.
[21] E.J. Colerick and L.K. George, Predictors of institutionalisation among caregivers of patients with Alzheimer's disease. *The Gerontologist* 34 (1986) 493-498.
[22] S. Zarit *et al*, Subjective burden of husbands and wives as caregivers: A longitudinal study. *The Gerontologist* 26, (1986) 260.
[23] L. Boydell *et al,* Report of a consensus Conference on Measures of Health Status and Well-being for the Elderly. Belfast, EPIC, 1993.
[24] Royal College of Physicians/British Geriatrics society (RCP/BGS,. Standardised Assessment Scales for Elderly People, Royal College of Physicians/British Geriatrics Society, London, 1992.
[25] R.A. Kane and R.L. Kane, Measurement of social functioning in long term care, in R.A. Kane and R.L. Kane (eds.), Assessing the Elderly: A Practical Guide to Measurement, Lexicon and Toronto, Lexington Books, (1981) 133-208.
[26] R.G. Morris *et al*, Factors affecting the emotional well-being of the caregivers of dementia sufferers. *British Journal of Psychiatry* 148 (1988) 147-156.
[27] J.L. Green and P.D. Coleman, Direct services for family caregivers: Next Steps for Public Policy. In: R.A. Kane and J.D. Penrod, Family Caregiving in an Ageing Society. Sage, Thousand Oaks, California, 1995.
[28] M. Nolan *et al*, Developping a typology of family care: Implications for nurses and other service providers. *Journal of Advanced Nursing* 2 (1995) 256-265.
[29] H. Jani-Le Bris, Family care of Dependent Older People in the European Community, European Foundation for the Improvement of Living and Working conditions, Loughlinstown House, Shankill, Co. Dublin Ireland, 1993.
[30] L.K. George, Caregiver burden and well-being: an elusive distinction. *The Gerontologist* 34(1) (1994) 6-7.
[31] J.C. Stuckey *et al*, Burden and well-being: the same coin of related currency? *The Gerontologist* 36 (1996) 686-693.
[32] R.J.V. Montgomery *et al*, Measurement and the analysis of burden. *Research on Aging* 7(1) (1985) 137-152.
[33] L.I. Perlin *et al*, Caregiving and the stress process: an overview of concepts and their measures. *Gerontologist,* 30 (1990) 583-93.
[34] M.J. Kinney and M. Stephens, Caregiving hassles scale: Assessing the daily hassles of caring for a family member with dementia. *The Gerontologist* 29(3) (1989) 328-332.
[35] S.W. Poulshock and G.T. Deimling, Families caring for elders in residence: issues in measurement of burden. *Journal of Gerontology* 39 (1984) 230-239.
[36] P.P. Vitaliano *et al*, Burden: a review of measures used among caregivers of individuals with dementia. *The Gerontologist* 31 (1991) 67-75.
[37] A.M. Warnes, Being old, old people and the burdens of burden. *Ageing and Society* 13 (1993) 297-338.
[38] M. Nolan *et al*, Understanding family care: A multidimensional model of caring and coping, Open University Press, 1996.
[39] S. Folkman and R.S. Lazarus, If it changes it must be a process: a study of emotion and coping during

three stages of a college examination. *Journal of Personality and Social Psychology* 48 (1985) 150-70.

[40] R.S. Lazarus and S. Folkman, *Stress, appraisal and Coping*, New York: Springer, 1984.

[41] W.R. Burr et al, *Re-examining Family stress: New Theory and Research*, Thousand Oaks, CA: Sage, 1984.

[42] L. Quine and J. Pahl, Stress and coping in mothers caring for a child with severe learning difficulties: a test of Lazarus' transactional model of coping. *Journal of Community and Applied Social Psychology* 1 (1991) 57-70.

[43] J.R. Edwards and C.L. Cooper, Research in stress, coping and health: theoretical and methodological issues. *Psychological Medicine* 18 (1988) 15-20.

[44] L. Spariol and H. Jung, Effective Coping: A Conceptual model. In: Hatfield, A.B.& Lefley, H.P. (Eds). Families of the Mentally Ill III: coping and Adaptation, Cassell, Londen, 1997.

[45] E.H. Thompson et al, Social support and caregiver burden in family caregivers of frail elderly. *Journal of Gerontology* 48(5) (1993) 245-54.

[46] P. Boss, *Family Stress Management*, Newbury Park, CA: Sage, 1988.

[47] P.G. Archbold et al, The clinical assessment of mutuality and preparedness in family caregivers of frail older people. In: S.G. Funk et al (eds.), Key aspects of Elder Care: Managing Falls, Incontinence and Cognitive Impairment, New York: Springer, 1992.

[48] L.K. George and L.P. Gwyther, Caregiver well-being: a multidimensional examination of family caregivers of demented adults. *The Gerontologist* 26 (1986) 253-259.

[49] J.C. Cartwright et al, Enrichment processes in family caregiving to frail elders. *Advances in Nursing Science* 17(1) (1994) 31-43.

[50] B. Almberg et al, Caring for a demented elderly person-burden and burnout among caregivers relatives. *Journal of Advanced Nursing* 25 (1997) 106-116.

[51] S. Astrom et al, Wish to transfer to other jobs among long-term care workers. *Aging* 3(3) (1991) 247-256.

[52] D. Kuremyr et al, Emotional experiences, empathy and burnout among staff caring for demented patients at a collective living unit and a nursing home. *Journal of Advanced Nursing* 19(4) (1994) 670-679.

[53] C. Maslach, Burnout: the cost of Caring, Prentice-Hall Inc., New York, 1988.

[54] A.M. Pines and E. Aronson, Career burnout causes and cures, The Free Press, New York, 1988.

[55] I. Fukunishi and K. Hosokawa, A study of psychological aspects of families living together with senile dementia. *The Japanese Journal of Psychiatry and Neurology* 44 (1990) 19-24.

[56] M. Fitting et al, Caregivers for dementia patients: a comparison of husbands and wives. *The Gerontologist* 26 (1986) 248-252.

[57] M. and C. Guest, Application of a multidimensional caregiver burden inventory. *The Gerontologist* 29 (1989) 798-803.

[58] I. Philp et al, Community care for demented and non-demented elderly people: a comparison study of financial burden, service use and unmet needs in family supporters. *British Medical Journal* 310 (1995) 1503-1506.

[59] M. Grafström et al, Caring for an elderly person: predictors of burden in dementia care. *International Journal of Geriatric Psychiatry* 9 (1994) 373-379.

[60] T. Drinka et al, Correlates of depression and burden for informal caregivers of patients in a geriatrics referral clinic. *Journal of the American Geriatrics Society* 35 (1987) 522.

[61] M.D. Pagel et al, Loss of control, self-blame and depression: an investigation of spouse caregivers of Alzheimer's disease patients. *Journal of Abnormal Psychology* 94 (1985) 169-182.

[62] M.L.M. Gilhooly, The impact of caregiving on caregivers: factors associated with the psychological well-being of people supporting a dementing relative in the community. *British Journal of Medical Psychology* 57 (1984) 35-44.

[63] R.A. Pruchno and N L. Resch, Aberrant behaviours and Alzheimer's disease: mental health effects on spouse caregivers. *Journal of Gerontology* 44 (1989) 177-182.

[64] S. Harper and D.A. Lund, Wives, husbands and daughters caring for institutionalised and noninstitutionalised dementia patients: toward a model of caregiver burden. *International Journal of Aging and Human Development* 30 (1990) 241-262.

[65] E.D. Rankin et al, Clinical assessment of family caregivers in dementia. *The Gerontologist* 32 (1992) 813-821.

[66] W.E. Haley et al, Stress, appraisal, coping and social support as predictors of adaptional outcome among dementia caregivers. *Psychology and Aging* 2 (1987) 323-330.

[67] S. Zarit et al, Relatives of the impaired elderly: Correlates of feelings of burden. *The Gerontologist* 20 (1980) 649.

[68] R. Schulz and G.M. Willliamson, A two-year longitudinal study of depression among Alzheimer's caregivers. *Psychology and Aging* 6 (1991) 569-578.

[69] I. Philp and J. Young, Audit of support given to lay carers of the demented elderly by a primary care team. *Journal of the Royal College of General Practitioners* 38 (1988) 153-155.

[70] I. Philp *et al*, Institutionalisation risk amongst people with dementia supported by family carers in a Scottish city. *Ageing and Mental Health* 1 (1997) 339-345.

[71] P. Boss *et al*, Predictors of depression in caregivers of dementia patients: boundary ambuity and mastery. *Family Process* 29 (1990) 245-254.

[72] C.J. Gilleard *et al*, Emotional distress amongst the supporters of the elderly mentally infirm. *British Journal of Psychiatry* 145 (1984) 172-177.

[73] M.P. Lawton *et al*, A two-factor model of caregiving appraisal and psychological well-being. *Journal of Gerontology* 46 (1991) 181-189.

[74] M. McCarthy Neundorfer, Coping and health outcomes in spouse caregivers of persons with dementia. *Nursing Research* 40 (1991) 260-265.

[75] L.W. Morris *et al*, Cognitive style and perceived control in spouse caregivers of dementia sufferers. *British Journal of Medical Psychology* 62 (1989) 173-179.

[76] J.G. Ouslander *et al*, Incontinence among elderly community-dwelling dementia patients. Characteristics, management and impact on caregivers. *Journal of the American Geriatrics Society* 38 (1990) 440-445.

[77] A.K. Motenko, The frustrations, gratifications and well-being of dementia caregivers. *The Gerontologist* 29 (1989) 166-172.

[78] A.P. Turnbull and H.R. Turnbull, Participatory research in cognitive coping: from concepts to research planning. In: A.P. Turnbull *et al*, (eds), Cognitive Coping, Families and disability, Baltimore, MD: Paul H. Brooks, 1983.

[79] J.M. Patterson, The role of family meanings in adaptation to chronic illness and disability. In: A.P. Turnbull *et al*, (eds), Cognitive Coping, Families and Disability, Baltimore, MD: Paul H. Brookes, 1993.

[80] R. Ingebretsen and P.E. Solen, Attachment, loss and coping in caring for a dementing spouse, Paper presented at III European Congress of Gerontology, Amsterdam, 30 August -2 September 1995.

[81] K.J. McKee *et al*, Coping in family supporters of elderly people with dementia, Paper presented at the British Society of Gerontology Annual Conference. Royal Holloway, September, 1994.

[82] R.S.Lazarus, Coping theory and research: past, recent and future. *Psychosomatic Medicine* 55 (1993) 234-47.

[83] V.A. Braithwaite*Bound to care*. Sydney: Allen and Unwin, 1990.

[84] M. Birchwood and J. Smith, Schizophrenia and the Family. In: J. Orford (ed), *Coping with Disorder in the Family*. London: Croom Helm, 1987.

[85] B. Beresford, Positively Parents: Caring for a Severely Disabled Child. London: HMSO, 1994.

[86] P. Boss, Boundary ambiguity: a block to cognitive coping. In: J.M. Turnbull *et al*, (eds.), *Cognitive coping, Families and Disability*. Baltimore, MD: Paul H. Brookes, 1993.

[87] Z. Stoneman and J.M. Crapps, Correlates of stress, perceived competence and depression among family care providers. *American Journal of Mental Retardation* 93 (1988) 166-73.

[88] C. Pratt *et al*, Burden and coping strategies of caregivers to Alzheimer's disease patients. *Family Relations* 34 (1985) 27.

[89] W. Bordon and S. Berlin, Gender, coping and psychological well-being in spouses of older adults with chronic dementia. *American Journal of Orthopsychiatry* 60 (1990) 603-610.

[90] A.M. Pot *et al*, Self-perceived pressure from informal care: construction of a scale. *Tijdschrift voor Gerontologie en Geriatrie* 26 (1995) 214-219.

[91] K. Hooker *et al*, Mental and physical health of spouse caregivers: the role of personality. *Psychology and Aging* 7 (1992) 367-375.

[92] M.R. Nolan and G. Grant, Regular respite: an evaluation of a hospital rota bed scheme for elderly people. Ace Books, Age Concern Institute of Gerontology Research Papers Series No.6, London, 1992.

[93] C. Dellasaga and K. Mastrian, The process and consequences of institutionalising an elder. *Western Journal of Nursing Research* 17(20) (1995) 123-140.

[94] J.P. Scott *et al*, Family of Alzheimer's victims: family support to the caregivers. *Journal of the American Geriatrics Society* 34 (1986) 348-354.

[95] P.G. Archbold *et al*, The PREP System of nursing interventions: a pilot test with families caring for older members. *Research in Nursing and Health* 18 (1995) 3-16.

[96] M.R. Nolan, and G. Grant, Helping new carers of the frail elderly patient: the challenge for nursing in acute care settings. *Journal of Clinical Nursing* 1 (1992) 303-307.

[97] M. Baumgarten et al, The psychological and physical health of family members caring for an elderly person with dementia. *Journal of Clinical Epidemiology* 45 (1992) 61-70.
[98] M.E. Dewis and H. Niskala, Nurturing a valuable resource: family caregivers in multiple sclerosis. *Axon* 13 (1992) 87-94.
[99] C. Dellasega, Coping with caregiving: stress management for caregivers of the elderly. *Journal of Psychosocial Nursing* 28 (1990) 15-22.
[100] F. Kiecolt-Glaser et al, Spousal caregivers of dementia victims: longitudinal changes in immunity and health. *Psychosomatic Medicine* 53 (1991) 345-362.
[101] S.L. Brotman and M.J. Yaffe, Are physicians meeting the needs of family caregivers of the frail elderly? *Canadian Family Physician* (1994) 679-681.
[102] C.K. Coleman et al, Influence of caregiving on families of older adults. *Journal of Gerontological Nursing* 20 (1994) 40-49.
[103] J. Cochran, Family caregivers of the frail elderly: burdens and health. *Nurse Practitioner* 91 (1994) 5-6.
[104] R,H, Fortinsky and T.J. Hathaway, Information and service needs among active and former family caregivers of persons with Alzheimer's disease. *The Gerontologist* 30(5) (1990) 604-609.
[105] H.S. Wilson, Family caregivers: the experience of Alzheimers's disease. *Applied Nursing Research* 2(1) (1989) 40-45.
[106] A.F. Jorm et al, The disabled elderly living in the community: care received from family and formal services. *Med Journal of Austria* 15 (1993) 383-385.
[107] B. Jerrom et al, Stress on relatives of caregivers of dementia sufferers and predictors of the breakdown of community care. *International Journal of Geriatric Psychiatry* 8 (1993) 331-7.
[108] T. Sharp, Listening to carers. *Nursing Times* 88(22) (1992) 29-30.
[109] B.A. Given and C.W. Given, Family caregivers for the elderly. In: J. Fitzpatrick et al,. *Annual review of Nursing Research*, vol.9. New York: Springer, 1991.
[110] M.P. Lawton, Measuring caregiving appraisal. *Journal of Gerontology* 44 (1989) 61-71.
[111] J.I. Kosberg and R.E. Cairl, The Cost of Care Instrument: a case management tool for screening informal care providers. *The Gerontologist* 26(3) (1986) 273-278.
[112] M. England and B.L. RobertsTheoretical and psychometric analysis of caregiver strain. *Research in Nursing and Health* 19 (1996) 499-510.
[113] S. Elmstahl et al, Caregiver's burden of patients after 3 years of stroke assessment by a Novel Caregiver Burden Scale. *Archives of Physical and Medical Rehabilitation* 77 (1996) 177-182.
[114] B.C. Robinson, Validation of a caregiver strain index. *Journal of Gerontology* 38 (1983) 344-348.
[115] K. Ellis, *Squaring the Circle: User and Carer Participation in Needs Assessment*. Joseph Rowntree Foundation, York, 1993.
[116] D.A. Loukissa, Family burden in chronic mentall illness: a review of reserach studies. *Journal of Advanced Nursing* 21(92) (1995) 248-255.
[117] J. Keady and M. Nolan, Behavioural and instrumental stressors in dementia: refocussing the assessment of caregivers need in dementia. *Journal of Psychiatric and Mental Health Nursing* 3 (1996) 163-172.
[118] D.J. Harper et al, Intervening to reduce stress in caregivers of impaired elderly people. *International Journal of Geriatric Psychiatry* 8 (1993) 139-145.
[119] E.M. Brody, Parent care as a normative family stress. *The Gerontologist* 25, 19-29.
[120] A. Opie, The instability of the caring body: gender and caregivers of confused older people. *Qualitative Health Research* 4(1) (1994) 31-50.
[121] I. Winoground et al, The relationship of caregiver burden and morlae to Alzheimers' disease patients' functioning in a therapeutic setting. *Gerontologist* 27 (1987) 336.
[122] S.M. Albert, Cognition of caregiving tasks: multidimensional scaling of the caregiver task domain. *The Gerontologist* 31 (1991) 726-734.
[123] S.M. Albert, Psychometric investigation of a belief system: Caregiving to the chronically ill patient. *Social Science and Medicine* 35 (1992) 699-709.
[124] A.H. Schene et al, Instruments measuring family or caregiver burden in severe mentall illness. *Social Psychiatry and Psychiatric Epidemiology* 29 (1994) 228-240.
[125] M.A.P. Stephens and J.M. Kinney, Caregiver stress instruments: Assessment of content and measurement quality. *Gerontology View* 2 (1989) 379-388.
[126] S. Hunter et al, The Interdisciplinary Assessment of Older People and Entry into Long Term Institutional Care: Lessons for the New Community care Arrangements. *Research, Policy and Planning* 11(1-2) (1993) 2-9.
[127] M. Wright, Taking care. *Community Care* 17 (1990) 14-16.

Chapter 2

France
(October 1998)

Judith Chwalow
*INSERM
Unit 341
Service de Diabetologie
Hôpital Hôtel Dieu
1 place de parvis Notre Dame
75181 Paris Cedex 04
France*

Andrea Bagnall
*I.U.H.P.E
2, rue Auguste Comte
92170 Vanves
France*

Christine Baudoin
*INSERM
Unit 341
Service de Diabetologie
Hôpital Hôtel Dieu
1 place de parvis Notre Dame
75181 Paris Cedex 04
France*

Fabienne Elgrably
*Hopital De L'Hotel-Dieu
Service de Diabétologie
1 Place due Paris Notre-Dame
75181 Paris Cedex 04
France*

Introduction

Policy and Practice

Over the past 40 years, the increasing proportion of older people within the French population has led to much reflection on the social and medical aspects of treatment of older people. Nonetheless, the systems of care for older people which have been developed remain difficult to understand and access, poorly coordinated, and therefore inefficiently utilised. In addition to this lack of coordination, there are regional and departmental differences throughout the country which also lead to varied access to services.

As is true in other industrialised countries, the demographic changes in France which are resulting in an increased older population are based on decreasing birth rates and increasing life-expectancy. Projections for the costs of caring for this growing older population have led to much political debate since the early 1960s, before which time there had been no specific social action policy for older people who, for the most part, lived with their families. However, several charitable associations during this period began a system of aid for geographically isolated older people which consisted of some medical care at home and help with domestic tasks (assistance in the home). Costs for these initiatives were covered by the departmental social aid fund (*Aide Sociale Départementale*) and later by the primary government health insurance funds (*CPAMs*).

In 1960 the French Prime Minister created a "Commission for the Study of the Problems of Old Age" (*Commission d'Etude des Problèmes de la Vieillesse*), presided over by Pierre Laroque, one of the founding fathers of the French Social Security system. The Commission was made up of specialists in the areas of gerontology and social sciences and was given, for the first time, the task of assessing the costs of demographic ageing and its consequences, as well as setting out directives for a national policy on ageing.

Through its work, the Commission's focus centred around redefining a new concept of old age which focused on autonomy and participation in everyday social life, with the goal of keeping older people active in society. This gave way to propositions aimed at preventing social exclusion (caused by placement in institutions), including measures geared to providing: better help at home, maintenance of social activities, actions for better conditions in the home, development of leisure activities and services, providing help with domestic tasks and care for physically handicapped people.

The Commission's Report of 1962, known as the Laroque Report, is the basis of all advances made in terms of policies for the elderly over the past 35 years. During the first ten years after the report's appearance, several advances were made concerning the provision of home care (mantien à domicile), the amelioration of the home environment, and the development of contracts signed between the state and a municipality or association which led to the implementation of multi-dimentional coordinated actions for "community care" or home care. However, despite these advances, a review of actions taken over the ten year period showed that, in the absence of a global policy, only services for household assistance (aide ménagère) had developed to a notable degree. Services of home care had not developed to a significant degree [1]. Other services depending on the goodwill of local communities and Social Security funds had developed unequally depending on geographic region.

In the area of collective housing, two categories of residential establishments were created, one medical, the other social, with different regulations, rates and personnel for the same types of clients. This contributed to the split between the health and social sectors and slowed the further amelioration of collective housing for older people. By the end of the

1970s services for medicalised care within the so called "social" establishments were still highly underdeveloped.

In 1978 a working group was charged with the task of establishing a report on an elderly policy for the years to come. The main recommendations from the group's 1982 report, "*Vieillir Demain*" (Ageing for Tomorrow) concerned:

- policy concerning housing and home environment, especially in rural areas;
- better coordination of services and legislation on required conditions for benefiting from household assistance;
- the management of residential establishments (avoiding unnecessary hospitalisation and "over-medicalisation" within these establishments, developing a medical sector in retirement homes);
- intermediate solutions between the private residence and group residences (i.e. temporary homes, and nursing homes for "dependent" people not needing major medical treatment);
- the distribution of responsibilities and financial charges (i.e. further engagement of the state in issues of housing;
- increased responsibility of communities in terms of social action for older people and in the coordination of decisions concerning provisions for long-term health and "social" residencie
- better integration of older people into social life (i.e. adapting urban and rural environments to older people with reduced physical capacities);
- facilitating family relations;
- ensuring the participation of retired people in the management of the services, equipment and policies which concern them) [1].

During the late 1970s and early 1980s the economic crisis led to a decrease in the legal age for retirement, thus leading to premature retirement for a large number of people. Spending was also curbed for several services and for care for older people. In order to control health costs related to older people, a new emphasis was put on reinforcing inter-generational solidarity and the role of "informal" carers to the detriment of investing in formal care [2]. During the same time period, several laws were passed, decentralising the responsibility for social and health actions to the department (a geographical division in France), which meant that the establishment of departmental plans for services and social institutions would be carried out at a local level.

More recently efforts have been made to reduce the insufficiencies in the provision of medical care at home and for medicalised housing in residential establishments. In 1997 a law was passed providing a *Prestation Spécifique Dépendance* (PSD), a temporary benefit to help pay for a service or carer in the home. This benefit is a transitory solution to the need for an "autonomy" benefit for older people which will better respond to their needs. It is allocated to dependent older people over 60 years of age subject to their level of income, as well as level of dependency. According to specifications, this level of dependency should be based on an evaluation carried out by a medical-social team within the department, who then implements a plan for care. Its creation was meant to facilitate the coordination of the diverse group of people intervening in the care of older people.

However it has failed to have this effect and has failed to integrate itself with the services and care from which older people may have already benefited (for example, it cannot be received simultaneously with other benefits for domestic help services). It is also very controversial as it is allocated at a departmental level, and creates an unbalanced level of care depending on geographical region. Furthermore, it is situated within the framework of social aid, or aid for the lowest socio-economic level of society. This means that some of the people who need it most (people with middle or lower-middle class incomes) are not receiving it. The level of dependency of the person in need is considered secondary to the issue of his or her income.

Who Provides Support?

Interventions for dependent older people in France are characterised by their diversity, in terms of financing, services and benefits. Under the current social protection system, dependency is not defined and managed as a social risk but in different and rarely coordinated forms, it has led to a system of care, for which the cost in 1989 was around 24 billion francs [3].

Financial responsibility for the different types of benefits and services is divided between the State, the Social Security fund and complementary insurance and retirement funds, and the Departmental Social Aid (*Aide Sociale Départementale*). In most cases the funding body does not directly provide the services it pays for. The various providers include:

- The Ministry of Work and Social Affairs (under the direction for social action);
- The local territories: the department represents the sum of medical and social aid provided for older people. Each local community has a budget and a system of social action in favour of older people (for things such as providing meals on wheels, creating senior-citizen clubs and restaurants, etc.).;
- Social Security: active mostly through health insurance which covers three types of costs:
  - expenses for the medical surveillance of residential establishments, (care provided by nurses and carers, as well as the medications and products necessary for care);
  - medical care for people who have lost the capacity to perform their everyday activities by themselves or who have a somatic or mental condition. This includes the remuneration of medical and paramedical personnel, the provision of medication, and financial support for the purchase of equipment;
  - professional care at home which includes medical care and hygiene for older people;
- The National Elderly Fund for Salaried Workers (*Caisse National d'Assurance Viellesse*), which is a national fund providing pensions. The fund is financed by a mandatory contribution of 9% by all salaried workers. This fund plays a fundamental role in providing services for assistance in the home. There are also a large number of supplementary funds and mutual insurance companies, all of which must spend 1% of their budgets on social action;
- A wide range of associations, volunteers and the families of the elderly themselves.

Legal Situation Concerning Responsibilities for the Care of Older People

In France, there is currently much discussion as to the division of financial responsibility between the State and families for the care of older people. Requests for social aid are awarded subject to the income of the person in need, which must not be greater than a certain amount per month. According to a survey of the fiscal income of households in 1984 [4], 82% of the essential income source for elderly households (over 75 years) came from retirement pensions and annuities. 11% of the income was related to property/real estate, 2% came from pay for work done, and 5% came from the old age minimum pension, which is a non-contributory scheme to provide older people with a minimum income [5]. It is made up of a range of basic allowances depending on retirement conditions and the family situation, to which a supplementary allowance can be provided where appropriate by the National Solidarity Fund.

In terms of the family, the maintenance obligation constitutes the legal basis of the family's liability to provide for the vital needs of its older members [3]. In essence, the maintenance obligation in France includes the idea of solidarity in the family, which for a long time was a value considered quasi-essential to the functioning of society [5]. Today, however, in an era of evolving family contexts and situations characterised by increasing life expectancy, decreasing birth rates, changing roles and employment patterns for women, greater geographical mobility within the family, increased divorce rates and an increase in the number of single parents, a number of questions are raised when considering the decision to substitute family solidarity with social solidarity.

It has been noted that there is often a cause and effect relationship between the socialisation of maintenance relations and the decline of familial solidarity [5]. By not allowing for a complete socialisation of the maintenance obligation, the State is caught between acting in the name of national solidarity while not being reimbursed by the family, and requiring the family to reimburse the money provided to the older person in need. The law is therefore highly criticised for its negative effects, as it authorises the State to recover from descendants, or even from an inherited estate, some or all of the social aid payments made to older people in need (except in cases where support is provided for assistance in the home). Many older people don't agree with the State "attacking their children" and would like to leave behind a material inheritance [3]. However, the State usually collects from the family an average of 40-45% of the money it spends on social aid for older people.

Specifically the law states that children have a maintenance obligation to their parents (natural or adoptive) or other ascendants in need. Children-in-law also have a maintenance obligation toward their in-laws, unless their marriage ends in divorce. In the case of death of the spouse linking a child-in-law to his/her parents, the obligation no longer exists unless there are legitimate children from their marriage [5]. There is also a maintenance obligation between spouses.

The sum of money to be provided to the older person in need of help may either be decided upon by the parties involved, or by a judge who will decide depending upon the income of the provider and the needs of the recipient. This sum can be re-evaluated if there is a change in the situation of either party's income (unemployment, inheritance, etc.) or if there is a change in the needs of the recipient (sickness, need for medical care, etc.).

Health and Social Care for Older People: Structures and Functions

Organisational Structures

Until the 1950s and 1960s the care of older people was mainly handled either by the family or, in the case of institutionalisation, by an establishment such as a hospice which housed large numbers of older people. Through the 1960s and early 1970s much emphasis was put on improving these institutions, and on creating retirement homes for older people in good health. Around the same time, a distinction was drawn between "social" establishments for people not needing major medical treatment, and medical establishments, which completely ignored the variety of needs of older people living in residential establishments, as well as the evolution of these needs with age. With the publication of the Laroque Report, the 1970s were characterised by a new emphasis on keeping older people active and at home. In order to advance these objectives of keeping

older people in their homes and avoiding placement in residential establishments, a specific administrative system was implemented in 1982, which relied on:
- the national committee and the departmental committees of retired and older people, which aim to help older people implement and participate in the actions and programmes concerning them; and
- the development of a departmental gerontological plan.

Because the needs of older people are so diverse, there is a range of institutions and services both private and public, national and local, non-profit and private, health related and social to meet their needs. These services, however, are very often poorly coordinated, dependent on several factors and varied according to region.

Funding for these establishments and services is also divided into two groups. Those involving treatment (at home or in an establishment) are covered by health insurance. The rest of the costs linked to housing are the responsibility of either the people receiving the services, their families, social organisations, social action of supplementary retirement funds and/or departmental social aid. With the sharp distinction between the health and social sectors, it is difficult to determine who pays for which forms of care, as some forms are highly medical, but some, such as daily hygiene and various types of psycho-social aid, are not. The system of financing in residential establishments, however, is currently being changed. There is also a reform concerning the distinction between technical medical treatments and care linked to dependency regarding the ability of the elderly person to carry out everyday activities. These reforms should be put in place by the end of 1998 and aim to reform the system of charges so that it will be based more on the level of dependency of the older person than on the type of establishment s/he is using [3,8].

The institutional system of care in France mainly addresses older people only when they have begun to experience difficulties with autonomy, whether these difficulties be economic, physical, or mental [6]. There is a clear separation between services providing home care, or "community care", and those providing accommodation and treatment.

Residential Establishments

The wide range of residential establishments in France provides accommodation and treatment to people no longer able to live at home. Among these there is a clear distinction between social establishments and health establishments, depending on the level of medicalisation, the degree of independence and capacity for self-care of the people living in them.

Health Establishments

Among older people in France hospitalisation in public and private establishments is frequent. This population represents 70% of the total number of hospitalisations [7]. The public sector provides the majority of housing, although the private sector has been developing residences for several years. In recent years, criticism of hospitalisation has included the fact that the concepts of private and social life are virtually non-existent. Also the majority of residents do not need major medical treatment, but rather paramedical care and help with activities of daily living, such as personal hygiene, eating, dressing, and walking. Therefore, hospitalisation in these cases is inappropriate and costly, and the presence of physicians is unsettling. Many hospitals are also geographically remote. These criticisms have led to recent advances in improving conditions in medical residential establishments.

Among the establishments categorised as medical or "health" establishments are:
- hospices, which since the hospital laws of 1970 and 1975, have been transformed into long-stay health-care units or medicalised retirement homes (nursing homes);
- long-stay centres, destined for people who have lost their independence and who need constant medical surveillance and treatment. Placement in such a centre often follows a period in a mid-term or short-stay centre when there are complications prohibiting the person's return home. This can have serious consequences on the mental health of the individual, as these centres are considered as "treatment" centres, and not social/residential establishments. These include:
- medium-term centres which function as a temporary residence for sick people, with the intention that after the critical phase of their sickness, they will readopt an independent lifestyle;
- geriatric services, largely populated with older people affected by mental deterioration;
- local hospitals, which provide the advantage of being close to the person's home, especially in rural areas; and
- psychiatric hospitals, within which there is often a well-adapted, multi-disciplinary team of geriatric psychiatrists.

Social Establishments

Among the residential establishments characterised as "social", there are several different types. These include:
- *Retirement homes:* These are the most common and widespread residential establishments for non-invalid older people. They provide a range of services and often take into account the gradual loss of independence while facilitating the maintenance of an active social and personal lifestyle. They often have a treatment component for those people not able to carry out their daily activities alone or for those who have a stabilised somatic or psychological condition requiring medical treatment, surveillance and paramedical treatment. These establishments may pose two problems: passivity which can lead to the regression of older people living there, and a care component which is not intensive enough, often leading to the hospitalisation of the tenants when they become sick.
- *Sheltered accommodation:* This type of accommodation has been closely developed with community activists and is essentially for older people in good health, capable of living independently but who would like occasional assistance and reassurance.
- *Temporary accommodation:* These are limited to 15-20 people and are for older people (dependent or not) needing a temporary residence either before or after hospitalisation, during a period where their family, friends or neighbours are not available to care for them, or simply wanting to spend the winter or a weekend in a warm, secure place. The service provided by this type of accommodation acts as a complement to other establishments and services and responds to situations of transition between the hospital and the home (in either direction). This type of accommodation is also often used to give family caregivers a break from their responsibilities as main caregiver.
- *"Maisons d'accueil"*, or adapted retirement homes: Characterised by their size and architecture, these are residential establishments which are meant to facilitate a community life with a number of social and cultural activities. Among them are "maisons d'acceuils" for dependent older people, which have a maximum capacity of 80 people, and rural "maisons d'acceuils" with a maximum capacity of 15-20 people. There

are also several dozen "cantous" throughout France, which lodge people experiencing mental deterioration and in need of surveillance, but in good physical health.
- *Small "proximity" structures:* these are still fairly undeveloped in France, with only a small number in existence. They are innovative, small residential establishments with a capacity for a small number of people (8-25), based on the idea that older people feel most comfortable at home. These structures therefore act as substitution homes for older people in their neighbourhoods and are well-adapted to their needs and to facilitating their autonomy and social links for as long as possible, without ignoring the medical and paramedical aspects provided by health-care providers. They often consist of several apartments or, in rural areas, can be set up within a house. There is a preventive focus to these structures, which includes the idea of preserving individual liberty, independence, and good physical condition. The tenants participate in daily tasks such as cleaning, cooking, and taking care of the house according to their capabilities. The personnel is coordinated by a "house mother", who manages a multi-disciplinary team. There is no internal medical component, rather outside services are called upon as needed. These structures are currently somewhat controversial, based on arguments around the absence of medicalisation and the importance of keeping older people within their social environment and not treating dependency as a disease.

Services

The range of services available for older people in France has developed considerably over the past 25 years, partly due to a dynamism on the part of locally elected politicians since the decentralisation of the responsibility for social and health actions, and partly due to greater awareness of the problems of an ageing population. However, this evolution is very varied in its success and, despite advances, there is an important lack of coordination. The changes have not reached and influenced all sectors equally and many advances are still only at an experimental phase [7].

Nevertheless, there is a wide variety of possible combinations of services, corresponding to the different stages of evolution of the loss of independence. The variety of services provided covers four types of needs linked to a partial loss of independence:
- information;
- entertainment, including senior citizen clubs and places providing community meals;
- help in the home, including things such as household assistance, improvement in the home environment, and meals on wheels; and
- home care/treatment through services such as hospitalisation in the home, or care from a visiting nurse.

Home care services, the most widespread component, can be divided into two main categories: household assistance (*aide ménagère*) and home health-care services (*services de soins infirmiers à domicile*).

Household Assistance

This is the principal and oldest existing service providing help in the home to people having difficulties in carrying out every day domestic tasks. Its mission is to carry out material, moral and social work contributing to the community or home care of older people. The first such services were created over forty years ago. These services are either provided by departmental social aid (if the recipient's income is low enough) or by various social security or retirement funds. Household assistance includes mainly domestic tasks such as all types of housecleaning, shopping, administrative tasks, and in a minority of cases includes cooking and personal care (hygiene). Very often, in fact, the person providing household assistance carries out tasks which the older person is capable of carrying out him/herself without difficulty. The national average for people receiving this help is around 16 hours of household assistance per month. In 1990, almost 500,000 people were receiving household assistance at this rate. Ninety-seven percent of the beneficiaries of this type of assistance are older people living alone [9]. The other beneficiaries are handicapped people, mothers of large families, and ill people.

Home Healthcare Services

Different from household assistance, but sometimes received in addition to the latter, this type of service began in 1978 to help older people who are sick or dependent and need medical care and help with activities of daily living such as personal hygiene, moving, eating, etc.. The costs of these health-care services are covered either by health insurance, or by default, by departmental medical aid. The objectives of this type of service include preventing, avoiding, or shortening the length of visits to hospital or to other medical or social establishments. These services are managed either by associations, community centres for social action, health or medical-social establishments, or diverse social organisations and they are coordinated by a salaried nurse, who employs a team of aides and visiting nurses. In addition to the family, friends, relatives, neighbours and independent nurses, these services play a important role in the care of dependent older people in the home.

In 1991 it was estimated that roughly .5% of people over 65 living at home or in sheltered accommodations were reached by this type of service [10]. In 1991, 26% of the people receiving this kind of aid were extremely dependent (confined to bed or in a wheelchair). 65% of them were in need of help with everyday tasks such as personal hygiene and getting dressed, while only 4% had no problems arising from a physical dependency [9].

Other Services

Several other types of services also exist (within or outside the home), in varying degrees, including:
- auxiliary nursing in the home (*auxiliaire de vie*), which can be carried out within a private residence to help a dependent person with everyday tasks;
- meals on wheels (funded by the department or community);
- home visits for people suffering from solitude and loneliness. Professionals may provide home visits to people needing someone to talk to etc.. This type of service is provided in addition to a psychological follow-up;
- tele-alarm systems enabling older people to keep their autonomy but at the same time have the facility to make urgent calls in case of need;
- financial assistance to improve the standard of comfort and/or accessibility within the home;
- special home restaurants, often set up in the neighbourhood for older people;
- geriatric day centres which are often used as a place for older people to meet and create social ties, and as a means for family caregivers to get a break from their responsibilities;
- home hospitalisation during which hospital services already undertaken may be continued in the home, if there is consent from the family;

- home supervision, which ensures the presence of a responsible person. This may provide a sense of security for an older person living alone, even though the supervisor is not required to have particular training;
- psychiatric homecare services which allow older people affected by mental disorders to stay in their homes;
- daily hospitalisation, during which a more specialised global therapeutic type of care can be carried out than in the home, and which may involve techniques, products and qualified personnel difficult to obtain outside a medical establishment. These very short-term periods spent in medical establishments avoid the disruption of the lives of older people, such as moving from their homes, etc.;
- senior citizen clubs, including vacation and leisure activities which are sometimes offered to older people in good health;
- senior citizen universities which provide training, with hours adapted to the lifestyles of older people;
- placement of older people within a "foster" family other than their own: this is a service which was reorganised by a law in 1989 allowing families to take one or two older people into their homes for a fee (in certain cases three people are allowed).

Despite the efforts and developments made over the years, this system of care suffers many insufficiencies:
- quantitative and qualitative insufficiencies of establishments and services which are unequally distributed throughout the country;
- a compartmentalisation of structures for which the costs are based on the type of structure and not the situation of the person receiving its services (this is changing, however);
- insufficient financial coverage for certain services for which the cost is often too high for those with middle-class incomes;
- a lack of coordination of services and a system of orientation for older people and their families.

Following the parliamentary mission on dependency of the elderly in 1991, it was emphasised that there is an absolute urgency to provide a measure to improve the conditions in which solidarity is exercised in favour of dependent elderly people and in providing trained personnel. The inadequacy or unsuitability of measures for providing residential and home care were also emphasised, particularly the fact that there were not enough homecare services, domestic assistance was not targeted at the most in need, and home supervision was rare. The lack of coordination of services was also highlighted, as was the fact that services are often poorly adapted to the level and type of dependency of the recipient [10].

The Relationship Between Formal and Informal Care

Non-remunerated family or "informal" care and formal (medical) care are interdependent, yet at the same time are independent systems of action. One cannot and should not substitute for the other.

Informal care is characterised by its adaptability, malleability, permanence, and diversity because it often covers the full range of needs of older people, with the exception of specialised care [11]. Formal care is standardised, specific and subject to a contractual logic. The former is generally based on social links, exchange, giving and symbolic debt, while the latter is often based on criteria of utility and economic efficiency [11]. Family support is seen as extremely important, as it extends far beyond the support provided by the formal system. It prevents and delays entrance into residential establishments and hospitals, it complements public services and financial aid, and it contributes to the institutional efficiency of the formal system [11]. It is also capable of adequately responding to "intermediary" situations, in which the older person is not really sick, but not completely independent either, and has needs which are not only medical, but social and emotional. Informal caregivers therefore often serve as the intermediary between older people and formal carers.

Formal and informal care work well together only if there is a relationship of partnership and respect. The acknowledgement that each system has its role and specific place is also necessary for the two to function in harmony. Formal care and specialised treatment cannot replace the family, and vice-versa. The challenge in France, as in other countries, is in articulating the two systems well, so that each works to its maximum effectiveness, each complementary to the other.

Practitioner's Roles

An older person's general practitioner should ideally play an essential role in coordinating the different services and care systems (including informal care) available to him/her. As practitioners often have regular contact with their clients, they would seem to be in a position to establish older people's needs and if necessary, to coordinate the different actors involved in providing care and improving their environments. This role should also be supported by a strong component of continual training on all aspects of ageing. This is rarely the case in France, even though the field of gerontology has greatly improved over the past 30 years.

In France, there is a need for a complete tool to assess the level of independence of older people, which can be implemented with the help of a common instrument for measuring dependency, a home visit in order to assess the daily environment, and the development of a concrete plan of assistance and orientation for older people and their caregivers. In addition to this, the practitioner should have a role in each step of the process, which would require him/her to adopt an attitude other than the prevailing traditional attitudes of intervention. There is a real need in France for practitioners to move toward a more social and cultural context of the treatment of older people [12].

Roles of Family Carers of Older People Living at Home

The changes in family structure and the changes in the State's role in caring for older people, have led to changes in the family's role in the care of its older members. Reflection on family solidarity, social and community support are some of the main components of the debate around the future of social protection and the welfare state in France.

The social security and social aid systems in France are in a financially difficult situation with increased unemployment, an increasing older population, increasing health costs, and a crisis within the retirement system. Several strategies have been implemented to respond to the financial crisis: reducing certain benefits, limiting access to certain services, decentralising their management, and privatisation. The State has also looked more toward the family, neighbourhoods, and communities to help respond to this crisis because they seem to be an economic and efficient solution when used in conjunction with the formal public systems of care [13].

Over the past decade, the role of informal care has been regarded as increasingly important, even to the detriment of formal care. Professional, formal care is very rarely the only care provided and is most often given in addition to informal care. In fact, informal care is more widespread than formal care. The impact of this is difficult for the family, however, which is often pushed to the limits of its capacities. Despite this, there is no real system of support for the family caregivers (financial or other), with the exception of scattered interventions throughout the country.

If the majority of older people in France are able to stay at home, it is because of their families, who complement the system of formal care. However, very few studies have been carried out concerning informal caregivers of older people in France. 90% of older dependent people living at home receive help from people around them [3]. For the most part, informal care is provided for older people living at home, although informal family care is also sometimes provided in residential establishments. According to a survey carried out by the National Elderly Fund for Salaried Workers (*CNAV*) in 1992, more than 80% of children of the "pivot" generation (aged roughly 45-55 years) said that if their parents or parents in law needed regular support in the future because of their health problems, they would provide it, either by housing them (25%), providing care and services without housing (23%), or providing partial care complemented by professional care (33%) [3]. It has also been shown that women are more concerned with the issue than men, no matter what their age, yet there is no difference between the proportion of men and women receiving care from informal caregivers [3].

The help provided by informal carers (either occasional or regular) is more frequently for activities external to the home (such as shopping) than for activities within the home (cleaning, cooking, laundry, etc.). Activities involving personal hygiene are the least common among informal carers [3]. However, the activities of a caregiver depend on several factors: the degree and nature of the dependency of the older person, their ability to carry out certain tasks themselves, the availability and extent of additional formal and informal assistance, and whether the caregiver lives with the person receiving care. The type of care provided also depends on the sex of the caregiver. Women are more likely than men to carry out household tasks such as laundry, cleaning, cooking, and personal hygiene.

Children as Caregivers

When possible, the spouse is the primary and most important caregiver. However, when a child is the main carer (or secondary carer when a spouse is capable) it is usually the oldest child who takes responsibility for the older parent.

For older parents receiving regular help from a child, in ¾ of the cases it is a woman, and more specifically a daughter (63%) or a daughter in law (9%) who provides the care. These daughters and daughters in law often live close to the parents they help-2 out of 3 live less than one kilometre away. When it is a son who is the primary care giver, he is most often single [3].

When the dependent older person lives with his/her siblings, there is a distinction between co-habitation and re-cohabitation. Cohabitation, or permanent co-residence, wherein the child who provides the care has never left home, is most often seen among unmarried sons in the agricultural milieu. This is also more common in certain regions, such as in the South-west of the country. In the case of re-cohabitation, it is most often the parent who goes to live with his/her children. In this case, it is often married, unemployed daughters with their own children who have their parents come to live with them. It is rare that parents go to live with an unmarried child [3].

How Carers are Affected

The responsibility for caring for an older member of one's family can have serious consequences on the lives of the carers in terms of psychological and physical health, social, professional, financial and family situations. These consequences can either be practical in nature (impacting on the everyday arrangements of the carer's personal time, physical environment, leisure activities, outings, holidays, work, marital and other social relationships, etc.), or psychological, involving mixed feelings of hatred and love, guilt, stress, fatigue, worry, isolation, sadness, etc. Also, communication with an older person (who may be ill) is not always easy. Studies show that families have a hard time tolerating and showing patience toward the people they care for, and also have a hard time setting limits and keeping distance. This often leads to feelings of frustration, failure, guilt and the loss of one's role as a family member, as opposed to caregiver.

Problems felt by informal caregivers differ according to several factors:
- the family ties involved (sometimes friends or neighbours provide care);
- the level of dependency of the older person;
- family history and composition;
- where the dependent person lives;
- socio-cultural milieu;
- economic situation;
- existing exterior aid (formal and informal); and
- capacity to communicate.

As far as carers' perceived rewards are concerned, there has not been much social research carried out in France on this aspect of informal care. However, it has been cited that contributing to family cohesion and family obligations may be rewarding experiences for the caregivers. Helping an older family member cope with his/her physical dependency and the psychological factors of the ageing process may also be rewarding for family members.

Assistance for Caregivers

Caregivers are currently inadequately informed when it comes to their options for assistance. The diversity of public finance sources, the sparse distribution of services providing information on possibilities for assistance, and the lack of coordination of services all contribute to this.

There are no real financial benefits from the State for informal caregivers, with the exception of certain small tax exemptions and a very limited and restrictive allowance for caring for one's parents in certain geographic areas. In fact, it has been noted that in France a decline has been seen in government assistance to informal carers. However, at local levels in certain areas of France, dispersed services and programmes are sometimes available for people caring for family members. These services do not begin to cover the needs of caregivers.

Assessment

Caregivers' Needs

Little study has been conducted concerning the needs of informal caregivers in France, although several points can be made concerning what support for caregivers should ideally include:

- information on various topics, such as dealing with the complicated administrative and care systems, coping with stress, guilt, etc. This type of information can be provided in a variety of ways (individual interviews, telephone exchanges, help groups, family associations, documents, videos, brochures, etc.);
- training on different aspects of caring for older people;
- more financial benefits;
- personalised interventions depending on: the older person's stages of dependency and illness, the psychological state of the dependent person, and the degree of involvement of the caregiver;
- better coordination with formal care services; and
- a stronger system of structures that can give the caregiver a break from time to time (geriatric day care centres, short-stay residential establishments, etc.).

Families are also in need of benchmarks concerning their aptitude to provide care and their relationships with their dependent family members. Personalised psychological support should be available on a systematic basis (especially for carers of older people affected by Alzheimer's disease or senile dementia) to help carers deal with their psychological problems and issues such as disease and death.

For measuring the psychological consequences of care for the carer, there are several quantitative tools in French, including a recently translated version of the "Burden Inventory" tool by Zarit, which has been used in several areas to synthesise physical, psychological and social dimensions of carers' situations.

Existing Programmes Intending to Provide Support to Caregivers

Dispersed and varied programmes and services exist for carers throughout the country, yet many carers remain uninformed of these services. Run by a variety of public, private and voluntary organisations, these programmes may include:
- help/discussion groups;
- seminars;
- training sessions on various health issues such as nutrition for the elderly, domestic accidents, use of the formal health care system, the rights of older people and their families, etc.;
- counselling sessions and home visits related to family relations, specific diseases;
- psychological and medical surveillance;
- networks; and
- temporary centres or residences where older people can go for short periods of time.

Fondation de France Since 1988 the Fondation de France has supported roughly thirty programmes providing support for family caregivers throughout the country. Their goal is to complement existing actions and services. In 1994 [14], the organisation carried out a survey among a sample of these programmes which provide one or more of three different types of interventions:
- individual or group psychological support;
- informational sessions within which the psychological component remains present;
- internships providing support and training.

Although the goal of these programmes is to meet the needs of family carers, the study showed that they are rarely developed "with" families, but rather "for" them.

According to the study and in terms of seeking support, the family caregiver, who is usually exhausted and very involved in the relationship with his/her older member, is not often in a position to request support. A recent study carried out by the Complementary Insurance Fund for Agricultural Workers and the Association of Rural Families has highlighted that it is also isolation and the heavy psychological responsibility which prevent families from participating in support programmes [15]. In rural regions, requests for help mostly concern access to information, an increase in the offer of household assistance services, and an increase in financial aid. In urban areas, requests are more often for long-term psychological support, although families in these areas do request information as well.

The *Fondation de France* study showed that evaluating their actions is not a priority for support programmes and they often go by intuition in maintaining that their actions are useful and necessary. However, even without formal quantitative evaluations, the sample of programmes which were surveyed expressed several commonalities in their experiences:
- the programmes provide a freeing of guilt for the families;
- the clients seem satisfied, even if their participation is irregular;

as well as several weak points:
- it is difficult to determine the needs of families and to measure their degree of satisfaction;
- it is difficult to find the best way to generate interest and participation of families;
- it is difficult to mobilise partners for distributing information; and
- it is difficult to integrate actions into a coherent process of treatment for older people and their families [14].

"Familes Rurales" and the "Mutalité Sociale Agricole" The decentralised network of the Complementary Insurance Fund for Agricultural Workers is highly active in rural regions. Since 1986 their Programme for Action Against Dependency has been adopted in thirty regions throughout the country. It is a global programme which addresses the issues of prevention, home care services, and support to residential establishments and which includes, in certain regions, interventions providing support to informal caregivers. This support may range from the provision of low-cost or free day care services and temporary residences, to the provision of forums for group help, information, training, etc.

Since 1993 the Complementary Insurance Fund for Agricultural Workers and the Association of Rural Families have also developed a programme for supporting informal caregivers in rural areas. This programme has as its objectives:
- helping families in their relationships with their parents;
- validating the central role of the family and contributing to its recognition in policies of social ageing actions; and
- interviews at home with families caring for older people in their homes in order to better understand their situations. (This last activity was carried out in 13 geographic departments).

The School for Parents and Educators Schools for Parents and Educators, which are non-profit organisations grouped under the National Federation of Schools for Parents and Educators, have been set up in several towns in France. Three schools in different regions ran a programme for family caregivers from 1989-1991 which addressed family carers aged 45-65 by providing an alternating programme of information and support for participants through verbal exchange [5]. The objectives of the programme included:
- helping family caregivers to have a better experience of their relationship with their elderly relative for whom they were responsible, by clarifying each one's roles;

- facilitating or re-establishing communication between the carer, the relative, other family members and care professionals involved;
- providing information on memory, sexuality, and clarifying values in order to help confront the psychological and physiological processes of ageing and death (for both the older relatives and the carers themselves).

Evaluation of the programme showed proof of the value of family support groups if they are led by personnel with specific training [5]. The mix of verbal exchanges and objective information appeared as main factors for the success of the programme. It also showed, however, that recruitment for participation was difficult, perhaps due to the fact that Schools for Parents and Educators are not specific structures for the elderly.

The "Green Door" Listening-Counselling-Orientation Programme This action, implemented in Versailles, is aimed at subscribers and beneficiaries of retirement institutions who find themselves having to cope with the loss of independence of an older relative (especially a spouse or parent) [5]. It serves as a structure for medical, social and psychological evaluation and addresses the whole family group, including the older person.

The assistance process, which is provided free of charge by the social section of the retirement fund, starts with a session in which the family situation is assessed in order to determine whether it is possible to keep the older person at home or whether admission to an institution is necessary. Although designed as support for the caregivers, the counselling and orientation provided through the programme aim to find a solution which meets the needs of both the carer and the older person, and to avoid unnecessary placement in establishments or hospitals. Decisions and responsibilities, however, remain the duty of the family. Other aspects of the programme focus on providing information on illnesses effecting the older person, home help, and possible psychological support for caregivers.

The experience of the programme has shown that the close linkage of its medical, social and psychological aspects matches the needs of carers and the complexity of their situations.

Experience has also shown that users of the service often contacted the service with an initial question concerning the administrative and care systems for their elderly relatives, but that this was usually a pretext, which quickly led to the uncovering of other psychological needs. Experience also shows that the programme has not made itself widely enough known and that the requests received for help do not match the actual need for assistance. It was also highlighted that the programme would be more effective if it were spread more broadly and if it formed part of an overall gerontological programme.

Despite the lack of complete evaluations for many of the above mentioned programmes, most of them could be rather easily reproduced in other regions of the country, although there is still much to be learned about the needs of carers as well as motivations for asking for support and participating in support programmes. It is known, however, that their needs are not being met.

Case Studies

In all of these cases, there is a large number of factors which contribute to the roles the family caregiver would play and to the benefits the older person may receive. Their exact level of income, the region in which they live, whether or not their children live in the same town, the complementary insurance fund they adhere to, etc. all impact on the way care would be provided. The following case-studies are therefore only examples of some of the possible situations, and are by no means represent "standard care". However, in all cases, medical care in France is a person's legal right, so any medical services or treatment used are always, at least in part, covered by the government.

It should be noted that in all of the cases for which the older person's income is sufficiently low, the "*Préstation Spécifique Dépendance*" (Specific Dependency Benefit) may be provided to help pay for a service or carer in the home, as all of the dependent older people in the case studies are over 60 years old. The benefit is distributed at the departmental level depending on levels of income and dependency which are also assessed at the local level. This level of dependency should ideally, according to standardised specifications, be determined based on an evaluation carried out by a medical-social team within the department, who then implements a plan for care. It is not provided for short-term needs, however (for example if the person is just recovering from a hospital visit). Also, if this benefit were provided, it would most likely affect the provision of other additional services.

The level to which the informal caregivers' needs would be assessed and the support provided to them would also very much vary from community to community depending on availability and quality of services.

Case 1

Female, aged 76 with osteoarthritis of the hips and knees, poor vision due to macular degeneration and hypertension. Mobile with a frame within her home, except for the stairs. Needs help with mobility outside, shopping, cooking and housework.

Situation 1- The daughter would probably play a large role in caring for her mother in this situation, especially with household tasks. The daughter would be receiving unemployment benefits and a large family allowance from the government, which would possibly help pay for her to have her own household assistance at home. She may also receive a small allowance for providing care to her mother and may have access to certain support systems, including geriatric day care centres allowing her to take a break from care occasionally. In rural areas, however, access to information and services for carers in often non-existent.

As this is a rural area, the Agricultural Mutual Insurance Fund (*Caisse Agricole*) would probably intervene by paying for household assistance (provided that the daughter lives in the adjacent town, and not the same town as her mother). Any home care provided by a nurse or other professional caregiver would be reimbursed by the National Health Insurance Fund (*CNAM*) and/or departmental social aid. As the older person has trouble with stairs, she may also be able to benefit from an allowance for home improvements (e.g. installation of an apparatus to help her with the stairs) and may benefit from the use of a tele-alarm, for emergencies.

Situation 2- As the daughter lives in the same town, she would probably be available to provide some help with household tasks, but her time would be limited due to her working full-time. Household assistance would also be provided, but the funding would depend on the older person's income. A tele-alarm may be provided by the community, as might various other services such as meals on wheels.

Since they are in town, the informal caregiver(s) may have better access to support programmes, such as help groups during which they may get together with other families to share their experiences.

Situation 3- The spouse would be the principle caregiver in this situation, with homecare services provided as needed and covered by health-care. As the couple in this situation is financially solvent, they could make improvements to their home so that the woman would be able to easily access her bedroom, bathroom and toilet. This may or may not be partially covered by aid from a retirement fund.

Case 2

Male, aged 80, facing discharge from hospital following a stroke. Expected to be confined to bed or a chair for several weeks with gradual recovery of mobility. Needs the help of one person for transfers, toileting, bathing, and dressing.

Care upon being discharged from a hospital largely depends on the hospital's recommendations. In certain cases, a nurse may be in contact with the family and may even make a visit to the home to see if home care is possible. If the family is well informed of the needs of the recovering person, they may take on the role as primary caregiver with professional help only when and if needed. Or, in certain cases, if the older person is not living alone and the family is in agreement, home hospitalisation may be provided, during which hospital services already undertaken may be continued in the home. If the family lives too far away to provide care, the older person would probably be hospitalised in an acute care hospital until s/he was able to return home without the need of constant supervision.

Situation 1- Since the children in this situation are unemployed and live close-by, one or more family members may temporarily go to live with the father to take care of him while recovering. Otherwise, homecare services would be covered by health insurance or the departmental social aid and would include daily help with hygiene and other technical needs.

*Situation 2-*This would be a difficult situation as the children both work full-time. Most likely the older person would be placed in a short-term hospital unit throughout the duration of his recovery period.

Situation 3- If well informed by the hospital, the spouse would be the primary caregiver, with homecare services provided as needed and covered by health insurance. If the spouse were not capable of carrying out the role of primary caregiver, home hospitalisation, or acute care hospitalisation may be provided.

Case 3

Female, aged 86, suffering from dementia. Frequent wandering by day and night. Frequent falls. Incontinent of urine and faeces.

Situation 1- The daughter in this situation would probably provide the majority of care, although permanent surveillance (perhaps by an auxiliary nurse) would be needed. The psychological and financial load (for products needed due to incontinence) on the family would probably be very heavy, and they may or may not have access to help groups for carers of older people suffering from dementia.

Situation 2- In this situation, as the children are both employed full-time, the older person would probably be placed in a residential establishment for people affected with senile dementia.

Situation 3- The spouse would be the main caregiver in this situation, with additional professional medical care provided when and if needed and covered by social security.

Future Developments

It is clear that there is much to do concerning the care of older people in France and even more in providing support for the caregivers themselves. The social security and social aid systems in France are being severely burdened with the patterns of increased unemployment, an increasingly older population, rising health costs, and a crisis within the retirement system, which only add to the challenges ahead. Support for dependency is costly and social risks are increasing for older people. Despite these challenges, there is some hope for development, especially at a local level.

The few studies carried out on the expectations of people over 75 show that they hope, above all, to maintain their independence and have equal access to services. Their main requests concern the improvement of their living environments and access to existing services [16]. Promoting healthy ageing and healthy lifespans must thus become a priority for medical and social professionals and policy makers if the needs of older people are going to be met and services are to be more effectively provided and coordinated. The state of health of the caregiver obviously affects the older person s/he is caring for. It is therefore critical to consider the caregivers in global policies concerning the care of older people.

Obstacles to the Implementation of Specific Policies for Older People

Several factors contribute to the existing gap between the definition of specific policies and their implementation. The first group of factors is linked to the fragmentation of responsibilities concerning the organisation and funding of the health care system. This fragmentation, aggravated by the decentralisation of social programmes, prohibits the provision of coordinated individual care for older people with multiple problems who are receiving different social benefits. It also prohibits the coordination between in-patient and out-patient services. The divisions found between health and social services, between help in the home and in institutions and between somatic and psychiatric care prohibit a system of integrated care which adjusts to the diverse needs of an older person and ensures that (s)he has a complete continuum of care. The current situation is so complex that not only older people and their families, but also health professionals, are not informed of what exists and have a hard time understanding and using available services [2].

At a national level there is competition among the different ministerial departments implicated in the implementation of social and medico-social ageing policies. The minister in charge of social programmes for older people has never had either the opportunity or the resources to coordinate the implementation of programmes from the different administrations working on the problems concerning older people. This has created an obstacle to developing a coordinated national policy.

Another set of obstacles is economic. In a period of slowing economic development, fewer resources are available for medical and social services for older people, unless they are taken from other sectors of care and social action, which means that a choice must be made. Without a strong political reference point in the area of gerontology, the issue has often been regarded as less important when compared to other social problems and groups.

Several cultural factors also contribute to the obstacles of implementing specific policies for older people. The biomedical concept of health and disease has contributed to the medicalisation of the social problems of older people with chronic diseases. There is a continuing rise in major medical treatment, and therefore in its costs, rather than increased emphasis on care given to diminish the functional and social consequences of chronic diseases [2]. The fact that the medical ideology in France is powerful and the fact that physicians have provided the dominant definition of "dependency", have contributed to the lack of solutions to problems such as the "dependency" of older people in need of coordinated multiple services, and not just medical care [2].

Recommendations

In terms of care for older people, recommendations for the future have appeared quite frequently in the literature. Some of the main recommendations include:
- further improvements for home or community care (providing more aid for improvements within the home environment, more financial assistance to family caregivers, better developments with small, well-adapted community residences, etc.);
- better provision of social services and networks for older people (opportunities for activities such as outings, school courses, clubs, etc.);
- better access to public services for older people (well-adapted public transportation, etc.);
- better coordination of health and social services and programmes;
- more equal distribution of services (among regions and socio-economic levels);
- unifying establishments into one single "medico-social" status to solve inequities due to the current billing system (this is currently changing);
- better (and mandatory) training for medical and social professionals on the multi-dimensional aspects of ageing and on the need to do away with traditional bio-medical attitudes;
- campaigns aimed at destroying the negative stigma of old age;
- better research (epidemiologic, needs assessments, evaluation of existing programmes, etc.);
- recognition by the social security system of a wider range of care providers and services (such as physio-therapists and certain technical services).

In terms of informal caregivers there is a need for:
- much more national research about who they are, how they contribute to the cost of health care, what they need, etc.;
- based on this research, better and more widespread programmes for providing support to them, which are well integrated with other gerontological actions in the community;
- a wide range of coordinated services and programmes, meeting all the caregiver's different needs;
- more governmental financial assistance, allowing for vacations, temporary caregivers to relieve them, and policies for informal carers who would also like to continue their professional lives.

Several lessons have been learned from the experiences of existing support programmes. Although still not very widely available, newly developed programmes are currently focusing more on:
- needs analyses and modification of actions to reflect on these needs;
- individualised and group support, with trained personnel;
- better and wider distribution of information;

- support for the family following the death of the person for whom they were providing care.

The issue of the care of older people in France, including the care of caregivers, is clearly a serious one which is increasingly affecting more and more people. With 1999 being the International Year of Older Persons, there is some hope that governments will be forced to participate and learn from one another and that a renewed focus on better policies for their care will result, yet it remains to be seen how these recommendations will be implemented.

References

[1] J.C. Henrard, Du Rapport Laroque à la Loi sur la Préstation spécifique Dépendance. *Gérontologie et Sociéte* **81** (1997) 43-55.
[2] J.C. Henrard, Les personnes âgées et la dépendance. In: *La protection sociale en France.* Paris: La documentation française; 1995.
[3] S. Renaut, and A, Rozenkier, A. Les familles à l'épreuve de la dépendance. In: Donfut-Attias, C. *Les Solidarités entre Générations.* Paris: Nathan; 1995.
[4] F. Granet, Créances alimentaires: les droits des personnes âgées. *Gérontologie et Société* **73 (1997)** 51-60.
[5] H. Jani-Le Bris, *Care for Carers of Dependant older elderly in France.* Dublin: European Foundation for the Improvement of Living and Working Conditions; 1993.
[6] G. Canceill, Ressources et niveau de vie des personnes âgées. *Economie et Statistiques,* **222** (1989) 3-12.
[7] Thévenet, Le Dispositif institutionnel pour les Personnes âgées. *La Santé de l'homme* **322** (1996) VI-VIII.
[8] Thévenet, Aide et services aux personnes âgées: le kaléïdoscope des prestations. *La Santé de l'homme* **302** (1992) 22-26.
[9] Alzon, Le financement de la dépendance des personnes âgées par l'assurance maladie. *La Santé de l'homme* **332** (1997) XVII-XVIII.
[10] M.R Joël, Le dispositif institutionnel. *Actualité et dossier en santé publique: revue trimestrielle du Hout Comité de la santé publique* **20** (1997) XII-XXVI.
[11] M.E. Joël, Dépendance et solidarité. Mieux aider les personnes âgées. In Expertise Paris: La documentation Française; 1991.
[12] F. Lesemann and C. Martin, Au centre des débats, l'articulation entre solidarités familiales et solidarités publiques. In: F. Lesemann, and C. Martin, *Les personnes âgées: dépendance, soins et solidarités familiales.* Paris: La documentation Française; 1993.
[13] D. Grizeau, La perception de la dépendance par le médecin généraliste. *La Santé de l'homme* **332** (1997) VI-VII.
[14] M.J. Guisset, Soutenir l'entourage des personnes âgées dépendantes: des initiatives d'aide et d'information en direction des familles. Bergerac: Fondation de France; 1994.
[15] Helfter, Aider l'entourage des personnes âgées dépendantes. *Le Monde*; March (1997) 23-24.
[16] J.L. Sanchez, Pouvoirs locaux et soutien au vieillissement à l'aube du prochain millénaire. *Gérontologie et Sociéte* **81** (1997) 111-119.

Chapter 3

Germany
(November 2000)

Hanneli Döhner
University Hospital Eppendorf
Institute of Medical Sociology
Martinstrasse 40, 1.Stock
D-20246 Hamburg
Germany

Christopher Kofahl
University Hospital Eppendorf
Institute of Medical Sociology
Martinstrasse 40, 1.Stock
D-20246 Hamburg
Germany

Introduction

To illustrate the role and situation of family carers in Germany, we first present an overview of the social security system and of the relevant legislation in Germany.

Today's German social security system is based on a social security act that was enacted by Chancellor Bismarck in 1883. It is in part financed through public revenues but mainly through contributions to social security. These contributions are paid in equal proportion by employers and employees. For civil servants, other forms of social insurance exist. The majority of employees and their families are compulsorily insured and thus members of statutory health insurance funds. Family members without income are insured jointly with those who receive an income. Only self-employed persons or employees with a monthly income of above 4,346 Euros (West Germany) or 3,681 Euros (East Germany) are exempt from statutory health insurance cover (status 2000). They are usually privately insured (approximately 10 % of the population). About 72 million of the 82 million inhabitants are compulsorily insured (1998) (Aktuell 2000). Today (November 2000), the social security system is based on six main pillars:

1. Old-age pension insurance (19.5% of the gross income).
2. Unemployment insurance (6.5 % of the gross income).
3. Health care insurance (in dependency of the individual statutory health insurance provider approximately 13.5 % of the gross income).
4. Accident insurance.
5. Long-term care insurance (1.7 % of the gross income).
6. Social Aid (taxes).

For the insured person, there is no difference between statutory health insurance provider and long-term care insurance body, since it is in fact always one and the same institution, i.e. the statutory health insurance provider automatically covers also long-term insurance care. In addition, further social benefits awarded to low-income earners, which are not covered by contributions to the social security system, are financed through public revenues within the framework of social aid.

In view of the demographic change, the enactment of the long-term care insurance law in 1995, as fifth independent pillar of the social security system (Pflegeversicherungsgesetz SGB XI), provided a new basis for both the persons requiring care and for family carers, as it allows to cover those risks which are associated with the need for care [1]. In 1995 the proportion of individuals aged over 60 years was 21.1 %. According to forecasts, it will increase to 24.9 % in 2010 and to 33.9 % in 2040 [2]. The long-term care insurance is part of the political goal to allow seriously ill patients and persons in need of care to live as long as possible at home, which is only possible if the provision of care by family carers is encouraged and thus maintained. To this end, a set of benefits which are financed through long-term care insurance were defined by law:

1. Benefits in kind (§ 36).
2. Benefits in cash for self-organised support (§ 37).
3. Combination of benefits in kind and benefits in cash (§ 38).
4. Professional domestic care in the absence of caregivers (§ 39).
5. Nursing aids and technical aids (§ 40).
6. Day care and night care (§ 41).
7. Respite care (§ 42).
8. Care in nursing homes (§ 43).

9. Care in homes for disabled people (§ 43a).
10. Benefits for the social security of family carers (§ 44).
11. Nursing courses for relatives and non-professional voluntary carers (§ 45).

These benefits were introduced in two steps: domestic care benefits as from April 1, 1995 and inpatient care benefits as from July 1, 1996. The social legislation expert Klie divides the most important norms underlying the law into six domains: self-determination, independence, dignity, activation, rights to freedom of choice and health care wishes, and religious orientation [3]. The long-term care insurance is not aimed at fully financing all long-term care benefits, but it is only supposed to reduce the financial burden on persons in need of care and to reduce the expenditures for social aid which is financed through public revenues [4]. According to estimates, the total spending for social aid could thus be reduced by 5 to 6 billion Euros in 1997.

According to estimates, a reduction in the 'misplacement' of people in hospital inpatient care settings led to savings of another 1.38 billion Euros. Furthermore, the average length of a hospital stay in 2,258 German hospitals (1997) decreased from 14.6 days in 1991 to 11.4 days in 1996 [5]. As a result, the legislation regulating hospital matters was changed: as early as mid-1996, measures intended to either reduce or reallocate hospital beds were taken. At the same time, the mean bed occupancy decreased from 83.8 % to 80.3 %. Besides, more and more health care services, formerly provided within an inpatient setting, have meanwhile become part of domestic care. This development also led to a marked increase in the need for domestic care and thus also in the number of domestic care services.

Moreover, long-term care insurance is aimed at maintaining the provision of care by family members on the basis of partial financial compensation for lost earnings and, thus, at improving the social status of the (mainly female) family carers, who, owing to the burden of care, had to put up with gaps in their old-age pension and therefore with lower pension claims in the past. Since the introduction of the long-term care insurance system, however, the time period during which care was provided by family carers has not only been taken into account, but it has also been cofinanced by long-term care insurance bodies within the framework of old-age insurance contributions for persons providing care (§ 44 SGB XI).

In Germany the Medizinische Dienst der Krankenkassen (MDK) (Medical Service of Statutory Health Insurance Providers) is responsible for the assessment of need for care. It acts on behalf of the different, actually competing, statutory health and long-term care insurance

Table 1: Long-term care insurance benefits in order of care categories in Euros (§ 15 SGB XI)

Care Category	Amount of care	Outpatient Benefits in cash (for non-professional care)	Outpatient Benefits in kind (for professional care)	Inpatient Benefits in kind (for professional care)
I	at least 90 mins a day	205	383	1023
II	at least 3 h a day	409	920	1278
III	at least 5 h a day *and* need of care during the night	665	1432	1432 (hardship case: 1687)

providers. Experts of the MDK exert a controlling function by investigating whether therapeutic indication and award of care benefits are correct, specifically with regard to the costs involved (for details, please see Section on Assessment).

Based on their assessments, the person in need of care is assigned to one of the three care categories. Table 1 lists the care category-dependent benefits. The long-term care insurance bodies themselves make the final decision on the award of benefits.

Pursuant to the health policy guideline 'medical rehabilitation before care', the expert assessment should also include recommendations on medical rehabilitation measures. It is, however, the responsibility of the health insurance provider and not of the long-term care insurance body to ensure the implementation of the recommended measures. Yet too little consideration has been given to rights to medical rehabilitation so far.

Persons in need of care at home can choose between benefits in cash for non-professional caregivers ("persons providing care") or benefits in kind for professional care, but they can also combine them. Persons requiring care can appoint any persons as carers. It is thus also possible to have non-family members registered as caregivers. In 1997 the contributions to long-term care insurance amounted to 15.94 billion Euros. Table 2 illustrates the distribution of expenditures amounting to altogether 15.14 billion Euros.

Table 2: Expenditure of the long-term care insurance 1997 in Euros

Expenditure for ...	Billion Euros
Benefits in cash	4.32
Benefits in kind	1.77
Care in nursing homes	6.54
Other benefits	1.7
Administration and other expenses	0.795

The fact that the expenditures for benefits in cash were higher than the expenditures for benefits in kind later turned to have a beneficial effect on the stability of the contribution rates for a longer period of time (compare Section 6). A more detailed English-language description of the long-term care insurance system and of its implications is provided by Evers [6].

Health and Social Care for Older People: Structures & Functions

In Germany domestic care takes principally a higher priority than inpatient care, as well as rehabilitation before care, not only because of the high costs that are associated with inpatient treatment, but also because of the importance to encourage domestic care for patients and persons in need of care. The provision of inpatient treatment is considered to be inadequate when domestic care could have been provided instead, - the same for nursing care instead of rehabilitation. Meanwhile, a wide variety of supportive services are offered to elderly people, but there are still many deficits in the provision of support and care. These are, however, less due to a lack of available support, but rather to a lack of transparency in structure and quality of the services offered [7]. Not only professional staff providing assistance to the aged, but also general practitioners, who play a central role in the German health care system, have difficulties in keeping track of the development in this sector [8]. The range of services that are (not only) offered to elderly people include:

- *Institutions for general information and counselling for:* seriously and terminally ill people, recreational activities, health, care, psycho-social problems, technical aids, addiction, accomodation, self-help, legal claims etc.
- *Recreational activities and social contacts:* day centres, senior citizen clubs, sport, cultural activities and further education, voluntary work incl. home visiting service
- *Mobile services:* meals-on wheels, pedicure, hairdressing, tele-alarm system, services for personal transport and accompanying
- *Housing:* senior citizens homes, age and disability adapted dwellings, sheltered accomodation, nursing homes, hospices
- *Outpatient medical and therapeutical care:* physicians, dentists, medical and dental emergency services and emergency practices, psychotherapy, occupational therapy, physiotherapy, speech and language therapy, massages, quack doctors
- *Domestic care services:* non-profit care services, private care services
- *Part-residential care facilities:* day care, night care, respite care
- *Hospitals:* Hospitals without geriatric departments, hospitals with geriatric departments, hospitals with gerontopsychiatric departments, day clinics

There is often no clear dividing line between the individual services. The major problem of providing efficient and comprehensive care is the aforementioned lack of transparency, which makes it difficult to find out where, when and how assistance can be obtained. The main difficulties in finding one's way through the German care system for the elderly and in coordinating care are primarily attributable to the different sources from which it is financed, such as social security contributions, public revenues and private funds. This diversity leads to the development of also locally different structures and to the establishment of various municipal, non-profit and private institutions. For this reason, elderly persons who need comprehensive care often receive a mix of services and benefits, which are, for example, financed through long-term care insurance, health insurance, social aid and possibly also through services provided by voluntaries and through support from family members. Depending on the nature of care, the person requiring assistance must therefore turn to different institutions. In many cases, relatives undertake this time-consuming task and often feel that they cannot cope with it.

Qualified personnel who have the exclusive task to assist persons in need of support with questions pertaining to the health care system and to help them find adequate supportive services (case management) are still hardly available in Germany [9,10]. General practitioners are mandated by law to coordinate health care services, but the coordination of care-related measures is often even difficult for them [11].

The individual institutions of the health care system are more or less dependent on one another. By virtue of their authorities, general practitioners can exercise power over care providers and therapists. For example, services provided by physiotherapists, occupational therapists, masseurs and speech and language therapists are only covered by health insurance providers if they are prescribed by physicians. Conflicts between these professional groups frequently arise when physicians, although not justified, refuse to prescribe or prolong medical treatment, because they are required by law to prescribe just a certain amount of services (capped budget). If they exceed the limit, they run the risk of becoming liable to recourse. The continuity of rehabilitation at home is thus threatened [12].

As the competing domestic care providers are partly under considerable economic pressure, it becomes increasingly difficult to achieve a cooperation between the individual institutions allowing the coordination of efficient community-oriented care [13]. It is hardly possible to realise financial gains through long-term care insurance, particularly since neither benefits in cash nor benefits in kind have been raised since the introduction of long-term care insurance. Therefore, professional care providers are forced to engage their employees on a part-time basis or to employ them to a minor degree in order to save non-wage labour costs. As a result, persons in need of care must put up with frequent changes in personnel. Care services requiring no qualification as a registered nurse are often performed by unqualified personnel at lower costs.

Roles of Family Carers of Older People Living at Home

At the end of 1998, 2.25 % of the German population required care. Altogether, 1.79 million people received long-term care insurance benefits. According to statistics compiled in 1997, almost 80 % of these benefits are awarded to persons aged over 65 years (Table 3). Three-quarters of the persons in need of care received home care, mostly from family members. Inpatient care accounts for about one-quarter of the benefits, but it constitutes about half of the total expenditures.

Table 3: Recipients of benefits in order of age, gender and nature of care received

	Care category I	Care category II	Care category III	Total	Proportion of all recipients of benefits in %
Age 0 - 64	144 627	139 067	61 117	*344 811*	21.6
Age 65 - 74	99 799	92 541	31 495	*223 835*	14.0
Age 75 +	422 903	438 769	165 279	*1 026 951*	64.4
Women	459 155	456 858	180 650	*1 096 663*	68.7
Men	208 174	213 519	77 241	*498 934*	31.3
Domestic care	532 011	490 401	143 369	*1 165 781*	73.1
Inpatient care	135 318	179 976	114 522	*429 816*	26.9
Total	*667 329*	*670 377*	*257891*	*1 595 597*	100.0

Source [14]

After introduction of the long-term care insurance, it turned out that, contrary to expectations, many individuals who were in need of care and lived at home preferred benefits in cash instead of benefits in kind (about 80 %; Table 4), although - depending on the respective care category - the amount of money is half that spent on benefits in kind. According to a study which was conducted to find out the reasons for this trend, the continuity of care arrangements plays a decisive role. Especially those persons who already benefited from a reliable health care safety net before usually want as few changes as possible and thus prefer benefits in cash as form of support, as the money awarded can be used for multiple purposes. The informal carers can now be paid for the care they provide, which was previously not or only partly possible. However, the study also shows that only in half of these cases family carers were in fact paid for the care provided, as a transfer of money within the family is presumably considered to be unnecessary. The comparison of the results of a study conducted by [15], reflecting the life situation of family carers in the time before the long-term care insurance, shows an only moderate influence of the long-term care insurance on the individual care arrangement.

The necessary requirements that must be fulfilled by carers in order to receive benefits in cash are defined by the long-term care insurance law. The definition of the term *caregivers* is as follows: *persons who do not provide professionally domestic care to a person as defined by § 14. According to § 44, the carer only receives social security benefits if she/he provides care at least 14 hours per week to the person in need of care (§ 19).*

Table 4: Benefit preferences of individuals receiving domestic care in order of care category (July to December 1996) in %

Type of benefits	Care category				Total
	I	II	III	Hardship cases	
Benefits in kind	8.8	8.7	8.7	99.9	*8.8*
Benefits in cash	83.7	77.1	67.0	0.0	*78.6*
Combined benefits	6.6	12.6	22.0	0.1	*11.3*
Day care / night care	0.2	0.3	0.4	0.0	*0.3*
Respite care	0.6	1.2	2.0	0.0	*1.1*
Total	*100.0*	*100.0*	*100.0*	*100.0*	*100.0*

Source [14]

Statistically, the exclusive use of benefits in kind is independent of the care category. The reason for a decision in favour of professional care is often rather based on the fact that the person in need of care lives alone and that informal caregivers are not available and less on the degree of need for care [16]. The combination of benefits in cash and benefits in kind shows that, depending on the degree of care needed, help offered by professional carers is increasingly accepted. Overall, though, professional care is still rarely used. When persons decide to make use of benefits in cash, supportive or substitutional services (day or night care and respite care) can temporarily be provided to ease the care-related workload and to maintain the provision of care at home. Some additional support is granted in the form of

Table 5: Main carers of individuals in need of care in private homes (%)

Relationship	Persons in need of care		
	All age groups	65 – 79 years	80 and older
Spouse (female)	24	39	12
Spouse (male)	13	22	5
Mother	14	0	0
Father	0	0	0
Daughter	26	24	44
Son	3	2	6
Daughter-in-law	9	6	17
Other relatives	7	6	9
Friends / neighbours	4	2	7

Persons in need of help or care in private homes = 100; care interval model: Infratest 1992, Source [18]

technical aids, and home adaptations up to an amount of 3,068 Euros may also be financed through long-term care insurance. However, the comparatively small number of persons using support in the form of day or night care shows that these opportunities for reducing the caregivers' burden are still rarely used, although they represent a considerable source of help.

The figures demonstrate indisputably that the family - despite high demands on flexibility in professional life - constitutes the largest group of carers in Germany. They also reveal that approximately 75 % of the family carers are most commonly females. Table 5 illustrates the typical division of responsibilities among family members in the German society and in many other social systems, according to which men usually earn a living and women provide care [17]. These data result from a representative study conducted from 1991 to 1992.

In 77 % of all cases, the main carers are the only persons providing care. In only 14 % the tasks are shared by at least two persons, and in 9 % non-family members provide help and support [18]. The caregivers assist with many activities of daily living, most of them every day (Table 6).

Table 6: Individuals in need of care in private homes with main carer in order of nature and degree of help received (%)

Type of care / help	Frequency of care			
	Nearly every day	2 to 4 times a week	Once a week or less	Never
Personal care (e.g. conversations)	90	3	3	4
Household activities	85	7	2	6
Hygiene care (e.g. washing)	83	5	4	8
Assistance with food intake	61	2	5	30
Treatment care	40	5	13	41
Help with activities outside their homes	28	7	38	26
Support in accompanying them to their training centres / workplaces	9	1	4	81

Multiple data; Persons in need of care in private homes with main carers = 100; care interval model: Infratest 1992, Source [18]

Table 7: Time period during which the main caregiver is available with regard to age of the individuals in need care or help (%)

	Persons in need of care		Persons in need of help	
	65 - 79 years	80 and older	65 - 79 years	80 and older
Constantly, round the clock	80	71	61	41
Daily, hourly	16	24	18	29
Several times a week	3	3	13	19
Once a week	0	1	7	7

Persons in need of care in private homes with main carers = 100; care interval model: Infratest 1992, Source [18].

The degree of need for care is closely connected with the carers' personal situation. Table 7 shows that many family members, together with the persons they care for, are often confined indoors. Consequently, they can rarely take part in social activities outside the home. As family members often do no longer have the opportunity of relaxing by taking part in leisure activities, such as talks with friends, their quality of life is often impaired [19,20].

As illustrated in Table 5, the main caregiver is often a close female family member. Table 8 includes all individuals who are in need of care or help in all age groups. However, it also shows that about one-third of the family carers are aged over 65 years and that they are frequently also the partners of the persons in need of care or help. Main carers of younger age are predominantly daughters or daughters-in-law.

Table 8: Age groups of the main carers in private homes (%)

Main carers	Persons in need of care	Persons in need of help
18 - 64 years	68	67
65 - 74 years	21	19
75 years and older	10	11
Missing	1	2

Main carers in private homes = 100; care interval model: Infratest 1992, Source [18]

Independent of the age of the individuals in need of care, more than 90 % of the main carers deem the workload to be a considerable or significant burden (Table 9).

Table 9: Main carers' burden in order of the age of persons in need of care (%)

Degree of burden	Persons in need of care in order of age groups					
	Total	0 - 15 years	16 - 39 years	40 - 64 years	65 - 79 years	80 and older
No burden	0	0	0	0	0	1
Light burden	8	6	1	9	9	9
Heavy burden	41	37	36	38	40	43
Very heavy burden	51	57	63	53	50	46

Persons in need of care in private homes with main carers = 100; care interval model: Infratest 1992, Source [18].

Investigations of 1911 caregivers revealed that their reported physical complaints such as exhaustion, pains in arms and legs, heart trouble and stomach pain are more severe in this group than in the general population. Moreover, these symptoms are found to be more pronounced in carers of demented patients than in persons who care for elderly people with largely unimpaired cognitive performances [21]. Yet carers of demented people do not make use of professional care more often than those who care for cognitively unimpaired individuals[16]. Schacke and Zank [20] investigated mental stress factors in 78 carers of demented persons and found out that the main factors impairing their quality of life were role conflicts and the feeling that they cannot provide adequate care. Interestingly, the degree of cognitive impairment was inversely related to the mental stress experienced.

In 1992, 77 % of all main carers were not employed, 5 % were employed to a minor degree, 7 % were part-time employed and 10 % full-time employed. Depending on the intensity of need for care, up to one-third of the carers gave up employment (Table 10).

Table 10: Main carers of individuals in need of care in private homes, aged 18 - 64 years, in order of employment status (%)

Employment status	Permanent need of care	Daily need of care	Need of care several time a week	Need of care in total
Unemployed when care was started	34	42	35	*38*
Employment discontinued	34	13	9	*16*
Partly employed	17	16	11	*14*
Employment continued	7	20	33	*22*
Other status	8	9	12	*10*

Main carers aged 18 – 64 years in private homes = 100; care interval model: Infratest 1992, Source [18].

Family carers tend to ask too much of themselves [22]. They often run the risk of becoming in need of care themselves, for which reason the demand for help and support has meanwhile become imperative.

As a consequence of this development, professional nursing staff visit carers every six months and conduct checks on behalf of long-term care insurance providers. These home visits are not only intended to avoid mistakes in care, but they should also enable family carers to learn and observe basic lifting and handling techniques that serve to protect themselves from health damage.

In addition, caregivers can receive counselling on home care from professional nursing staff. Assistance is also offered by self-help groups and advice centres. If family carers want to go on holiday or take part in social activities to increase the quality of their own lives, respite care facilities, day-care centres or professional carers offering day and night care can provide help to their caregivers.

With the enactment of the long-term care insurance law, insurance providers, often in cooperation with other experienced institutions such as charitable institutions, have conducted training courses for family carers throughout the country, which are intended to support them in their efforts. It soon turned out that it is not only important to take different target groups into account [23], but to allow also for the fact that different care situations determine the interests of the family carers [24,25]. In view of the increasing number of services offered, systematic guidelines with particular attention to psychosocial problems were developed for these courses [26,27]. Furthermore, it also proved to be necessary to combine the offered services with other supportive measures [28] such as self-help groups for family carers or separate courses dealing with selected topics. Interviews with 1118 course participants and 112 instructors showed that the most frequently requested supportive measures are: respite care/day care, substitute carers (58.3 %), information on home care (50.6 %), financial support (28.1 %), comfort/encouragement (26.3 %), domestic care services (23.6 %) or active help in providing care (19.8 %) [29].

These services are offered free of charge, because most of them are financed through long-term care insurance or by municipal institutions. There are many reasons why these supportive measures are not used despite the aforementioned requests for support. Specifically two reasons should be mentioned.

On the one hand, it is known that family carers are principally not well informed about supportive measures and thus rarely take the initiative to look for adequate help. It is therefore necessary to ensure that information on preventive and supportive services is brought to the attention of family carers. As has also been observed in the provision of care to the elderly, efficiency can only be achieved if information on supportive measures or services is actively distributed to family carers.

On the other hand, carers frequently perceive the symptoms of excessive stress only when the patient-carer relationship has already reached a difficult point at which they are too much involved with the situation and hence are hardly able to think about help from outside. Typically, the burn-out syndrome is not perceived until the first signs and symptoms have already developed and are manifest.

Before introduction of the long-term care insurance, a study was conducted on behalf of a health insurance provider [30], which was aimed at obtaining additional information with respect to the law-defined task of counselling carers that goes beyond the semi-annual home visit by a registered nurse. In the course of the study, the avoidance of burnout in family carers, which represents a central problem in this context, was investigated. It was also a goal of the study to find out the reasons for burnout, on the basis of which possible solution-oriented approaches were defined [31]. One health and long-term care insurance provider has meanwhile implemented these recommendations.

Considering the significant burden of physical and mental stress experienced by family carers, which often even causes them to give up their employment, it is amazing that only few people make use of professional care. Several reasons account for this phenomenon. The traditional moral obligation of the families to care themselves for their members in need of help is considered by many people to be natural, even in an industrial state such as Germany. Many families try to arrange for support within their own family, as the presence of unfamiliar persons is often associated with concerns about loss of privacy for the person in need of care and for themselves and with feelings of shame and loss of integrity. Also, relatively few professional carers are able to guarantee continued provision of care by not more than three different persons per patient, which makes it even more difficult to establish a confidential carer-patient relationship. The most common criticism expressed by patients and their families is the frequent change in personnel [32].

Moreover, potential clients of these domestic care providers are often also unsure about the quality of the services offered. Particularly at the time when the number of these services increased rapidly after long-term care insurance had been introduced, this development was a subject of considerable debate in the media. Irregularities in the billing of services and mistakes in care reported in the media were detrimental to the reputation of the professional home care system. The overall satisfaction with professional caregivers expressed by patients was, unfortunately, less a matter of discussion in this context [33].

Regional differences, too, influence the decision as to whether or not professional home care should be accepted. Owing to the high population density in large conurbations, a wider range of domestic care services is available. Hence the number of alternative home care services in the event of dissatisfaction is also higher. Compared to rural areas where the choice of providers is restricted and the distances to be covered are long, urban domestic care providers can work more efficiently because of shorter driving distances.

Overall, the experiences of family carers with support services are positive. However, representative longitudinal studies allowing the assessment of possible concrete effects have not yet been conducted in Germany.

Assessment

In order to assess the nature and amount of care needed, the health insurance providers entrust experts of the MDK with the assessment. Based on their results, the long-term care insurer assigns the patient to a care category. Paradoxically, the information obtained from these expert assessments is not made available to general practitioners or professional carers, making it impossible to plan supportive measures on the basis of these data or to evaluate the effectiveness of care measures. A major drawback in the assessment of need for care is that the expertise of general practitioners is not taken into consideration. They even do not receive a copy of the assessment protocol. Although according to the health care insurance law the general practitioner plays a pivotal role in coordinating health care services, his role is not allowed for in the long-term care insurance law [4].

If the persons requiring care receive benefits in kind, the care provider is responsible for *nursing care planning and care documentation*, which exclusively relate to the care provided. Uniform planning and documentation standards do not exist, which means that no comparisons can be made and that no multidimensional and multiprofessional assessment procedure is used. Currently, the use of such a standardised assessment method in community care is only realised in research projects [11,34-36].

Expert assessments including information on the amount of support needed by family carers [37] are even more difficult to find. When assessing the need for care, the experts of the MDK are also asked to find out whether family members can provide support, but the failure to ask about the family carers' resources and constitution has often been criticised in this context [22]. The family's situation is also discussed with the domestic care provider when planning nursing care, but this assessment is not based on standardised procedures.

The planning of intervention measures using standardised assessments could be improved and, in individual cases, also contribute to a better old-age care reporting system within the scope of health care reporting, which is more than insufficient in Germany [38]. The availability of such data would represent an important basis for the adequate planning of care for the elderly and substantiate quantitatively the demand for a better support for family carers.

The experts appointed by the MDK are mostly physicians, although professional carers have also increasingly been appointed to act as experts in recent years. There are differences in the composition of expert teams in the individual German federal states. Initially, profession-related differences in perspectives and different experiences led to problems [4], but as result of changed practice the situation has improved. Depending on the circumstances of the case, the assessment of need for care is now mainly performed by only one of the two profession groups. Nevertheless, in any case a physician has to be involved in the report for the insurance company.

The home-visit-based expert assessment only includes the time period during which help is provided in coping with daily *physical* activities. In the planning stage of the long-term care insurance, relative time units were calculated for the provision of individual care services such as washing, positioning of the patient, toileting, bandage change, administration of medication and other services such as disposal of rubbish. On the basis of these time units measured in minutes, the time period during which care is provided during the day, one of the three care categories is assigned. The use of these time units is hotly disputed, particularly since there are considerable variations in the time needed for the provision of care. The functional health status of the patients, the quality of the carer-patient relationship and the layout of the flat as, for example, size and furnishings, markedly influence the amount of time required. These time limitations, as defined by long-term care insurance, have proved to be especially inappropriate when care is provided to demented persons. However, the need for support in cases of dementia is not taken into account, which is not only severely criticised by family members and all other caregivers, but also by social legislation experts.

Apart from determining the respective care category, the experts of the MDK are also asked to find out whether protective, alleviating or preventive measures or domestic rehabilitative measures can be taken and, if so, to make appropriate recommendations. Furthermore, they must assess whether home adaptations are necessary in order to allow adequate care and whether technical aids could ease the provision of care or increase the mobility and independence of the patient. As a result of these assessments, the experts recommend to long-term care insurance providers that benefits should be awarded in accordance with one of the three care categories, or they come to the conclusion that the eligibility criteria for receipt of care are not fulfilled.

In the latter case, many persons requiring only little care or help are often disappointed when, based on expert assessments, no benefits are awarded, although there is objective need for help. This shows that the criterion for receipt of care according to the lowest care category (90 minutes of care per day) is rather inadequate and that need for help in social-domestic domains such as shopping, cleaning, cooking etc. is not at all considered by long-term care insurance. Moreover, the classification of need for care into only three categories allows just an approximate assessment and does not reflect the actual need, which often leads to underestimation or overestimation in borderline [12]. Among other aspects, this may be one reason why the recently enacted adaptation of the Japanese long-term care insurance meanwhile differentiates between six care categories [25].

Case Studies

The role of family carers in Germany will be made more explicit by the description of three standardised cases which vary in the nature of the illness and disabilities of the older person. Additionally for each of the three cases there are three variations of the older person's and their family carers' social circumstances. For each of the nine different situations resulting from these combinations, three questions will be answered:

- What role(s) would the family carer typically occupy on caring for the older person?
- What services would typically be provided to support the older person?
- How would the family carer's needs typically be assessed and what support would typically be provided for the carer?

It is nearly impossible to generalise typical situations due to the fact that provision of care is influenced by individual personal and living circumstances, e.g. level of education, quality of relationship between family members, local specifities according to differences in the infrastructure as well as different attitudes of the persons in need of care and their carers. Since the long-term care insurance has been implemented, the individual situation is closely determined by the result of the assessment, conducted by the MDK, as the basis for the care category decided by the long-term care insurance body.

The development of the following nine scenarios has been supported by two nurses with comprehensive experience in the care for older people.

Case 1

Female, aged 76 with osteoarthritis of hips and knees, poor vision due to macular degeneration, and hypertension. Mobile with a frame within her home except for the stairs. Needs help with mobility outside, shopping, cooking and housework. In this case, it must be assumed that no long-term care insurance benefits will be awarded.

Social circumstances (A): Older person living alone in an isolated farmhouse. Widowed. Little money. Daughter and son-in-law unemployed with four children, aged 9 months to 7 years, and live 5 kilometres away. Two other children of the older person live over 100 kilometres away.

The role of family carers Typically, the daughter and the son-in-law, who are both unemployed, will be the closest contacts for the elderly mother, although they have four small children. They will undertake housekeeping and shopping of bulky articles that can be stored. The daughter will do all other housework once or twice per week, especially house cleaning. Since she lives five kilometres away from her mother and does not have a car - due to unemployment the family had to sell it – she will try to do the work on certain days. Neighbours will also help in buying fresh products and all other everyday household essentials. The two other children can only provide financial support, as they live too far away and thus cannot visit her regularly.

Professional services Due to limited mobility outside her flat, she will depend on social contacts and social integration. Another important factor is the size of the community. In this case, the eligibility criteria for the award of long-term care insurance benefits are not met, as she is able to perform all physical activities of daily living on her own. However, in view of her limited financial resources, it would be possible to turn to the local social aid bodies and apply for supportive services (domestic help and technical aids such as walker and tele-alarm system). As the network of domestic services in rural areas is poorly developed, the community nurse, the pastor and conscientious objectors doing community work will usually provide help. Three times per week, the elderly lady will receive meals–on–wheels. Blood pressure measurements performed by professional home care providers are paid by most health insurers only in combination with other health care services. Therefore, the general practitioner will have to visit the patient at home or relatives or neighbours will have to arrange for a means of transport to the physician.

Assessment and support of family carers Typically, the family carers' need for assistance will not be assessed. The family will usually turn to the general practitioner and enquire about possibilities of support, or the physician will offer help on his own initiative. In general, it is very important that informal and family caregivers are well informed about existing supportive services. In this case, too, they will play a decisive role in ensuring that any possible help is provided to the 76-year-old lady. Sometimes, health insurance providers offer advice as well.

Social circumstances (B): Older person lives alone in a ground floor flat in town. Widowed. Daughter and son-in-law are both teachers in full-time employment, with 2 children aged 7 and 11, and live 1 kilometre in the same town.

The role of family carers In this case description, the children of this elderly person are employed full-time and, therefore, have little time. However, as they earn good salaries, they could afford to pay for private domestic care services. Occasionally, the older grandchild would assist with shopping or with other things she has to do in town. Considering the educational level of the children, they would certainly be able to obtain information on the different forms of support from the competent advice centres. The availability of informal help to the elderly lady, especially from her neighbours, depends on the time period during which she and the informal carers have lived in the same part of the town. Furthermore, age structure and friends living in close proximity play an important role.

Professional services For the aforementioned reasons, the eligibility criteria for the award of long-term care insurance benefits are not fulfilled. In view of the good income earned by the family members, social aid benefits will also not be awarded. Since the elderly person lives in a city, it is assumed that a large network of private and municipal domestic services exists. Here, the family members would probably pay for professional help, as, for example, private care, domestic services, a window cleaner or pedicure. In addition, enough money would be available to buy, for example, a reading aid with magnifier or a hand-held blood pressure measuring device.

Assessment and support of family carers Typically, the amount of help needed by informal helpers and family carers will not be assessed. They will not receive support in providing care to persons with this disease. Pertinent information could be obtained from advice centres, long-term care insurance or health insurance providers or possibly from the general practitioner, who, however, is often not sufficiently informed about available assistance.

Social circumstances (C): Older person lives with spouse in 2-storey house. Retired with savings. Spouse is fit and well. No children. Bedroom, bathroom and toilet are upstairs.

The role of family carers In this case, the husband will normally provide the care needed. Outside their home, he will take her to all places (e.g. shopping or visit to a physician). He will also assist her with housework and meal preparation. Sometimes, help offered by neighbours will also be accepted, but only rarely.

Professional services For the above-mentioned reasons, the eligibility criteria for the award of long-term care insurance benefits are not fulfilled. The husband will probably employ a domestic help to support him. The physician could issue a prescription for a cane, a walker or wheeled walker, physiotherapy and maybe also for a wheelchair. Despite considerable costs, the elderly couple may put their savings into buying and installing a stairlift connecting ground floor and first floor.

Assessment and support of family carers Typically, the amount of help needed by informal helpers or family carers will not be assessed. The husband might find support in senior centres, but he would have to ask for information on his own. He could turn to the long-term care insurance or health insurance provider, to the medical equipment company or to the general practitioner.

Case 2

Male, aged 80, facing discharge from hospital following a stroke. Expected to be confined to bed or chair for several weeks with gradual recovery of morbidity. Needs the help of one person for transfers, toileting, bathing and dressing.

Here, it can be assumed that the Medizinische Dienst der Krankenkassen (MDK) (Medical Service of Statutory Health Insurance Providers), based on the assessment will recommend care category 2, which will also be accepted by the long-term care insurance body.

Social circumstances (A): Older person living alone in an isolated farmhouse. Widowed. Little money. Daughter and son-in-law unemployed with four children, aged 9 months to 7 years, and live 5 kilometres away. Two other children of the older person live over 100 kilometres away.

The role of family carers In view of the severity of the case, the family members, who live in the vicinity of the elderly man, would probably not be able to provide the needed care unless the family would move to the farm. However, this would almost be impracticable, since the daughter and son-in-law have four small children. Moreover, the search for a new job when living on a remote farm would be very difficult. Theoretically, the three children could alternately spend 14 days in the house of the father. Alternatively, the children who live far away could provide care to the father by taking him to their homes. In the end, though, the result of all these theoretical considerations will usually be that the children will place their father in a nursing home.

Professional services During hospital stay, the hospital social service will investigate possibilities for the provision of care after discharge and, as far as possible, initiate all necessary steps from there. The classification of the need for long-term care into a care category will be applied for but not be performed before discharge. Since the elderly man lives alone and not in proximity to his children, the hospital social service will enquire about the existence of a respite care facility, where the mobility of the patient could be improved and gradually restored during a short-term stay. This scenario is unlikely, though. The family members will be asked whether private domestic care services should be organised. After discharge, a domestic care provider will visit the patient three times per day. In general, the first four weeks of care are covered by statutory health insurance. By then the patient ought to be assigned to a care category so that the long-term care insurance body can bear all further costs. The community nurse will usually undertake the provision of care, the pastor will occasionally visit him, and the general practitioner will prescribe physiotherapy.

Assessment and support of family carers The hospital social service will support the relatives by preparing the discharge of the patient (see above). At a later stage, it will be suggested that the elderly person should be placed in a nursing home. The nursing home – which should be located in proximity to the family members – will assist them with all formalities.

Social circumstances (B): Older person lives alone in a ground floor flat in town. Widowed. Daughter and son-in-law are both teachers in full-time employment, with 2 children aged 7 and 11, and live 1 kilometre in the same town.

The role of family carers It is rather unlikely that the children of the elderly man will decide in favour of providing the required care themselves, except in the case of a higher level of physical independence after respite care or rehabilitation stay. With the support of professional carers, the family members would have to look after their father several times per day to make sure that he is all right. This would be possible before or after work. The oldest grandchild could possibly also assist. Typical care-related tasks of the family would be to do the shopping, to keep house, to talk with the professional home care provider about a disability-adapted bed, technical aids, a tele-alarm system and necessary home adaptations, to have keys made, to arrange for appointments with the physiotherapist and physician and to assist with food intake. Either the daughter or the son-in-law could temporarily give up teaching and apply for unpaid leave.

Professional services The hospital will usually recommend respite care facilities, rehabilitation hospitals or domestic care services. After consultation with the hospital social service and the general practitioner, the patient will be transferred to a geriatric department.

After five weeks, the patient will be discharged home. In the beginning, care category 2 of the long-term care insurance can be assigned and is often already applied for during the hospital stay. A domestic care provider will visit the patient three times per day. In addition, physiotherapeutic services will be offered. A conscientious objector doing community work and a private domestic help will care for the elderly man. The daughter will make the switch from full-time to part-time employment.

Assessment and support of family carers Typically, the amount of help needed will not be assessed, but the hospital social service will include the family members in the subsequent planning of patient care. Most commonly, only professional nursing staff offer further assistance. Help from general practitioners is usually only available if good contact has been maintained consistently. The family can also contact the rehabilitation counsellor of the respective health insurance provider. Moreover, health insurers increasingly offer courses that are intended to help their insured in providing care free of charge.

Social circumstances (C): Older person lives with spouse in 2-storey house. Retired with savings. Spouse is fit and well. No children. Bedroom, bathroom and toilet are upstairs.

The role of family carers In this case example, the spouse will care for her husband at home. Provided that her husband had not suffered a severe stroke, the spouse will presumably provide the needed care by herself, since she is fit and healthy, and her husband will probably consider help from "unfamiliar" persons as unnecessary. She will therefore help him with hygiene care, toileting, dressing, food intake, etc. To restore his mobility and to reduce the difficulties in climbing stairs, she will arrange for physiotherapeutic treatment at home. She will participate in the organisation of the required care and supervise the work of helpers. Together with her husband, she will consider the sale of their house, as sheltered accommodation would make their lives much easier.

Professional services Domestic care services would be recommended either by the hospital or by the general practitioner. The hospital staff would probably inform her about the possibility of applying for long-term care insurance benefits (benefits in kind or in cash). A so-called A-Verordnung (treatment care) ensures that a domestic care provider will visit the patient three times per day during the first four weeks after discharge. After that time, the long-term care insurance body will bear all further costs. Professional nursing staff will see to it that sufficient technical aids such as a toilet chair are available. The general practitioner will issue a prescription for physiotherapy at home. A conscientious objector doing community work and a private domestic help will support her in providing care to her husband. Should the elderly couple decide against sheltered accommodation, the installation of a stairlift will probably be taken into account.

Assessment and support of family carers Normally, the amount of help needed by family carers will not be assessed. Before discharge of the patient, the hospital social service will inform the family about existing supportive services. Most commonly, assistance is also offered by self-help groups (for family carers) but frequently not used. When experts of the MDK visit the patient for assessment of need for care, the spouse of the patient could enquire about supportive services for herself. However, this is less likely, since the attention will be focussed on the patient. Theoretically, the rehabilitation counsellor of the health insurance provider, the medical equipment company, the domestic care provider or the general practitioner could advise the family members of the patient on supportive measures. However, counselling frequently only takes place when the family carers establish contact on their own initiative.

Case 3

Female, aged 86, suffering from dementia. Frequent wandering by day and night. Frequent falls. Incontinent of urine and faeces.

In this case, the elderly lady will presumably be assigned to the lowest category (care category 1), even though the family members will certainly consider the need for care to be significantly higher. This example clearly demonstrates a major weak point of the long-term care insurance, as mainly physical handicaps are taken into account.

Social circumstances (A): Older person living alone in an isolated farmhouse. Widowed. Little money. Daughter and son-in-law unemployed with four children, aged 9 months to 7 years, and live 5 kilometres away. Two other children of the older person live over 100 kilometres away.

The role of family carers In view of the family's own difficult situation, the family members who live in proximity to the mother will not be able to provide sufficient care to the mother, specifically not in her familiar environment. The other children living far away could care for their mother by taking her to their homes. Alternatively, the daughter and son-in-law could move with their children to the mother's farm. It is, however, more likely that the mother will be placed in a nursing home.

Professional services In this case example, nursing home placement will typically be recommended, since, from the family's point of view, the elderly lady can no longer live on her own. Her children cannot or do not want to take her to their homes or move to her farm. Long-term care insurance benefits for inpatient care will be applied for. If the family is in a bad financial position, it will also apply for social aid.

Assessment and support of family carers The general practitioner will strongly advise the family members against asking too much of themselves, but the community nurse will only be able to provide the required care with additional help of the family. She will therefore recommend nursing home placement as well.

Social circumstances (B): Older person lives alone in a ground floor flat in town. Widowed. Daughter and son-in-law are both teachers in full-time employment, with 2 children aged 7 and 11, and live 1 kilometre in the same town.

The role of family carers Considering the severity of her disease, permanent nursing care will be necessary. The elderly lady cannot be left alone. Her daughter could apply for unpaid leave and give up teaching for a longer period of time to be able to care for her. The household of the mother will be dissolved, and the elderly lady will move to her daughter's home. Later the family members will have to decide whether she can live with them on a long-term basis. They will arrange for the provision of day care in a day-care centre, where she will stay five days per week. In the evenings and at the weekends, the family members will care for her themselves. They will prepare the meals and assist her with toileting and incontinence care. All necessary home adaptations will be made to protect her from falls.

Professional services Domestic care alone will not be sufficient, as the woman cannot be left alone. For this reason, day care will be applied for within the framework of long-term care insurance. In addition, a private domestic help will be employed who will also stay overnight when necessary. Sooner or later, with increasing severity of dementia, the elderly lady will be transferred to a nursing home.

Assessment and support of family carers Normally, the family carers' need for help will not be assessed. In this case example, day care and self-help group participation as additional means to exchange experience and to better cope with the situation, will be recommended by the professional care provider, who will also give them the address of a competent advice centre. There too, it will be recommended that the family members should participate in a self-help group. However, for reasons of time, the daughter and son-in-law may not make use of the services offered. The advice centre will provide them with information on patients with dementia. Furthermore, they will try to obtain additional literature. From time to time, they will talk with their general practitioner about the health status of the mother, possible disease progression and the workload associated with care.

Social circumstances (C): Older person lives with spouse in 2-storey house. Retired with savings. Spouse is fit and well. No children. Bedroom, bathroom and toilet are upstairs.

The role of family carers Apart from the provision of professional help (basic care, incontinence care), the husband will perform all other domestic chores during day and night. He will do the shopping, prepare most of the meals, constantly remind his spouse to take her meals and assist her with toileting. As the elderly couple lives in a two-storey house, it will be very difficult for the husband to watch over her all the time.

Professional services The husband will decide for a combination of benefits in kinds and benefits in cash. In the morning, a professional carer will provide basic care, and a conscientious objector doing community work will take her out for a walk once per week. A private domestic help will assist the husband in doing the washing and ironing and in cleaning the house. Twice per week, meals-on-wheels will be delivered to the elderly couple.

Assessment and support of family carers The amount of help needed by the husband will not be assessed. Occasionally, the nurse of the domestic care provider or the general practitioner will talk with him about how the future care of his spouse can be ensured, specifically with a view to a possible deterioration in her but also in his health status. Based on these considerations, the elderly man will plan their future. Should his health deteriorate, he will arrange for 24-hour care or at least for night care so that he will be able to sleep. He will care for his wife at home as long as possible and, only when inevitable, think about the possibility of day care. If he is in need of care himself, he will move with his wife to a nursing home.

Future Developments

Health Care System

Currently, there is much hope that, within the framework of the Health Care Reform 2000, the quality of health care will improve with respect to a stronger orientation towards patient and family care, comprehensive care and deregulation measures on the basis of newly introduced remuneration systems and co-operative agreements concluded between the different institutions. By enabling health care institutions to develop and implement new concepts, which, as a result of regional framework agreements concluded with the insurers, are less impaired by a lack of interaction between the different institutions and providers, health care and nursing care services can be offered more efficiently and in accordance with the individuals needs.

To achieve the overall goal of *integrated care*, physician networks are currently being established in cooperation with hospitals, which is primarily aimed at coordinating the respective regional health care services on the basis of decentralised budgets for self-management. However, expenditures are not expected to decrease as a result of this measure, as the economic interests of the individual institutions will not change, but it may be assumed that there will be an increase in the number of direct professional services provided to patients by qualified personnel. This, in turn, will improve the quality of care.

Another chance of avoiding inefficient care due to 'misplacement' of patients in inadequate care settings is the establishment of health care centres, which, in co-operation with hospitals, would provide domestic care services. All providers offering professional home care, rehabilitation at home and other medical and social services 'under one roof' could then offer *integrated care* packages. This approach would also allow the integration of hospitals into the concept of comprehensive care. "If this goal is not achieved, medical ethics and publicly financed health services will be determined by strictly economic considerations. As a result, the system would continue to fall apart, and a fragmentation into even more uncoordinated care areas would be the inevitable consequence" [39].

Assessment

The assessment of need for care by experts of the MDK is a mere cross-sectional assessment, which takes about 45 minutes per case to complete. The Medical Service of the leading associations (umbrella organisation of the different MDKs) is aware of the problem that the non-availability of the general practitioner's expertise causes a loss of important information, especially with regard to recommendations on rehabilitative measures and their potential implementation. Possibilities for the inclusion of the general practitioner's valuable patient data in the expert assessment and appropriate ways in which to keep the general practitioner informed are currently under discussion. In addition, greater attention will be given to the assessment of possibilities for medical rehabilitation. The health policy guideline 'medical rehabilitation before care' should be supplemented by the guideline 'medical rehabilitation in addition to care'. These approaches should be implemented with the help of general practitioners. A variety of investigations revealed that rehabilitation will contribute to an up to 20-fold reduction in long-term care expenditures and thus to considerable care cost savings [39]. However, successful rehabilitation also means that the individuals in need of care will probably be awarded less benefits than in the past (lower care category), which may be problematic for the recipients.

The MDK which is financed by health and long-term care insurance providers cannot be deemed to be a neutral institution and is criticised on the grounds that it represents the interests of the insurers and that the assessment criteria are not always appropriately applied. However, plans according to which the MDK would act as an independent institution are currently not under discussion.

Supportive Services for Family Carers

The provision of support to family carers by the society as a whole will always represent a major challenge not only to the national economy, but also in each individual case. In this context, it should be mentioned that about 80 % of all family carers are women and that 68 % of all family carers of working age (16 – 64 years) are not gainfully employed, although the number of persons who must manage both is increasing [40]. There are several reasons why care provision is at least partly incompatible with full- or part-time employment, especially when family members care for demented individuals. Supportive measures are needed to promote part-time employment, financial compensation for the time period during which gainful employment was not possible because of care, or the adaptation of already existing regulations, such as the possibility of parental leave when children are ill. Specifically in enterprises employing a high proportion of women, there is urgent call for action. Realistically, financial support for financial risk sharing is needed to implement adequate regulations in these enterprises, as these cannot bear all care-related risks and costs alone.

The low number of family carers accepting supportive measures such as respite care or day and night care shows that alternatives must be offered which are more suitable for their families. According to investigations conducted in 1995 by several research facilities, competent and professional care would have been better suited to the individual needs of about 150,000 patients than care provided by nursing homes or family members [2]. On the other hand, the availability of just 7,000 respite care and about 5,000 day-care places in Germany is considered as definitely insufficient [2]. For these reasons, only about 7,000 demented individuals made use of day-care services in 1998 [41].

There are currently no signs indicating that the additional expenditure of time and energy needed to provide care to persons with cognitive impairments is taken into account. However, this is no lack of appreciation of the family carers' additional workloads. Socio-economic data show that long-term care insurance services could no longer be financed if care for demented persons would be fully covered, at least not without raising long-term care insurance contributions. Two federal states suggested that a maximum of 40 minutes of additional care per day should be rewarded financially. In view of a total number of about 500,000 demented individuals in Germany, this would result in an additional financial burden of approximately 1.92 billion Euros [41].

A draft bill which is currently under discussion in parliament is aimed at expanding day and night care in order to ease the family carers' workload. According to this bill, demented persons could make use of day- and night-care services once per week without a reduction in their benefits in cash or [41]. However, this suggestion is criticised as being inappropriate, as it is not tailored to the different individuals needs. It has also been proposed that additional financial means (e.g. an annual budget) should be granted to family members caring for demented persons, which would enable them to choose the services or assistive devices which are best suited to their needs and care situation. These additional financial means could also be used for financial compensation for care provided, prolongation of normally time-limited respite care, or for partly financing cures for caregivers [42].

The workload reduction achieved by combining family and professional home care is also not at all [43]. To allow for efficient and coordinated care arrangements in the future, even higher flexibility and psychosocial competence will be necessary on the part of professional home care providers [44]. Coordinated care arrangements, which are adapted to the individual needs and care situations, can help avoid hospitalisation of patients or shorten their hospital stays. Good cooperation with the general practitioner is a prerequisite for all this, which, however, cannot always be presupposed. Domestic care providers criticise that general practitioners often undervalue the quality and performance of their services. As a result, help offered by them in providing terminal care, for example, is hardly ever used, even though most patients want to die at home. At present, nursing care plans including information on family and professional resources are not developed on a systematic basis since, as yet, coordinated case management represents rather an exception to the rule.

Counselling for Family Carers

Irrespective of the nature of the supportive services offered, it is also important to think about appropriate ways in which persons in need of help can be informed about the different forms of support and how care-related tasks and questions can be best explained and clarified. Indisputably, qualified and specially trained personnel are needed to increase the acceptance of these services among patients and caregivers. Ideally, – and here the already mentioned structural problem of financing care from different financial sources becomes again apparent – these persons should be independent observers, i.e. they should not work on behalf of long-term care insurance bodies or professional home care providers. As soon as patients or caregivers assume that recommendations are made on the basis of financial interests – as, for example, savings in expenditures on the one hand or earnings from the provision of care on the other hand – the level of acceptance will decrease.

During the past years, an increasing number of advice centres were established for elderly people and family carers, which merged into one organisation at federal level (BAGA 1996). Members of this organisation have set guidelines for psychosocial counselling of elderly individuals and their family carers. "When caring for their family members, caregivers perceive psychic stress as being significantly harder than physical stress or expenditure of time or money."

Based on the experience with investigation models developed by two long-term care insurance providers, another currently discussed future model envisages the formation of an association of qualified and independent care and rehabilitation counsellors, who, immediately after assessment by experts of the MDK, provide counselling to the patients and their family members in the home of the family. The long-term care insurance providers would in part bear the costs, but they would not be authorised to influence the counselling process [44].

Health Economy

During the first years following introduction of long-term care insurance, receipts exceeded expenditures. Due to a reduction in receipts caused by unemployment and demographic changes in the population, these reserves (about 5.6 billion Euros early in 1999) will be spent in the first years of this century. Long-term care insurance contributions will therefore have to be raised earlier than expected [39]. In comparison, statutory health insurance expenditures (taking private health insurance and long-term care insurance not into account) amounted to 127 billion Euros in 1998. From this results that care-related costs account for 10.5 % of the (direct) health care costs within the statutory social insurance system.

Although health care costs, in relation to the gross national product, have remained constant (about 10 %) over the years, statutory health insurance faces a permanent financial crisis owing to eroding basic wages, which, after a long-standing debate on efficiency measures, has meanwhile sparked a debate on rationing measures. Obviously, the opportune time to discuss openly about restrictions of services (denial of services) has not yet come for German politicians. Age limits or "age discrimination" [43], a criterion sometimes used in European countries, should be mentioned in this context. However, from the point of view of a gerontologist, the use of age as sole criterion is definitely inadequate and does not make sense. Nevertheless, rationing measures have already been taken for years, as insured persons must partly pay the costs of ambulatory therapies, medication, dentures, hospital stay, cures etc. themselves. Given the globalisation process and the present situation in Germany, it is, however, very unlikely that social security contributions will be raised further. Although the German solidarity principle has found high acceptance by the majority of employees in this country so far, the level of acceptance will certainly decrease in the event of a further increase in contributions. For this reason, discussions are focussing more on 'sharing' the financial resources. This already vigorously debated topic will be even more heavily and controversially discussed in the future. One of the major challenges faced by our welfare state is therefore to avoid that the financial burden will finally rest on the shoulders of the families in our country.

References

[1] T. Klie, Pflege im sozialen Wandel: Wirkungen der Pflegversicherung auf die Situation Pflegebedürftiger. *Zeitschrift für Gerontologie und Geriatrie* **31** (1996) 387-391.

[2] Statistisches Bundesamt Gesundheitsbericht für Deutschland: Gesundheitsberichterstatung des Bundes. Stuttgart; Metzler-Poeschel, 1998.

[3] G. Igl, Die Leitprinzipien des neuen Pflegeversicherungsrechts. *Zeitschrift für Gerontologie und Geriatrie* **28** (1995) 67-70

[4] G. Igl, Zum Stand der Dinge: Die Pflegeversicherung kurz vor der Einführung der zweiten Stufe - Versuch einer sozialpolitischen Zwischenbewertung. *Zeitschrift für Gerontologie und Geriatrie* **29** (1996) 159-162

[5] Statistisches Bundesamt Statistisches Jahrbuch 1998 – CD-ROM. Stuttgart; Metzler-Poeschel; Röbel: Optimal media production GmbH, 1998.

[6] A. Evers, The New Long-Term Care Insurance Program in Germany. *Journal of Aging & Social Policy* **10(1)** (1998) 77-98

[7] H. Döhner and B. Schick, Gesundheit durch Kooperation - Die Rolle der Hausarztpraxis in der geriatrischen Versorgung. Gerontologie Band 6, LIT Verlag, Münster und Hamburg, 1996.

[8] C. Kofahl and H. Döhner, Kooperation in der Primärversorgung. Erfahrungen aus dem Projekt Ambulantes Gerontologisches Team PAGT. In: Organisationsgruppe Studentische Fachgruppe Bremen (Hg.) PflegekultTour 2001. Impulse und Perspektiven. Fünftes Jahrbuch der Studentischen Fachtagung Gesundheits- und Pflegewissenschaften. Frankfurt am Main: Mabuse-Verlag, 1997 107-131

[9] P. Wißmann and M. Langehennig, Durchblick für die KundInnen im Pflegemarkt. Die Berliner Koordinationsstellen: Auf dem Weg zum bleibenden Angebot. In: *Häusliche Pflege* **1** (1998) 21.

[10] M. Wissert, Wer ist der richtige Case Manager? Anforderungs- und Handlungsprofile bei der Hilfeplanung für die ambulante Pflege und Versorgung alter Menschen. In: Gesellschaft für Soziale Gerontologie und Altenarbeit Deutsches Zentrum für Altersfragen e.V. (Hrsg.): Neue Steuerungen in Pflege und sozialer Altenarbeit. Transfer verlag, Regensburg, 1998, 322-323.

[11] H. Döhner *et al*, Interdisziplinäres Case-Management in Kooperation mit dem Hausarzt: Verbesserung der Versorgung und der Lebensqualität geriatrischer Patienten. In: Deutsche Gesellschaft für Public Health e.V. (Hg) Public-Health-Forschung in Deutschland. Verlag Hans Huber, Bern - Göttingen - Toronto - Seattle, 1999, 324-329.

[12] H. Döhner and C. Kofahl, Versorgungsmanagement – eine Angelegenheit nur der Profis? Die Gesundheitsmappe in der Hand des Patienten. Schriftenreihe Forum Sozial- und Gesundheitspolitik Bd. 14; St. Augustin: Asgard, Hippe, 2000.

[13] C. Kofahl and H. Döhner "Die Menschen wissen, es ist jemand für sie da!" Care- und Case-Management durch das Modell PAGT in Hamburg. *Häusliche Pflege* **9** (1996) 638-646.

[14] U. Schneider, Die soziale Pflegeversicherung in Deutschland: Gestaltung, Implementierung und erste Bewertung. *Internationale Revue für soziale Sicherheit*; **52** (1999) 37-89.

[15] H. Döhner *et al*, Family Care of the Older Elderly, Germany. European Foundation for the Improving of Living and Working Conditions. Working Paper No: WP/93/18/EN, 1991.

[16] E. Gräßel, Häusliche Pflege dementiell und nicht dementiell Erkrankter. Teil I: Inanspruchnahme professioneller Pflegehilfe. *Z Gerontol Geriat* **31** (1998) 52–56.

[17] M. Veil, Der Beitrag der Familienarbeit zum Sozialstaat – umsonst und grenzenlos? In: U. Behning (ed.), Das Private ist ökonomisch. Widersprüche der Ökonomisierung privater Familien- und Haushaltsdienstleistungen. Berlin 1997 89-102.

[18] U. Schneekloth U *et al*, Hilfe- und Pflegebedürftige in privaten Haushalten: Endbericht. Bericht zur Repräsentativerhebung im Forschungsprojekt "Möglichkeiten und Grenzen selbständiger Lebensführung", Band 111.2, Schriftenreihe des Bundesministeriums für Familie, Senioren, Frauen und Jugend. Stuttgart; W. Kohlhammer GmbH, 1996.

[19] L.I. Pearlin *et al*, Caregiving and the stress process: An overview of concepts and their measures. *J Gerontol* **30** (1990) 583–593.

[20] C. Schacke and S. Zank, (1998) Zur familiären Pflege demenzkranker Menschen: Die differentielle Bedeutung spezifischer Belastungsdimensionen für das Wohlbefinden der Pflegenden und die Stabilität der häuslichen Pflegesituation. *Z Gerontol Geriat* **31** (1998) 355–361.

[21] E. Gräßel, Häusliche Pflege dementiell und nicht dementiell Erkrankter. Teil II: Gesundheit und Belastung der Pflegenden. *Z Gerontol Geriat* **31** (1998) 57–62.
[22] L. Decker *et al*, Die Verantwortung für die Anleitung der Angehörigen liegt bei den Pflegenden. *Pflegezeitschrift* 7/99 Jg. **52** (1999) 474-477.
[23] A. Buhl, Den richtigen Kurs bestimmen. Anforderungen an Schulungs- und Pflegekurse für pflegende Angehörige im Rahmen des § 45 Pflegeversicherungsgesetz. *Häusliche Pflege* **2/95** (1995) 129-131.
[24] C. Siedhoff, Qualität sichern heißt Wissen weitergeben. Ein konzept zur Durchführung von Pflegekursen für pflegende Angehörige. *Pflegen Ambulant*, 8. Jg. **6/97** (1997) 28-30.
[25] E. Richter, Ist die japanische Kopie der Pflegeversicherung besser als das Original? *Ärzte Ztg*, 2000.
[26] I. Mauritz, Für andere dasein - ohne sich selbst zu vergessen. Bausteine zur Bildungsarbeit mit pflegenden Angehörigen. Arbeitshilfe. Hrsg. von der Evangelischen Erwachsenenbildung Niedersachsen. Hannover, 1995.
[27] M. Tampl, Pflegekurse planen und leiten. München, Hans-Weinberger Akademie der Arbeiterwohlfahrt e.V, 1996.
[28] H. Faßmann H, "Regionale Service-Zentren für häusliche Altenpflege - zur Entwicklung und Sicherung von qualitativen Standards in der privaten Pflege. München, Verlag der Hans-Weinberger Akademie der Arbeiterwohlfahrt e.V, 1998.
[29] R. Meierjürgen, Hilfen für pflegende Angehörige. Das Schulungsprogramm "Zu Hause pflegen". *Konzeption und erste Praxiserfahrungen*. Ersk. **2** (1995) 52-58.
[30] R. Wasilewski R *et al*, Pflegeberatung zur Sicherung der Pflegequalität im häuslichen Bereich. Nürnberg; Schriftenreihe des Instituts für empirische Soziologie, 1995.
[31] U. Mattmüller and G. Vogel, Die Profis sind gefordert. Burnout bei pflegenden Personen in Privathaushalten. Häusliche Pflege, **10** (1995) 739-742.
[32] P. Zeman, Häusliche Altenpflegearrangements. Zum Aushandlungsgeschehen zwischen lebensweltlichen und professionellen Helfersystemen. Diskussionspapiere Nr. 4; Berlin: DZA, 1996.
[33] T. Klie, Qualität in der häuslichen Pflege. DAK Versicherten-Befragung. Hamburg: DAK, 1999.
[34] V. Garms-Homolová, Qualitätssicherung in der ambulanten Pflege. Erste Erfahrungen mit dem RAI HC-System in Deutschland und Österreich. *Pflegen ambulant* **9,2** (1998) 18-20.
[35] H.P. Meier-Baumgartner, Modellvorhaben: Ganzheitliche Betreuung und medizinische Therapie geriatrischer Patienten. Zwischenbericht. Albertinen-Haus Hamburg, Hamburg, 1998.
[36] H.P. Meier-Baumgartner, Modellvorhaben: Ganzheitliche Betreuung und medizinische Therapie geriatrischer Patienten. Zwischenbericht 1998. Albertinen-Haus Hamburg, Hamburg, 1999.
[37] M. Nolan and I. Philp, COPE: towards a comprehensive assessment of caregiver need. British Journal of Nursing **8(20)** (1999) 1364-1372.
[38] P. Gitschmann, Altenpolitik und Altenhilfepolitik im Wandel in Bund, Ländern und Gemeinden. In: Tews HP (Hg) Altern und Politik. Melsungen: Bibliomed, 1996.
[39] F. Schulz-Nieswandt, Zur Zukunft des Gesundheitswesens. *Z Gerontol Geriat* **31** (1998) 382–386.
[40] G. Naegele, In: Ärzte-Zeitung 29.6.2000.
[41] Bundesministerium für Gesundheit, Eckpunktepapier zur Förderung der Tagespflege als erster Schritt für eine bessere Versorgung demenzkranker Mitbürgerinnen und Mitbürger. www.bmgesundheit.de Stand: 21.7.2000.
[42] H.J. Ahrens, AOK. *Ärzte Zeitung* 21.6.2000.
[43] A. Walker, Ageing in Europe – challenges and consequences. *Z Gerontol Geriat* **32** (1999) 390–397.
[44] B. Matthies, Angehörigenarbeit in der häuslichen Pflege. Vortragsmanuskript, 2000.

Chapter 4

Greece
(September 1998)

Judith Triantifillou
SEXTANT Co
Irakleous 40
Kallithea 176-71
Athens
Greece

Elizabeth Mestheneos
SEXTANT Co
Irakleous 40
Kallithea 176-71
Athens
Greece

Introduction

Overview of policy and practice towards older people and family carers of the dependent elderly

Although there has been a growing awareness amongst Greek governments of the possible problems associated with the rapidly increasing numbers of elderly people in the Greek population, there has been no overall national plan for the development of health and social services for older people, though some piecemeal activities have been initiated[i] and wider policy measures are currently under review by the Ministry of Health and Welfare. Even though discussion on the need for public policy to support family carers started at the end of the 1980s [1], very little priority has been given to this issue and as yet support for family carers has not been incorporated on a systematic basis into public policy. There is a lack of data on the extent of family care and on the health or well being of family carers [2,3] and the applications for disability allowance from those requiring someone to care for them does not provide even a rough estimate of the numbers of family carers.

The main axis of Government policy towards older people for most of the previous decades has been the emphasis on providing pension support, with a large percentage of the welfare budget being spent on this one item[ii]. Very little of the public budget has been spent on providing social assistance or social services for the elderly and there are no statutory services. Only since the 1980s has there been some change in the direction of public policy with the development of the Open Care Centres for Older people (KAPI) in over 230 local authority areas, a description of which is provided later. Also during the same period various experimental and pilot projects were set up which were designed to provide a variety of social and health care and help to older people in the community. Some of these programmes, while primarily focusing on the isolated elderly, also served family carers who needed support with the care of elderly family members.

In the field of health care the main development in the 1980s was the introduction of the National Health Care system, though resources have been devoted to hospital rather than primary health care. What was written in 1993 still holds true:

"There are no statutory services either for the carers of the elderly or the elderly themselves to support them in the home; district nursing, day care centres, meals on wheels, home helps, hospices, chiropodists and sheltered housing do not exist as public services."[4].

The system of national health care is financed and organised in a similar form to the system implemented in other continental European countries where rights to treatment, other than emergency hospital care, are accessed through the social insurance fund to which individuals contribute. Although there are numerous insurance funds[iii], the main fund for urban workers (IKA) covers about 70% of the population. IKA runs extensive primary health care centres in all the major urban centres which are, however, overcrowded. In the rural areas, given that the Agricultural Workers Fund provided pensions and services on a non contributory basis, the main system of primary health care is built around the long established agricultural rural surgeries manned by newly qualified doctors who are required to undertake a period of service in the countryside, and the newer Health Centres, established in the late 1980s and strategically placed in rural areas, which are supposed to provide far more comprehensive health services. As regards tertiary or long term institutional care for the older disabled and chronic sick, state provision is again minimal with only 2500- 3000 beds[iv] to serve an estimated 10,000-20,000 (1-2%) of the population of all ages in this category. The majority of these beds are occupied by over 65 year olds. Private and philanthropic (NGO) residential care homes slightly increased in number (to approximately 10,000 beds) over the past decades but for many reasons are generally considered only as a last resort by both older people, their family carers and formal social services. Only in the case of luxury residential homes may they be perceived as a positive choice by well off older people and family carers[v].

Since under 1% of those aged 65 years and over are in residential homes, the numbers of disabled and dependent elderly living in the community is high. The lack of comprehensive primary health and social care services means that the overwhelming majority of the elderly are being cared for by family members who are thrown back on their own resources and have to provide or fund virtually all forms of care. Those who are fortunate enough to have financial resources can usually pay for some care and a considerable section of those with good incomes have increasingly turned to the use of foreign migrant care workers in recent years, mainly women, as a solution to providing care in the home of the elderly person. Hospitals, the only statutory service available, are sometimes used by family carers and elderly persons as a form of emergency respite care though even in these, if the elderly person is in need of actual nursing care, the family has to take on responsibility for giving or finding private nursing services since the public ones are inadequate. Public and private residential homes do not formally offer respite care.

The welfare triangle

A political policy development that is very slowly being implemented and that is likely to have implications for the development of health and welfare support services for the elderly and their family carers concerns the political decentralisation of governmental powers. Until very recently Greece was a highly centralised state, with all decisions being made and finances allocated from the centre. The devolution of powers and the capacity to raise and administer their own funds is beginning to change the face of local government. The needs of local elderly people and their family carers are far better known to the local authorities than to central government. The Open Care Centres were devolved to the local authorities about 3 years ago, though not always with the necessary funding. However since then some municipalities, recognising the needs of their local populations, have supported a few initiatives e.g. training and employing Home or Family Carers, which were designed to help the elderly, though also to generate new employment. In 1998 the government obtained funding through the European Union to finance a pilot program for two years of home care services for older people in over 140 municipalities, to be organised and run by each municipality. Only a few of these are yet fully in operation and there are both ethical problems about starting a program with funding that is only available for two years, as well as organisational problems concerning the running and staffing of these services. More importantly few people at the local level are yet aware that the problem of care of the elderly does not concern only the elderly on their own but also family carers who need support.

Voluntary work in Greece for older people has long been practiced in what can be described as traditional forms i.e. philanthropic and church associations. This still constitutes a major element in the care of the dependent elderly outside the family. Such organisations, mainly run on a community, parish or specific origins basis (e.g. villages, areas with Asia Minor refugees) have often provided help to family carers in practice, even if this was not perceived as their primary function, which was usually the care of the isolated dependent or needy elderly. The Hellenic Red Cross with a long, and for many decades, an almost unique tradition in training volunteers, began services with joint funding by the Ministry of Health and Welfare, on a pilot basis from the early 1980s. These were designed to provide nursing services, voluntary visiting and support and home care services and were extended to cities other than Athens. Funding difficulties have been the main reason why these services have not been extended throughout all the major cities.

Organized private service initiatives to support elderly people in their homes are minimal: there has been no development of private domestic and home care services, few organized nursing and para-medical services, no meal delivery service for older people, no accompanying services. These remain entirely the province of the older person and the family carer to either arrange for individually or to provide personally.

Country specific context

The rapid urbanisation of the Greek population since the 1950s has had the effect of skewing the population structure so that in many rural areas of Greece there are overwhelming numbers of older people and many of those from the younger generations are 'missing'. In certain islands and mountain villages the percentage of those over 65 years of age rises to over 27% e.g. Samos island. The care needs of many older people who do not have their children in their neighbourhood and village is thus problematic, remembering that a large amount of family care is given by other older people (as spouses, siblings and older children) and that thus the general lack of young people can be a significant problem in the care of elderly dependent people. Additionally despite the existence of rural surgeries and Health Centres, many villages have no easy access to medical services of all kinds, not only doctors but also physiotherapy and nursing services. Lower incomes, poorer housing, a difficult physical environment and geographical remoteness, have repercussions for family carers, while local authorities do not have the resources to set up extensive and expensive medical or social care facilities in every village. There have been various attempts to overcome these difficulties through the creation of volunteer support networks, the mobilisation of local organisations and institutions, e.g. the local authority, governmental bodies, the churches, women's groups, and even the institutionalisation of telemedicine in some areas. However all these projects and programmes are experimental, partial and relatively rare and older people remain dependent in many rural areas on old fashioned neighbourliness and the care of whatever family is left. This is often quite inadequate and family carers may experience great stress. One result is that elderly people who become dependent may suddenly have to leave their village home so that they can stay with their child /children in the major cities and be cared for there. In a follow up study in 1986 of the rural elderly originally surveyed in a WHO study in 1980, it was found that a considerable percentage had moved away from their village (17%) apparently as a result of growing disability and the need they had for care [5]. Such relocation may result in considerable strain both for urban families, who suddenly find themselves having to make room in small urban flats for their elderly relative, and for the older person who is taken out of his/her familiar context and environment. However, as already indicated, the problems of the urban areas are also acute since there is a general lack of organised home care services or facilities.

Legal situation concerning responsibilities for the care of older people

The Greek constitution makes the child of an elderly dependent person responsible for his/her welfare and support. However this responsibility comes second to their responsibilities to their own children, and thus effectively if a child does not wish to look after his/her parent s/he can usually claim exemption by virtue of these other responsibilities. The Greek Constitution, Article 21, para.3. states that the State has responsibility for the welfare of its citizens and that it should take special measures for groups such as the elderly or the disabled. However the enforcement and implementation of this legal provision is extremely rare.

There is a department in the Ministry of Health and Welfare for the Protection of the Elderly and People with Special Needs. The head of this department is a civil servant whose training and experience may have little relevance to this area, and in addition they may have been political appointees. Nevertheless, one or two people occupying this position have exhibited great enthusiasm and vision in their work and managed to create a significant change in attitudes and approaches to the care of older people i.e. development and rapid expansion of the KAPI centres network during the late 1980s and early 1990s.

Health and Social Care for Older People: Structures and Functions

Organisational structures and division of labour

Health care for older Greeks is provided in the context of general health care provision for the adult population. There are no university medical departments of gerontology and geriatrics is not a recognized medical specialty. There is some pressure from doctors in the Hellenic Association of Gerontology and Geriatrics for this to change but interviews with hospital specialists indicate that there are mixed feelings within the profession about how positive this would be as a development for older people themselves. As one doctor said wryly : "There is no discrimination against the elderly... they suffer the same vagaries of the health system as the rest of the Greek population!" There is no specialised geriatric nursing although this is just being instituted in the Nursing Department of the TEI Athens.

As indicated above, the major change in the health system in the past 20 years was the introduction of the National Health Service by the PASOK government in 1983 with Law 1397/1985 (Gov.L.J.143 7th Oct.Vol.1.) This provided access, for the first time, for all Greeks to medical care regardless of their ability to pay. However the NHS was implemented initially at the hospital or secondary care level.

The primary health care centres which were planned for the rural areas were built at a later stage and although designed to provide comprehensive services, from the outset suffered from understaffing leading to the unequal and inadequate provision of primary health care. These centres are supplemented in very remote areas by newly qualified doctors serving their obligatory year of rural service without which they are unable to obtain a licence to practice. This experience is frequently a baptism by fire with inexperienced young doctors living and working in primitive conditions with virtually no equipment and back up services some distance away. A recent report in a Sunday newspaper indicates that this situation remains virtually unchanged at the present time. (Eleftherotypia "Epsilon" 9th August 1998). However it can be argued that the high proportion of elderly served in these areas provide the doctors with invaluable first hand experience of caring for older people in the community with no other access to health care.

In urban areas the provision of primary health care services varies according to the patient's health insurance and pension fund which are numerous and linked to occupations. Attempts by successive governments over the past 30 years to unify these into a single system have failed, mainly due to the resistance by the richer, smaller funds to relinquish their superior services to a lower common denominator. The major urban workers insurance fund, IKA, has the most extensive and comprehensive primary health care provision through a system of polyclinics which provide specialist services for 12 hours a day. They also contract the services of general practitioners working from their own medical offices, who provide a minimum of 5½ hours a day to IKA patients. The IKA system is increasingly in debt, overloaded with bureaucratic red tape, underpays its doctors and is denigrated by doctors and patients alike. The time needed to negotiate the system means that it is frequently avoided by busy working people who prefer to pay for quicker, private health care services and is heavily overused by pensioners.

Roles of practitioners

General practice has only been introduced as a specialty in Greece during the past 15 years and is still not a popular option amongst doctors, being seen as a second class specialty. Thus most older people visit a variety of specialists according to their health problems and few have a doctor with an overall view of their health status. Even more importantly the public sector does not give doctors the overall responsibility for their patients' health care so that the public, including older people and their family carers, use medical and health care services as *consumers* according to their needs, their insurance and their ability to pay. For emergency and out of hours services, patients have the choice of attending hospital emergency services, which provide a 24 hour rota, or requesting and paying for a private visit at home.

Despite some de-centralization[vi], hospital beds are still heavily concentrated in the 2 main urban centres of Thessaloniki and Athens and these tend to be overused, especially by older people who have higher rates both of admission and length of stay compared with younger age groups [6].

In a study of the use of an Athenian general hospital emergency department by over 70 year olds it was found that, for the three Emergency Department clinics most used by older people (General Medicine, Cardiology and Surgery), over 70 year olds attended with more than twice the frequency of the younger age groups and were significantly more likely to be admitted to the hospital via this route. In the absence of alternative forms of care the use of the hospital as a form of "respite care" was reported by most of the hospital professionals interviewed who were aware of the increased admissions of dependent older people during weekends and holiday periods when family carers needed a break from their caring responsibilities. The staff were often sympathetic to this need although they disliked being manipulated into a medically unnecessary admission.

The lack of easily accessible primary care services was reflected in the fact that 41% of the sample of older people arrived at the Emergency Department without prior consultation with a medical practitioner. Only 12% of the sample subjects were unaccompanied, reflecting the importance to older people of the informal care network.

Social care for older people — the KAPI centres

The KAPI (Open Care Community Centres for Older People), begun originally as pilot centres by volunteer groups using public financing, were incorporated into government policy in 1982 and developed to form the present extensive network of KAPI centres under the auspices of the local authorities throughout rural and urban Greece. The main objective of these centres is to help maintain the elderly as active and participating members of their local communities. The services offered are primarily recreational in character but include those of a full time social worker with some medical services provided by a full time health visitor, a part time doctor and, in some cases a physiotherapist, the emphasis being on preventive health care. Chiropody and occupational therapy services are available in some KAPIs, as are washing machines which can be used by elderly members or their carers. The medical services are not integrated within the National Health system, though attempts have been made to combine them with those of IKA and there is cooperation with OGA insurance for drug prescriptions etc. It should be noted that the services of the KAPI are oriented more towards the well elderly. Although the KAPIs are supposed to provide home helps, there have been difficulties in the implementation of this program resulting in the bedridden, the housebound, and the dependent elderly in the community being those least likely to benefit from the KAPI. Whilst the KAPIs are aimed at the elderly, they frequently work closely with family members in such matters as drug prescription and provision, advice and counselling, while also providing some relief care through limited supervision of elderly members on weekday mornings, or holiday care for those elderly who go on annual camping holidays organized by the majority of KAPIs in association with the Ministries of Tourism and of Health and Welfare. It should be emphasized that the KAPIs do not undertake responsibility for the care of the dependent elderly in their area and in any case not all people choose to join a KAPI.

Home care services

As outlined in the introduction, 1998 has seen the introduction by the Government of an EU funded 2 year pilot project to provide home care services run by the municipalities for dependent older people. Many of these teams are working in close cooperation with the local KAPI centres but it is too early as yet to report on the results of this program. The home care services run for the past 10 years by the Hellenic Red Cross alone or in association with the Ministry of Health and Welfare (Gerontological Unit, Help at Home, Nursing at Home) use both professional and trained volunteer services to support older people at home. Although these services were developed initially to support the isolated elderly, interviews with the staff and service organizers in 1992 indicated that they were already extending their work to support family carers e.g. counselling services, training carers in home nursing techniques etc [7]. For example the Help at Home services working from three bases in Central Athens consist of a team of three social workers, a visiting doctor, physiotherapist, nurse, psychologist and home helps plus the volunteer network, and provide services to approximately 600 households, 350 of these with regular support (over a one year period).

Recent developments or interesting new schemes designed to support family carers. Any evidence of impact?

The role of the family carer of an older person is still not recognized in Greek society as a distinct social role separate from normal family obligations. Although there has been some progress in this area amongst professionals working with older people in recognizing the problems faced by family carers, there has been no public debate on the subject and carers have no public voice. The recently formed organization for the support of family carers of people with Alzheimer's disease, under the auspices of the Hellenic Association for Gerontology is a first step but it is too early to report any evidence of impact. There is an obvious need for a more general Carers' Association to promote issues of importance to family carers of older people.

Roles of Family Carers of Older People Living at Home

Financial aspects

In Greece poverty is still strongly related to age[vii] with older people far more likely to be living in poverty than younger people, reflecting their low levels of pension and capital resources, though there are considerable inequalities in income and resources amongst older people [8,9]. As in other Member States women live longer than men (on average 5 years more) though in worse health and with less income. There is no financial data on the situation of family carers of older people, though the fact that many are themselves older people suggests that a considerable percentage of older carers do not have the resources either to buy in help and support or sometimes even to have access to facilities which might make their caring work easier (e.g. washing machines, modern houses). There are large inequalities in the financial situation of carers. It does appear that the care of older people may be directly influenced by financial considerations. Higher levels of pension are correlated with the probability of an older person maintaining their own household but there are also indications of some correlation between the provision of family care and higher pension levels i.e. those who were on the lowest level of pension were less likely to be in receipt of care from a member of their family [10]. This finding needs to be examined in greater detail but some reflections on reciprocity, outlined below, suggest why this may occur.

The direct financial costs of care vary with the resources of the carer. Those families or individual carers who have few resources tend to depend almost entirely on their own labour for care. Where a couple are available to care for an elderly parent, the woman's labour tends to be used for personal and home care, while care outside the home tends to be done by the man. Where more than one child is available to provide care another financial arrangement is for the older person to "circulate" between carers -each child taking the elderly parent for a fixed period of care. This is based on the assumption that any existing property or capital will be distributed in an equitable and determined fashion at death between the children who provide the care. Brothers and sisters may agree, in the case of one of them being the main carer, that this person will receive a larger share or all the assets of the older person on death.

Working carers, typically children between the ages of 40-65, are faced by difficult choices with respect to caring since this age is important with respect to seniority and earning pension entitlements. Thus the relative financial advantages and disadvantages of a family member giving up paid employment have often to be carefully calculated - not an easy task given the unknown time period for which care will be needed, and it is more usually married women in the paid labour market who tend to have to make such choices unless early retirement is offered or available at the critical moment. Choices depend on the degree to which the household is dependent on their income, their career expectations, their potential loss of pension entitlements and their level of earnings since those with high earnings may decide to use their income to pay for care. Those on low or insecure incomes may give up work more easily and in a small percentage of cases a heavily dependent person may be able to receive a disability allowance which enables them to pay for care[viii]. Until recently women with children under 15 years of age and with 15 years of employment service were sometimes able to leave their employment early with a lower level of pension. Where this entitlement coincided with the need to care for elderly parents or parents in law, the incitement to leave the work place was high[ix]. Part time employment, especially of women, in many European countries is often perceived as allowing the combination of caring duties with staying in the labour market. However the very low percentage in part time employment in Greece does not correlate with the high dependency on family care.

Part of the explanation for working carers lies in the fact that especially amongst Greek older workers there is a very high percentage who are self - employed or in family employment (47% amongst those 45 years and over) which may allow greater flexibility in time schedules. Finally the tax system provides a certain limited tax relief on expenses involved in the care of a dependent relative.

As already indicated in the Introduction, family carers with an adequate income typically pay for domestic and care support, though mostly in recent years this is non registered labour. People offering such care vary from female neighbours who undertake such work, to foreign migrant workers. The cost is high (e.g. 120,000 Dracjma for full time assistance[x]) but still less than the direct cost of putting an older person in residential or nursing homes or using private nursing services[xi].

Family carers report that the main caring costs lie in the special needs of the elderly dependent person for medicines, doctors, nurses, disposable incontinence pads, which can stretch the budget of lower income family carers.

Social relations and reciprocity

A strong influence on care in old age is the notion of reciprocity. During their lifetime it is a very common form of behaviour for parents to transfer significant capital resources to their children in order to help with the setting up of their children's new families e.g. a house, furniture, land, as well as to pay for extended years of education. This generation of parents has often sacrificed its own comforts and life style in order to ensure that the children manage to get an education and move out of poverty. It is not only the immediate parental generation that may do this but also other relatives such as childless uncles and aunts. The success of children, measured in educational achievement, civil servant appointments and own housing, is interpreted as reflecting positively on the parents and wider kin group. The 'investment' in children thus brings social status recognition. However it is also understood that this kind of 'investment' may have to be repaid in arrangements for the care of a dependent elderly parent or relative. While not all children fulfill these filial obligations, most do. Elderly parents, until the onset of dependency, frequently continue to act as net transferrers of small services and resources e.g. child care, pocket money and help with the studies of grandchildren, cooking.

Thus many carers have already been beneficiaries of an older person's gifts which set up obligations of reciprocity with respect to care[xii]. Rarely are such obligations resented. However those parents who did not or could not behave in this culturally approved way i.e. were unable or unwilling to make particular efforts to help their children (with capital and/or services) , run the risk of being ignored when dependency occurs. Their "moral" capital is inadequate - they have in some sense failed their children and thus the obligations to reciprocate are not particularly felt by the child nor necessarily enforced from social pressure. Those with the least resources (pensions, capital, property) and who have not been particularly helpful to their children (services) are at risk of being abandoned. Older people who have no children, recognizing their potential future need for care, can also make provision for this e.g. by gifts to cousins, nieces and nephews, especially if the latter are single persons or persons with whom they have a good relationship. These gifts are designed to set up obligations for reciprocity later. In the case of someone without any family or close kin, then neighbours and co-villagers can also be the object of wills and gifts[xiii] on the understanding that they will offer care when necessary.

The fact that the Greek family is both in ideological and relative terms the central social institution of Greek society helps to explain why generalized reciprocity of gifts, services, information, support and practical help does not occur only in the context of the narrow nuclear family, but to some degree extends as a form of behaviour into many areas of Greek social life. Additionally the absence of alternatives - in the form of welfare state support and services - also explains why not only the family but many people in the wider society are willing to enter into gift relationships that set up bonds of reciprocity and obligation. Although Greek society is conscious of age and ageing, intergenerational relationships do appear easier and more frequent by virtue of the centrality of the family and kinship.

Despite reciprocity and a greater ease in social relations between generations, this does not mean that fulfilling care obligations is easy- as already indicated, small urban flats quickly become overcrowded when an older person needs to move in to receive care and where the family's income is not enough to allow additional space to be rented or purchased. This leads to real role conflicts where the family carer has obligations to offer care and attention to his or her own children. Some of the older urban generation foresaw this problem and made housing provisions for themselves and their children in the same block of flats.

However attention needs to be paid to the fact that social changes are occurring rapidly and there are significant differences within families which relate to generation, education, income and location [11]. The fall in the birth rate, the entry of women into the paid labour market[xiv], the increase in individualism and consumerism will all act to redefine the family and family obligations. Already it is not uncommon for 4 elderly parents to have just 2 married children responsible for any care they may need. In such a situation where physical dependency sets in, the carer is under tremendous stress and without any money can find no real support from the state. Hardly surprisingly, given the lack of social and practical support for carers, some carers reach the end of their tether and may abandon the older person in a hospital[xv].

A further positive sanction for carers in their work is that of religion; although not generally passive in their everyday lives, Greeks have a fundamental belief that God has his own will and that one cannot fight against this but must live it out. Acceptance of one's lot - whether as an older person or as a carer - both resigns people to their fate and stops them resenting it. The best medical care and advice can be sought incessantly to improve the health of the older person, but the acceptance of death as being outside human control and meaning also acts to reconcile carers to their task.

Personal

The domestic role of women in Greek society, especially those from the older generation, as well as the rural origins of so many Greeks of the older generation - whether carers or cared for - helps to explain why individual carers accept the hard role that they face in providing total care without state or welfare support or any services[xvi]. Research suggested that for many carers the greatest help they could envisage from the state was financial aid, almost no-one could imagine having practical assistance in the work of caring except for those who had been in receipt of the few pilot services. The personal relationship pre-existing between carer and older person was another key to satisfactions in the caring role.

Age / gender

There is no national or representative data on the age or gender of carers. The high marriage rate amongst men aged 75 years and over reflects the fact that in the older generations age differences at marriage were large - it was common for men to be 10 years older than their wives. However even looking at the data for the marriage rate amongst older women, despite having older husbands, their rate is the same as for the European average. This suggests that more couples can care for one another and that older men are available as carers both of their wives - since older women tend to have worse health than men - and their parents.

The high levels of longevity in the Greek population indicate that when dependency does set in, many of the carers from the children's generation are themselves older people. This has repercussions for their own health and capacities to care.

Stresses and rewards

Given the extensive care needed by many older dependent people and the lack of support services, it is obvious that many carers are under considerable physical and psychological stress. Not surprisingly some of this stress may take the form of violence against the older dependent person [12]. In a study of such violence [13] of 757 older persons interviewed, 117 suffered from abuse but only 1% from actual physical violence. Part of the tolerance for the heavy load of caring lies in the expectations of families and carers. Caring is seen as an inevitable element of family life, part of the duties one has as a family member. Here the term ' duty' (kathikon, ypokreosi) is not a word with a negative meaning in Greek, unlike English, but involves a strong sense of positive moral satisfaction and rightness, of a debt repaid. It is this, along with the idea of reciprocity, which makes family care feasible for many carers despite the enormous difficulties under which they labour.

Attitudes towards practitioners

As suggested Greek carers are not passive when considering the appropriate treatment for their dependent elderly person. Though there is great respect for good doctors, few of the latter are able to exercise any kind of absolute control over diagnosis or treatment. Families frequently consult a number of doctors, if they have the financial resources, or call on kin who are doctors, for second opinions. There is a far greater realisation of the fallibility of medical doctors and this perception is aided by the fact that unlike other countries where medical terminology often acts to confer a sense of mystique and incomprehension amongst patients, much of the medical language used is Greek. Thus, as emphasized in Structures and Functions, older people and their family carers act as *consumers* using a mixture of public, private and voluntary health and social services as their circumstances demand.

Assessment

How it operates in practice for older people and family carers; which methods are used. Any evidence of effectiveness.

There are no payments made directly to family carers for the services they perform in looking after their older dependent relatives. Assessment of older people for disability benefits takes place through the Welfare department of the Ministry of Health. An application is made accompanied by a brief medical report from a State hospital and the older person is requested to appear before an assessment committee of 3 persons, usually doctors, who assess the degree of disability using strictly medical criteria. The guidelines for these assessments however lead to many anomalies both in the awarding and in the rejecting of claims e.g. one of the medical criteria for which a disability allowance is awarded is paraplegia; hemiplegia, however severe following a stroke, does not qualify. Disability is assessed on a percentage basis with x% scored for each disability and the total score must exceed 67% for an allowance to be awarded. The amount varies between 30-67,000 drachmas per month (90-203 ECU). Disability pensions are only awarded before normal pensionable age so that if disability occurs when the older person is already in receipt of a pension this latter can only be supplemented by a disability allowance. If an allowance is awarded, the long bureaucratic procedure has to be repeated at least every 3 years when the case is reviewed. In practice the procedure can be so daunting that many carers of highly dependent older people are either deterred from starting the bureaucratic process or fall by the wayside and give up at some stage. One practical difficulty frequently encountered is in the transportation of the disabled applicant who has to appear in person before the committee. This in itself can prove an insurmountable obstacle and whilst there is theoretical provision for the committee to perform home assessments in such cases, in practice this takes place mainly in the larger urban areas and rural home assessments seem to be rare. There are no payments made directly to carers. On the contrary disability pensions form a relatively high proportion of total pensions in Greece particularly between the ages of 40-60 years; this is probably due both to the awarding of them in the past as "favours" in dubious cases, and their being used to replace non existent social security protection for the long term unemployed, especially amongst older workers who become redundant and can't find work again in the labour market [14].

The Red Cross Home Care services perform home assessments on all older people who apply to them for support. This is done during one or more visits by the social worker in charge and supplemented as required by other members of the Home Care Team e.g. doctor, nurse, physiotherapist. Thus a composite picture of the older person's physical, mental and social states is built up and services supplied according to availability and frequency of requirement e.g. daily, weekly etc. Whilst the clients serviced are mainly isolated older people, predominantly women, as part of the assessment process the contribution of any family carers is taken into account and their needs informally assessed with a view to co-operating with them in the support of the older person and where necessary supporting them e.g. by "throwing out of the house" an elderly husband carer in the mornings when the nurse and home help attend his disabled wife and providing volunteers to "granny sit" while the carers have a break. No formal assessment instruments are used by these services for the assessment of the older person or the carer and although they are aware of and sometimes use EASY-Care, this is not on a systematic basis. Interest was expressed in the use of such instruments as it was felt that they would simplify and standardise their work to a large degree. The home care pilot programmes being developed by the local authorities are not yet in a position to provide any data on their assessment processes.

Finally, during the Family Carers Study carried out in Greece in 1990-92, from information given by the 24 carers interviewed, a list of carers' tasks was developed which can be used to provide a rough assessment of the degree of disability of the older person and the support needed from the carer's point of view, although no attempt was made to assess the hours of care provided. This "instrument" has been demonstrated in training programmes for unemployed women to develop services for older people but no information has been received as to whether this has ever been used in practice.

Carer's Assessment of help needed

Tasks	Full help needed	Partial help needed	No help needed
i. Toilet			
ii. Feeding			
iii. Lifting			
iv. Bathing			
v. Dressing			
vi. Cooking			
vii. Housework			
viii. Shopping			
ix. Laundry			
x. Representing			
xi. Company			
xii. Nursing			

Case Studies

Questions : For each of nine combinations the following questions have been answered.

1. What role(s) would the informal family carers typically occupy in caring for the older person?
2. What services would typically be provided to support the older person?

3. How would the informal/family carer's needs typically be assessed (if at all) and what support (if any) would typically be provided for the carer?

Case 1

Kyria Maria is aged 76, with osteoarthritis of the hips and knees, poor vision due to macular degeneration, and hypertension. Mobile with a frame within her home except for the stairs. Needs help with mobility outside, shopping, cooking and housework.

Situation 1. Kyria Maria, living alone on the outskirts of a remote mountain village in an isolated farmhouse, is widowed and lives on the OGA (Agricultural Organization's) pension which is very low. Her daughter and son-in-law are both unemployed with four children, aged 9 months to 7 years, and live 5 kilometers away. Her other two children live over 100 kilometers away.

1. The family carer would be either her daughter or one of her children in the city. Whoever it was would take on full responsibility for her medical, physical, psychological and social care. Thus if Kyria Maria has a reasonably good relationship with her daughter who lives 5 km away, the most probable scenario is that she would go to live with her daughter and her family despite their financially difficult circumstances. Her pension, albeit small, plus her house, are resources for negotiating her care, not necessarily explicitly, but implicitly. However her other two children might also wish to be involved in a rotating system of care since by law they will also inherit part of her property. Thus she might be transported to the homes of her other children at various times during the year. The least likely scenario is that she would be left on her own. This would happen if she were a particularly difficult old lady who either insisted on living on her own until an inevitable catastrophe, or her children refused to take her. In case of dire need she might be sent to a local public or church residential home, inhabited mainly by those without families or the very poor and the abandoned.
2. In the case where Kyria Maria stayed in the village she would find no public services to support her in her home. Neighbours would help with some shopping and also would bring in meals both on a paid and unpaid basis.
3. There would be no assessment of the family carer's needs and the only support would be informally provided by neighbours and kin.

Situation 2. Kyria Maria lives alone in a ground floor flat in town. Widowed. Daughter and son-in-law are both teachers in full-time employment, with 2 children aged 7 and 11, and live within 1 kilometer in the same town.

1. Kyria Maria's daughter and her family would be responsible for providing support with shopping, cooking and housework. They would try and support her in her own home, willingly or unwillingly, depending on their relationship and if they had a car she would probably be included in family excursions. However teachers are not well paid and to some extent her ability to help her daughter's family economically or even to a limited extent within the home might mean that she would be taken in by them. If her family were having to contribute to her household expenses, another common strategy would be to take her into their house and rent out or sell her flat if it was owned by her.
2. If Kyria Maria had been a member of the local KAPI (Open Care Community Centre for Older people) before she became disabled, then she would continue to receive some

services from the KAPI e.g. rudimentary medical care, drug provision and visits from the social worker. Some KAPIs also provide home help although mostly for the isolated elderly. If she was fortunate enough to live in one of the areas where there are pilot home care programmes run by the Red Cross and some Local Authorities, and her carers were able to influence decision making, she might get some home help.
3. If the daughter made contact with a Home Care Service some assessment of her situation would be made by the social worker to judge her mother's eligibility for services. The Red Cross Home Care service provides a very limited counselling service for family carers and occasionally volunteers who provide some respite day care.

Situation 3. Kyria Maria lives with her spouse in a 2-storey house. Retired with savings. Spouse is fit and well. No children. Bedroom, bathroom and toilet are upstairs.

1. In this case the husband is the main carer. Since finance is not a major problem they would most likely employ live-in help in the form of a foreign female migrant worker who would undertake household duties and personal care on a full time basis for a salary of 3-400 ECU per month depending on her knowledge of Greek, her experience and her country of origin. If they did not want to employ anyone to live in, they might pay for domestic help and help with personal care from a Greek woman or a foreign migrant worker.
In the house, consideration might be given to installing privately a chair lift if money permitted this investment. It is unlikely that Greeks living in villas (2 storey modern houses) would not have a downstairs lavatory and wash basin at least. Facilities are usually available on the same floor.
2. None.
3. They would not. The family carer, especially being a man with means, would make his own assessment of the situation and buy his own solutions.

Case 2

Kyrios Georgos, aged 80, is facing discharge from hospital following a stroke. Expected to be confined to bed or chair for several weeks with gradual recovery of mobility. Needs the help of one person for transfers, toileting, bathing and dressing.

Situation 1. Kyrios Georgos lives alone on the outskirts of a remote mountain village in an isolated farmhouse is widowed and lives on the OGA (Agricultural Organization's) pension which is very low. His daughter and son-in-law are both unemployed with four children, aged 9 months to 7 years, and live 5 kilometers away. His other two children live over 100 kilometers away.

1. Following discharge from hospital Kyrios Georgos would be taken to stay with one of his three children. Which child this would be initially would probably be determined by their proximity to the hospital where he had been treated, since they would have been the main carers while he was in hospital and would have to organize any follow up treatments that he needed e.g. physiotherapy, hospital and medical visits, drugs. They would have a vested interest in rehabilitating him as quickly as possible. His children and their spouses would take turns to supervise him at home but physical care e.g. toiletting, bathing, dressing, would be undertaken preferably by his own daughter/s unless he was living with a son who would then take some responsibility for these tasks

together with the daughter-in-law. He would not be sent back to his daughter in the countryside, 5 kilometres away, until he was more mobile and while there were still fears that he would need hospital care. She would then take responsibility for him probably by taking him into her own home where his pension would help the family finances. In the situation where none of the children want to be involved in Kyrios Georgos' care and rehabilitation, they might choose to abandon him in hospital, temporarily or permanently, and in this case the social workers would try to contact them. If they then refused to take any responsibility for their father, the social workers would have to try and find a residential home prepared to take him, despite his low income. The problem would be that the criteria for admission to such homes usually specify that the older person is self caring. In this case he would have to stay in hospital, blocking a bed, until he was self caring. However this situation - especially as he has three children - would be exceptional.
2. None.
3. If the children actively sought the advice of the hospital social worker before discharge from hospital, they would be able to discuss some of the caring options but this would be oriented to what was best for the father (and hospital). The carers' needs would not be assessed formally.

Situation 2. Kyrios Georgos lives alone in a ground floor flat in town. Widowed. Daughter and son-in-law are both teachers in full-time employment, with 2 children aged 7 and 11, and live within 1 kilometer in the same town.

1. His daughter and son-in-law would undertake responsibility for Kyrios Georgos on discharge from hospital. They would have been closely involved in his medical and nursing care during his admission, if necessary taking time off from work for this, calling on various relatives and friends for informal support with the children during this time. Since it is often the case that older urban Greeks give their family house in exchange for flats in a new block (behaviour that began in the early 1960s) it is highly probable that Kyrios Georgos has his daughter living in the same block of flats. This would enable her to let him live in his own ground floor flat while under immediate and easy supervision. She and her husband would organise a rota but since both would be busy teaching for part of the day, they would probably employ a neighbour, if available, or temporary live in help. (again typically a foreign migrant worker). However if they lived up to one kilometre away from Kyrios Georgios they would probably take him into their own home following discharge, until his final level of independence was apparent. The 11 year old child would probably participate significantly in supervision of grandad, running errands, taking meals to him etc. The daughter and her husband would also be frequently checking up by telephone concerning his care and well being with each other, with him and any paid carer.
2. If Kyrios Giorgos was a member of the KAPI he might be visited by the medical personnel, social worker or other members. The doctor would provide some medical supervision and drug provision, the social worker would coordinate with volunteers and the home help, if available, although the latter would be unlikely since it would be known that he had a family to care.
3. As employees they would have the right to take unpaid leave of absence for the care of Kyrios Georgos.

Situation 3. Kyrios Georgos lives with spouse in a 2-storey house. Retired with savings. Spouse is fit and well. No children. Bedroom, bathroom and toilet are upstairs.

1. His younger and fit wife would care for him devotedly at home, waiting on him hand and foot and probably even delaying his recovery of independence. She would in any case have a domestic cleaner and arrange extra hours if this was felt to be necessary. In the unlikely event that the bedroom, bathroom and toilet were only upstairs she would nurse him upstairs until he was mobile enough to negotiate the stairs with help. She would have called on neighbours or other family members e.g. nephews and nieces, for help when he first returned home and these younger kin would usually be only too willing to help partly because they would be aware that they would be likely to inherit.
2. None are provided.
3. Nothing.

Case 3

Kyria Anna, aged 86, suffering from dementia. Frequent wandering by day and night. Frequent falls. Incontinent of urine and faeces.

Situation 1. Kyria Anna lives alone in an isolated farmhouse. Widowed. Little money. Daughter and son-in-law unemployed with four children, aged 9 months to 7 years, and live 5 kilometres away. Two other children of the older person live over 100 kilometres away.

1. Kyria Anna, if still living in a village house alone and in an advanced state of dementia with incontinence, appears to have been abandoned by her family, which may happen usually when the previous relationships had been bad. In this case the village neighbours or president might contact the daughter who lived 5 kilometres away to see if she could help. Under the circumstances there may be low expectations of a satisfactory solution and the situation might be left to resolve itself i.e. she would fall without anyone knowing and die. The villagers would keep an eye on her and even take her meals but would be unwilling to undertake personal care and responsibility.
2. In some cases the village officials or her children might arrange for her to be taken to a state or church home for the aged and infirm - basically an asylum.
3. None

Situation 2. Kyria Anna lives alone in a ground floor flat in town. Widowed. Daughter and son-in-law are both teachers in full-time employment, with 2 children aged 7 and 11, and live within 1 kilometre in the same town.

1. Her daughter would have tried initially to look after her in Kyria Anna's own flat but as the situation deteriorated she would have looked around for a private clinic or home willing to take her mother, despite her incontinence. Many private homes are inhabited by a number of people with dementia, but the additional problem of incontinence would make placement very difficult. An alternative solution might be to find someone to live in with her i.e. a paid carer. This might be a Greek woman - which is highly unlikely - or a foreign migrant worker, a solution which has grown over the past 5 years, solving the problem of residence for the illegal migrant and care for the old person. The daughter and son in law would retain constant supervision and look after her one day a week when the migrant worker had her day off. They would

have to pay her between 90,000 and 120,000 drachmas (300-400 ECU) per month with all found, but without insurance and no tax declaration.
2. To manage her wandering, the daughter might obtain sleeping tablets or tranquillisers from their own doctor in their Civil Servants' Insurance Fund or from Kyria Anna's insurance doctor, if he was amenable. To manage her incontinence they would use disposable incontinence pads, popularly known as BabyLino and advertised widely for older people. If she fell badly they would arrange for a doctor to come to see her and assess her at home, paying privately for the home visit. Who to call would be a problem since there are very few GPs and most doctors are reluctant to take responsibility for such cases. Thus if they used a neurologist to look after her dementia, he would not necessarily be called if she fell. No doctor has statutory responsibility for Kyria Anna's care.
3. If the fall involved a fracture they would call the Emergency Ambulance Service who would take her to hospital where she would be treated for the fracture and either admitted or sent home. If she arrived unaccompanied at the hospital and the social worker was unable to contact her daughter she would legally have to be admitted until further arrangements could be made.
4. If she lived in Athens, Patras or Thessaloniki her daughter may have contacted the Red Cross home support service to see if they could help with home help, although the personal care would be problematic i.e. it is not in their work contract. If she had been a member of a local KAPI then typically at this stage of dependency the best that they could offer would be suggestions about which homes would take her i.e. they would act as a channel for information.
5. If her daughter was aware of the existence of the newly formed association for carers of people with Alzheimer's disease, she might contact them for advice and information. She would receive their newsletter and obtain some moral support.

Situation 3. Kyria Anna lives with spouse in a 2-storey house. Retired with savings. Spouse is fit and well. No children. Bedroom, bathroom and toilet are upstairs.

1. Kyria Anna's husband would gradually have learned to take on the care of his dementing wife and to some extent the management of the household, probably with paid domestic help. They would pay to a greater or lesser extent for medical advice and personal interest in her case by a doctor, if possible working with their insurance company. They might pay for a specialist opinion and then obtain her drugs through the insurance (her husband would pay 25% of the real cost). For Kyria Anna's personal care and constant supervision he would probably eventually get live-in help as in Situation 2. Given that he has savings, when his wife reached the stage of no longer recognising him, he might eventually consider a good private nursing clinic where he would pay 300,000-400,000 drachmas per month. He would visit frequently to ensure that the standards of care were adequate.
2. None.
3. The Alzheimer's society is the only possibility for obtaining information and support - and this is in Athens and Thessaloniki. He might contact the help-at-home service and a volunteer from the Red Cross might occasionally come and sit with Kyria Anna at home when he had to leave the house.

In summary, no-one wants to be responsible for cases of dementia because the problems of care are so complicated, usually long term, and without many satisfactions.

Future Developments

Likely direction of change

With respect to services for older people which help and support family carers, the development by local authorities of home care services is still too recent to evaluate likely outcomes. If the LAs can establish a more stable economic basis for all these service departments then local pressure groups could lobby successfully for particular services. However if the present trends in social inequalities continue unchanged or even increase, then it is unlikely that the better off middle classes will press for LA services, as they will probably prefer to buy in their own services i.e. pay for cheaper private solutions to care. One point made by a carer who was paying for care services was their lack of supervision or recognized standards so that there was no guarantee of reliability or quality. The multiplicity of different training programmes for home helps, family aids and social helpers (mainly for unemployed women), implemented over the past few years, have produced no notable improvements in this direction, probably due to their lack of clear objectives and co-ordination. Both national and European funding obtained for such programmes could be better used if formal evaluation of outcomes was incorporated into the original proposal and the results used for policy planning. However since the Ministry has not been able to develop any kind of effective standards of care for residential homes, which are legally under its remit, the probability of them developing training standards and ensuring the quality of home care services is limited. However still another fundamental difficulty lies in the preference of Greek women for other kinds of work.

Increasing incomes will, over time, see more of the middle classes paying for the newly developing private insurance programmes which will cover the costs of home care and even residential care. Again this will not help those who are unable to or are unaware of the need to protect against such eventualities. The provision of other services to aid family carers by the state either on a more extended basis or as new services is highly unlikely e.g. rehabilitation centres, hospices, holiday facilities.

Main challenges

Within two years the main challenge for many local authorities will be how they can continue to *finance* their newly developed home care services as well as their established Open Care Centres. The initial funding from the European Union is allowing these services to start, without deliberation being given to their longer term financing and to fair systems of payment. It is true that those most in need of support i.e. the poor and isolated, will be primary recipients of care but if LAs devised fair systems of payment and subsidy for services, they could also extend home care services to other dependent older people who currently are reliant on family carers.

The *management* of these home care services will be a particular problem given the poor management skills generally in the public sector, the lack of professionalism in many public care services, the low expectations of both clients and those working in the service, and to some extent the negative attitudes to the care of the elderly who do not belong to one's own family, which exist especially amongst less educated women typically employed for some of the work of home help.

The reliance on foreign labour by so many family carers with adequate incomes is likely to continue well into the next century. The continuing inequalities in the world will provide an ever ready supply of women willing to undertake care work in return for an income which is "good" by their home standards, which allows them to save and send home remittances. Despite moves to tighten up immigration into the country, illegal and legal migrant women will continue to arrive for as long as job and life opportunities are so much worse in their own country. Social and political pressure on successive Greek governments will ensure that the supply will continue. This in turn will mean that family carers will continue to use private solutions, if they can pay. If they cannot pay, they bear the cost of their own and the older person's poverty through their own exclusive contribution to care work. The challenge here is to find effective methods of supporting those most in need who cannot resolve their difficulties through private market solutions.

[I] This included Law 1483/1984 with an amendment in 1988 to cover the public sector, which in Article 7 provides that working people caring for a family member who is chronically sick, disabled, old or dependent has the right to 6 working days leave per calendar year without pay, with an addition of up to 10 working days where care is for more than 2 dependent persons. Dependants may include spouses, parents, unmarried brothers or sisters; in the case of parents or siblings this entitlement occurs when the latter have a lower income than the average annual unskilled wage - which would cover the situation of most Greek pensioners. This entitlement is part of the normal work contract and entitles the employee to full employment rights such as holiday leave, pension contribution entitlement and compensation payments. An employer cannot break the work contract with an employee who takes such leave, and additionally these entitlements are the minimal legal ones and if better conditions have been negotiated between an employer and employee then these hold.. However few employers appear to be aware of this legislation while employees needing time off for caring tend to use their paid holiday leave first.

[II] 62% of social insurance funds were paid out in pensions

[III] There are over 200 insurance funds, the majority covering specific occupations. Some of them have been heavily subsidised by the state and have considerable resources; others are virtually bankrupt as a result of changes in employment and the large numbers of pensioners. Currently there are attempts to slim down the numbers of pension funds but those in the more privileged funds are very unwilling to lose their privileges.

[IV] The exact number is unknown since many small residential homes are unregistered.

[V] Amira [15] in a small sample of better off Athenians found that amongst the frail, demented and disabled aged 75+ , approximately 17% of the men and 29% of the women ended up in some kind of residential home, clinic or nursing home.

[VI] University hospitals exist in Ioannina, Alexandroupolis, Hrakleion, Patras.

[VII] This contrasts to the situation in Northern Europe where single parent families and unemployment are strongly linked to poverty.

[VIII] In a study in 1991 (Triantafillou, Mestheneos) of the 15 subjects over 75 years of age with high rates of disability being cared for, only 3 or 4 were in receipt of a disability allowance.

[IX] Those joining the labour force since 1993 do not have such an entitlement and pensionable age is now fixed for men and women in the younger age groups as 65 years of age.

[X] This is without insurance and involves a 12-24 hour day coverage 6 day per week in the case of migrant women paid carers.

[XI] The cost of private often semi-trained nursing aides is 140,000 for a 7 - 8 hour day, 5 days a week, extra for holidays and an additional sum for insurance contributions. This amount almost exceeds average earnings and does not makes such a service a viable choice for most people.

[XII] Evans-Pritchard (1953) following M.Maus pointed out that "gifts are the chains along which social relations run"; a plethora of gifts (in services and kind) indicates a stronger social relationship.

[XIII] This can be badly abused in some cases where unscrupulous people have set up exploitatory circles

[XIV] Women have long worked as unpaid family members assisting in agriculture and other forms of self employment and this allowed them considerable flexibility in caring for older parents.

[XV] The Council of Europe (1992) in a report on cases of abandonment of elderly persons over a 4 month period in an Athens general hospital, said that of the 225 cases 35,5% had family who would not look after the patient while 24,4% the family couldn't look after them because of hardship.

[XVI] In the majority of cases the total care provided is excellent.

References

[1]   KEPE (Centre of Planning and Economic research), Social Welfare Report for the 1988-92 Athens, (in Greek) 1989.

[2]   J. Triantafillou and E. Mestheneos, 'Pathways to Care for the Elderly in Greece'. *Social Science and Medicine* **38(7)** (1994) 875-882.

[3]   J. Kavounidi, 'Older people and informal help networks: the circulation of goods and services amongst the generations.' In: Old Age and Society : The proceedings of the Panhellenic Conference of EKKE. EKKE, Athens. (in Greek) 1996.

[4]   E. Mestheneos and J. Triantafillou, 'The support of Family Carers of the Older Elderly in Greece'. In J. Twigg (ed.), Family Care of the Elderly in Europe. University of York, 1993.

[5]   J. Triantafillou *et al* 'Health Related Quality of Life in Rural Elderly Greeks'. In: L. Ferrucci *et al*, (eds.), *Pendulum: Health Related Quality of Life of Older Europeans* 1996, WHO, Florence, 1996.

[6]   I. Yfantopoulos, *Health Planning in Greece: Some Economic and Social Aspects."* National Centre for Social Research, Athens, (in Greek), 1981.

[7]   J. Triantafillou and E. Mestheneos, '"Professionalizing" the work of family carers of dependent older people'.In: *Health and Social care in the Community*. Pp..257-260. Blackwell. Oxford, 1994.

[8]   I. Emke-Poulopoulou, *Demography* , Ellin, Athens. (in Greek) 1994.

[9]   P. Tsakloglou and G. Panopoulou, 'Who are the Poor in Greece? Analysing poverty under alternative concepts of resources and equivalence scales.' *Journal of European Social Policy* **8(3)** 1998 213-236.

[10] P. Tinios and S. Zografakis 'Family and the Economic Position of Older people in Greece'. In: I. Kyriopoulos *et al*, (eds.), *Health and Social Protection in the Third*. Centre for Social Science and Health, Athens. (in Greek), 1993.

[11] H. Kataki, The Three Identities of the Greek Family. Athens, Kedros (in Greek) 1984.

[12] Dritsios *et al*, Unpublished research report on violence towards the elderly in Greek families, 4th Panhellenic Gerontological and Geriatric Conference, December 1995.

[13] K.D. Spinelli and E. Pitsiou, 'The Elderly : Victims of Violence and Neglect'. *Eklogi,* 1991 No. 89.

[14] A. Petroglou, 'Âge Discrimination at Work'. Greek Report for EuroLinkAge, London, U.K., 1993.

[15] A. Amira, 'Family Care in Greece'. In A.Jamieson and R.Illsley (eds.), Contrasting European Policies for the Care of Older People. Aldershot, Avebury, U.K. 1990.

Chapter 5

Italy

Giovanni Lamura
Istituto Nazionale di Riposo e Cura Anziani
Dipartimento Ricerche GerontologicheVia S. Margherita, 5
60124 Ancona
Italy

Maria Gabriella Melchiorre
Istituto Nazionale di Riposo e Cura Anziani
Dipartimento Ricerche GerontologicheVia S. Margherita, 5
60124 Ancona
Italy

Sabrina Quattrini
Istituto Nazionale di Riposo e Cura Anziani
Dipartimento Ricerche GerontologicheVia S. Margherita, 5
60124 Ancona
Italy

Massimo Mengani
Istituto Nazionale di Riposo e Cura Anziani
Dipartimento Ricerche GerontologicheVia S. Margherita, 5
60124 Ancona
Italy

Alberto Albertini
Accademia Italiana Medici di Famiglia
Via Circo 18
20123 Milan
Italy

Introduction

Ageing, disability and demand for care in Italy

Italy is going through an impressive process of demographic ageing, owing to which in 1996 the number of 60 year old residents in the country was among the highest in the world [1], estimated as high as 22,6% of the total population [2], which may reach the ratio of one elderly person out of four of the population by 2004 (see figure 1). This ageing process has been extremely fast, since in 1951 the number of people over 60 was just half the present number [3]. This trend is even more marked if we think that the over 65 population[1] has more than doubled from 8.2% in 1960 to 16.8% in 1996, which means that the number of Italian families with at least one elderly member has reached today 38.2% of the total [4].

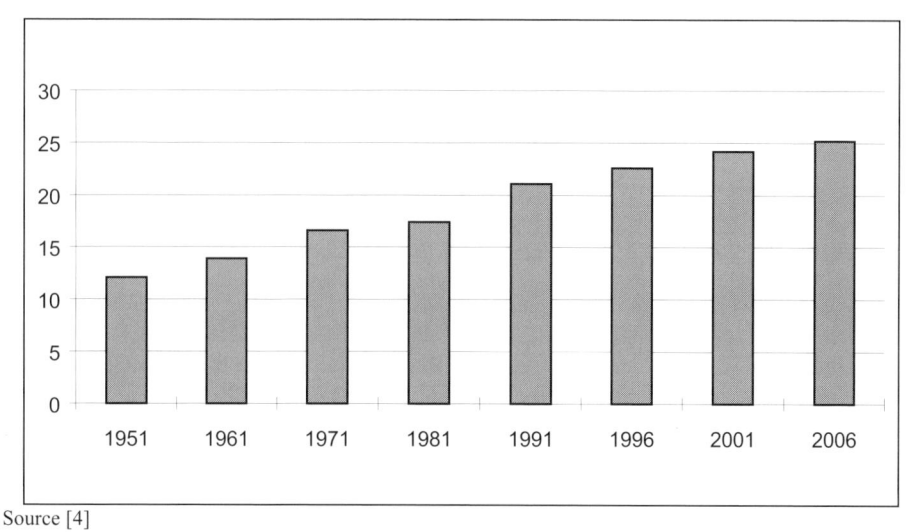

Source [4]
Figure 1: Over 60 Year Old Population in Italy

However, being an elderly person does not necessarily mean needing to be cared for. In order to analyze the demand for social and health care for elderly people, we must consider only the part of the elderly population which shows a sufficeintly high loss of self-sufficiency to warrant intervention by another person or persons to satisfy their own vital needs. For this purpose, the Italian National Statistical Institute (ISTAT) has used the Activities of Daily Living (ADL) indices to calculate that in Italy in 1994 more than one elderly person in five (20.9%, equal to 1,875,000 people) was disabled in at least one ADL, 4.5% (409,000 people) were confined to their home and 2.0% (176,000 people) were bedridden. These data refer only to those living at home and are therefore an underestimate, as they exclude people admitted to nursing homes or hospitals, where the quota of disabled persons is higher [5,6]. An attempt to take this institutionalised population into account is therefore illustrated in Table 1. On the basis of current prevalence coefficients, the number of disabled elderly - which reaches today over two million people if we consider the mildest disability form, but drops to below 200.000 if we consider only the bedridden elderly - is expected to increase by nearly 50% in the next 25 years, when disability will affect nearly three million people in at least one ADL and make about 270,000 of them nearly totally non self-sufficient. For the organization of social and health care services it is also relevant to note that one disabled elderly out of three lives alone - in 1990 (the last year of available data) about 511,000 persons, or 31.1% of the over 65 year old disabled residing at home.

Table 1: Disability degree of the elderly population in Italy, projections 1994-2024

Years	Over 65 year old population	Disabled in one ADL (22%)*	Disabled in three ADL (9.8%)*	Completely disabled (2%)*
1994	9.203.500	2.024.770	901.943	184.070
1999	10.127.600	2.228.072	992.505	202.552
2004	10.994.000	2.418.680	1.077.412	219.880
2009	11.767.500	2.558.850	1.153.215	235.350
2014	12.551.100	2.761.242	1.230.008	251.022
2019	13.107.500	2.883.650	1.284.535	262.150
2024	13.570.100	2.985.422	1.329.870	271.402

*: these coefficients indicate that 22% of all elderly subjects are unable to carry out one ADL, 9.8% are unable to carry out three ADLs and 2% all ADLs. [7]

Overview of health and social care policy for the elderly

Bearing in mind this general situation, and in particular the fact that the rapidity of the process makes the reorganization of the intervention in favour of this group of population more difficult and at the same time more urgent than in most other European countries, it is important, first of all, to point out that in Italy the law divides care of the elderly into two sectors: health care and social care.

Historically and until the early 70s, it was the Central Government which tried to satisfy and respond to the needs of this sector of the population, through the provincial branch offices of the Ministry of the Interior as well as through numerous public "assistance and charity" institutions working at a local or national level [8]. During the 70's there was an attempt to rationalize and decentralize the so called "territorial institutions" - i.e. the 20 Italian Regions and the over 8,000 Communes - the social and health functions, through the abolition of many public institutions which became redundant, and the concentration of all the functions concerning social care in the Communes under the control of the Regions (Decree of the President of the Republic - or DPR - n. 616 of 1977). At the same time those concerning the health sector were concentrated in the Local Health Units (Aziende Sanitarie Locali: ASL) which constitute the Italian National Health System (Sistema Sanitario Nazionale: SSN) (law n.833 of 1978).

This operation was successful only for the health function, since it joined tasks and functions previously fragmented among different Ministries and institutions under the care of the Health Ministry. Social care, on the contrary - despite any attempt at parliamentary level [9] - never succeeded in being organized in a general reform Bill, though this had been planned in the same DPR n. 616 of 1978 [10]. This fact has impeded the process of transference of all the functions to the territorial institutions and has virtually blocked a great part of the regional legislative activity in this field, thus contributing to a continued high degree of uncertainty about the tasks and modalities of intervention in the field of social care [11].

The main consequence of this state of affairs which has characterized the Italian Welfare State since the end of the 70s is a lack of integration between health and social care services. This integration, which was clearly stated in the normative, has never found recognition in the national laws promulgated after the creation of the two sectors, leaving the Region with the burden of adopting provisions on this matter. This has resulted in great territorial variability, since a unitary and integrated management of health and social services can be found mainly in a limited number of regions in Northern and Central Italy - e.g. Emilia Romagna [12], and Liguria [13] - and much less frequently in the South [14], where there is a degree of uncertainty about the financing of the interventions, and about the distinction between expenses in the health care and social care sectors. In fact, while the SSN is responsible for health costs, responsibility for social care services rests with the Commune: a situation which often results in an attempt by both institutions to shift reciprocally the responsibilities for management of the single interventions, with negative effects on the cared for and their families, not only from a financial point of view, but also in terms of practitioners' attitude, timeliness and quality of care in [15].

While the social care sector has been facing a sort of standstill situation, the health care sector has, in the last few years, been going through a more dynamic phase, at least on a theoretical level. As a matter of fact, towards the end of the 80s the idea began to take ground of establishing so-called *Residenze Sanitarie Assistenziali* (Health Care Residences, or HCRs), "mixed" structures providing medical and social care together, in order to support the growing number of non self-sufficient elderly who could not be cared for at home for "proven lack of suitable family support allowing necessary continuous medical treatment and care to be supplied at home". This proposal, formally included in the financial law of 1988, established that - at an overall cost of about 30,000 billion lire (about 20 billion U.S. dollars of that time) over a period of ten years - 140,000 beds would have to be supplied in new structures or reconverted ones, covering a demand equal to 2% of the over 65 year old population [16]. Today - at the expected deadline for the ten year plan - it can be seen though that, of the 2,8 billion lire allocated for these measures in the first three years, only 26% has been authorised so far, corresponding to only 180 HCRs and 11,000 beds, equal to 8% of those planned [17].

This result is even more disappointing considering that another legislative push for the establishment of HCRs was given by the "the Health Protection Plan for the Elderly" passed by the Italian Parliament in 1992 [16]. This Plan specified how to organize and manage the HCRs, proposing furthermore some innovative systems of primary elderly care, preferable to institutionalisation, such as "Integrated Home Care" [18] - which includes social, psychological, nursing and rehabilitation support - and the "Home Hospitalisation" [19] - consisting of nursing care, medical visits and specialised advice - both to be provided at the home of the cared-for person [16]. At the same time, in the last few years a campaign has been started, within a global reorganisation of the Italian SSN - mainly operated through legislative decrees n. 512 of 1992 and n. 517 of 1993, as well as the National Plan 1994-1996 - to improve care quality and promote a "service culture" meant to offer health care which is both more efficient and more respectful of the users, by increasing the importance attributed to the Regions and the ASLs and by reorganising their functions.

It has to be admitted that, more than five years after the Plan was adopted, the results attained are well below those expected. In fact, the anticipated unification of care levels and of health provision has been realised only partially, since not all Regions have implemented the home services provided for by law, and only some of them have adopted a three year plan specifically for the elderly [13]. As a result, Integrated Home Care is today carried out in only a few hundred of the over 8,000 Italian [17] - mainly highly urbanised ones [20], reaching less than 0.3% of the over 65 year old population [13] - and Home Hospitalisation is practised in very few small experimental units [21,22], thus being absolutely insufficient to cover the existing care demand [23]. All this, despite the fact that recent studies have pointed out the positive impact of home help for non self-sufficient elderly patients on the health of their care-givers. These data show in fact that the caregiver's stress level tends to substantially decrease when the cared for person takes advantage of a home hospitalisation service, especially if compared to those who have an institutionalised relative, among whom an increase in stress level is [24].

Legal situation concerning responsibilities for the care of elderly people

From a juridical point of view, in Italy a non self-sufficient elderly person still has the legal right to choose whether to ask for external help, whatever his/her age [25]. When this capacity disappears partially or totally - and the assessment of this condition is far from easy - the responsibility to assist a person who has become "disabled" is given by the "probate judge" to a guardian (who may also be a relative), who has the task of representing the cared-for person in the decision-making concerning acts of ordinary and extraordinary administration [26]. In reality, in the current praxis - somehow contravening the strict and old laws in force, which are actually more aimed at the defence of the possessions of the tutelated person rather than of the person himself - many people who have been declared "incapable" are still left a small margin of freedom to carry out some functions (such as, for example, the administration of a monthly or weekly amount of money or consultation about decisions concerning the sale of goods or the choice of where to live). Even this limited amount of freedom of action plays a positive role in terms of the psycho-physical health of the elderly person. A frequent alternative to this consists of appointing a "temporary public guardian", who has the role of providing administrative and managerial support to the non self-sufficient person who is no longer able to carry out some tasks either by himself or through other people but who, according to the law, is not incapable of acting.

Another measure which has been adopted in Italy in the last few years - but which appears to be detrimental to the rights of the elderly (in fact most of the people involved are elderly people) - is the praxis adopted by the Communes which require a contribution towards the quota, often substantial, which is not covered by the elderly person's resources. A clear example is given by the fees which have to be paid in Italian nursing Homes for non self-sufficient elderly people. These fees usually vary from a minimum of three to a maximum of five million lire or more every month (depending on the residential area and the person's self-sufficiency degree), while the average amount of a retirement pension for people who retired in 1996 is between 1,2 and 2,7 million lire a month [27]. Even considering a possible companion payment - which amounts to 783,000 lire a month (see next paragraph) - it is easy to realize that not many Italians are in a position to pay for their admittance to a Nursing Home themselves. Thus, the current laws (art. 38 of the Italian Constitution and the above mentioned DPR n. 616 of 1977) oblige the Communes to supplement the fees with public means. In an attempt - certainly illegal but unfortunately rather common - to recover at least a part of the money spent in this way, many Communes ask the relatives of the non self-sufficient elderly person to sign an "agreement", by which they undertake to cover personally the costs of the fee which cannot be covered by the cared-for person and which should otherwise be borne by the Commune. However, the only person entitled to ask for the so-called "maintenance fee" from his/her relatives - in the following order: spouse, children, parents, sons and daughters-in-law, father and mother-in-law, brother and sister, (art. 433 and 538 of the

Italian Civil Code) - is exclusively the elderly person him-/herself, who, if he/she doesn't want to, is not obliged to do so [15,28]. Some Communes prefer therefore to transfer the possessions and estate of the cared-for elderly to themselves, always with the purpose of reimbursing the Commune for the expenses borne to supplement the fee of the institution where the elderly person has been admitted [29].

Health and Social care for Elderly People: Structures and Functions

As has already been said, in Italy a distinction is made between health services and social services. Assistance to the elderly is carried out on the one hand through State measures - mainly consisting of State allowances and general legislative schemes - and on the other hand through the activity of local Authorities (Regions and Communes) and of the SSN branch offices: the ASLs. While the territorial organization and the planning of health services and social services rest on the Regions, the Communes and the ASLs guarantee their actual implementation, by fixing modalities, times, costs, and management. In particular services to the elderly can be divided, according to their contents, into three different categories:
- health care services only;
- socio-health services;
- social services only.

Health care services - usually guaranteed by the ASL or certified health centres - as well as socio-health services are funded by SSN and are therefore generally free of charge for the people whose pathology and whose income fall within the limits stated by law. The ASL is, however, responsible for both kinds of service. As far as social and financial services are concerned, it is the Commune which is responsible, through its own municipal budget, possibly with a contribution from the beneficiaries. Municipal services do not usually undergo qualitative and quantitative audits, so they vary greatly depending on the tradition and the sensitivity of each single municipal administration.

As the following paragraphs will show, some of the interventions in the field of elderly care reveal the existence of overlaps between different institutions, to which it has been tried to find a remedy through the setting-up of so-called Geriatric Assessment Units (Unità di Valutazione Geriatrica: UVG). These are interdisciplinary teams made up of health and social personnel together, supposed to guarantee the coordination among the different services, in order to provide an adequate response to the multidimensional needs of the elderly. However, the elderly and his/her family often still find themselves alone in the search for proper care solutions, because in Italy monetary transfers are the most common form of help provided by public institutions - instead of direct services - so that the beneficiaries enjoy not only the freedom but also the burden of deciding how to use the amount received in the form of allowances.

Health care sector

In Italy health services are mainly offered through three "poles", ideally separated but operatively integrated: the General Practitioner, the ASL District and the Hospital.

The three main poles of the Italian SSN: the MMG, the ASL district and the hospital

The General Practitioner (MMG) is the professional institutionally responsible for supplying free, continuous primary care (except from 10 a.m Saturday. to 8 a.m Monday, when the Emergency Care Units are on duty) - in his/her surgery, at home or by phone - to any Italian patient of any age. Specialist Treatment and laboratory services are supplied by ASL - which operates through the ambulatorial structures of ASL Districts - and by the Hospital where patients should go for admittance and for ambulatorial out-patient services.

The SSN normative scheme is centered around the MMG as sole referent - and therefore sole responsible - for the patient, both for primary care and the activation of specialist treatment and laboratory services [30]. In particular, it is the MMG's task to supply elderly people with so-called Scheduled Home Care (Assistenza Programmata Domiciliare: ADP) (see next paragraph), as well as care when they are residents in nursing Homes, in cooperation with the ambulatorial services of Hospitals and the ASL District. The latter, in fact, according to the law, is responsible to the MMG who, if he agrees with its opinion, prescribes the treatment they suggest. Hospital Admittance, on the contrary, is to be considered separately, because of the wide legislative and operative freedom: in fact - even if, theorically, Admittance should be activated by the MMG - the Hospital can independently open access to its facilities through the Emergency Care Unit.

Normally an Italian MMG can treat 1,500 patients - the maximum number allowed by law - with an average of about 12,000 ambulatorial visits a year, most of which concern over 65 year old patients. The MMG becomes therefore the natural confident of the problems of the elderly patient and of the ways used to deal with them. While the MMG's intervention is liable to be controlled and is controlled by the ASL, the MMG doesn't have any legal and institutional instruments to allow him to evaluate the quality and efficiency of interventions offered by other socio-sanitary operators (specialist consultants, social workers, paramedical staff, clerks of the Health structures etc.) nor can he take measures against them since they respond to the Managers of the Districts and the Hospitals.

Finally, it should be pointed out that in Italy the location of Hospitals and Districts is quite inconsistent, not only as far as their number and size is concerned, but also from the point of view of the efficiency the quality of the services offered. This situation has always produced an overlapping of roles and a conflictual atmosphere - with a consequent lack of coordination between hospital and territorial practitioners [30] - which is in contrast with the optimization of health care promoted by the World Health Organisation, and which does not always provide a suitable response to the care needs of different local cases.

The main forms of health care for the elderly

In Italy health care for elderly people is mainly offered in the following forms:

- in the district:
  a) care in the MMG's surgery;
  b) Home Care Services upon request;
  c) Scheduled Home Care Services;
  d) Integrated Home Help Services;
- in institutions:
  e) Assistance in Nursing Homes;
  f) Assistance in Hospitals;
- mixed:
  g) Home hospitalization.

a) Care in the MMG's surgery: the self sufficient older person who needs medical care goes to the MMG, who examines him and gives him medical prescriptions, if required. If the older person is not able to go to the MMG and only needs a "bureaucratic" prescription, it is often a relative who goes in his place.

b) Home Health Care upon request: if the older person is affected by an acute condition which does not allow him to go to the MMG, he can ask for a home visit. If the request is received before 10 a.m., the visit will take place on the same day; if not, the visit will take place by 12 o'clock of the following day.

c) Scheduled Home Care (Assistenza Domiciliare Programmata: ADP): The DPR n. 484 of 1996 defines as "scheduled" any home assistance offered to those patients who cannot go to the MMG but who are not suffering from acute conditions. It is meant for those patients who, though needing frequent monitoring, cannot go to the MMG by standard means owing to health problems or for socio-environmental reasons. ADP aims to check the health conditions of a particular group of patients at regular intervals. The MMG plans the visits on a weekly or monthly basis. The motivated request for the intervention must define the diagnosis and the care programme and must be sent to the Doctor in charge of the Health District who must give an answer within 15 days. The sphere of the MMG's intervention within the ADP concerns: an inspection of hygienic and living conditions; suggestions to the carers (nurses, family members, volunteers) with particular reference to feeding and to cooperation with the Social Services personnel; the planning, implementation and verification of the care and rehabilitation programmes; the updating of the clinical records. The ADP is a relatively new intervention procedure but it is widely used in the field of general medicine.

d) Integrated Home Help Services (Assistenza Domiciliare Integrata: ADI) (DPR n. 484 of 1996. The ADI provides, at the patient's home, the necessary interventions of general and specialist health care, of nursing, of rehabilitation care, of social care with a view to creating a valid alternative to institutionalisation for mainly social reasons or to enable completion of an intensive therapeutical programme already started elsewhere, for example in a Hospital. The service activation is authorized, subject o the approval of the Geriatric Assessment Unit (UVG, see below) by the Doctor who is in charge of the District within 48 hours of receipt of a special request form. The health care interventions are agreed with the MMG who is the sole responsible for the patient, who updates the clinical records at the patient's home, coordinates the operators and activates the eventual specialist advice. The District must guarantee 365 days a year of ADI service, 24 hours a day; nurses on call 24 hours a day; the supply of health care equipment; contact with the Care Community; specialist advice, especially for physiotherapy treatment, pain therapy, chronic oxygen therapy and nutritional assistance; adequate information. This type of assistance is avaliable for terminally ill patients, patients with acute disease, temporarily disabled patients or patients discharged early from hospital. As a matter of fact ADI, unlike ADP, is meant for non self-sufficient patients who need a more continuous and multidisciplinary care: the frequency of the MMG's visits is therefore agreed upon without any limits and according to the needs of the patient. The fee for each visit of the MMG is 35,000 lire and includes only treatment from the standard list: the cost of other treatment is calculated separately. A social worker works with the MMG who, according to art. 9 of law 404 of 1992, can activate the social services of the Commune to supply: social and financial assistance; meals and help with feeding; laundry service, shopping and administrative services. Family members, publicly employed hospice workers, volunteers and specially trained consciencious objectors provide these services.

The UVG is a multidisciplinary specialist commission whose task is a multidimensional assessment of the elderly patient to establish a plan for individual assistance to be implemented within the network of territorial health and social care services and rehabilitation services, to guarantee continuity of care between the hospital and the district, to decide admission and dischasrge to/from nursing homes and the services of the district. The UVG are usually made up of a MMG, a geriatrics specialist, a doctor from the Health District, a professional nurse, a social worker and, according to need, other specialized doctors, physiotherapists, speech therapists, entertainers etc. The UVG evaluates the patient's psycho-physical condition, his residual functional capacities, his social and financial state, and then devises a working plan.

e) Assistance in nursing Homes (artt. 69-70 of DPR n. 484 of 1996): assistance to patients in nursing Homes is regulated by regional agreements, while the payment of the fees for the poor is borne by the Commune of residence (sentence of the Tribunale Amministrativo Regionale of Brescia n. 787 of 26/06/92). Nursing Homes for elderly people can be divided into two main categories on the basis of different levels of assistance acknowledged by the Regions:
   – Homes for non self-sufficient elderly patients (Residenze sanitarie Assistenziali: RSA);
   – Homes for self-sufficient or partially non self-sufficient elderly patients (Community Homes, Hotel Houses, Polifunctional Collective Homes).

RSAs, as it has already been said in paragraph 1.2, were set up by law in 1988 with the purpose of offering accommodation to non self-sufficient elderly people and supplying health care, rehabilitation, socialization and entertainment. On the basis of Regional laws - such as L. R. n. 13 of 1995 of Friuli Venezia Giulia - they also accept patients discharged early from hospital and who need rehabilitation treatment for up to 3 months. RSAs generally contemplate the presence of a Doctor on site, while in the Homes for self-sufficient patients health care is offered ad personam by the MMG. As a matter of fact, though, the minimal requirements for consideration as an RSA remain a problem, since many traditional nursing homes still do not have such pre-requisites [16,31].

f) Health assistance in Hospitals: assistance offered to elderly patients in Hospital does not differ, from a juridical point of view, from the assistance offered to other patients and which is guaranteed by the Italian Constitution (art. 32) and provided according to the MMG or through the Emergency Care Unit.

The difficulty experienced by hospitals in taking care of the increasing number of non self-sufficient elderly patients affected by a chronic illness [32] - a phenomenon which, as already seen, was one of the reasons for the setting up of RSAs, even if so far only partly implemented - causes frequent conflicts with the relatives of the elderly patients who do not always find a satisfactory solution [33], despite the law and the jurisprudential orientation which clearly go in their favour [22,34,35].

g) Home Hospitalisation (Ospedalizzazione Domiciliare: O.D.): According to its definition in the "Health Protection Plan for the Elderly" adopted in 1992, OD means "the activation of the main diagnostic and therapeutical interventions at the patient's home which are normally carried out in a hospital, eventually integrated, for particular assistance, with a short stay in hospital through facilitated admittance and transport".

The Service, envisaged and encouraged by the law, is seen as "an integrating function of each Geriatric Operative Unit" and can be activated only when relatives live in the same home as the patient. Its main health care aspect can be integrated with social care. The team and the hospital equipment intervene upon request at the patient's home to support the MMG. They also facilitate protected hospital discharge [19]. It must be remembered that the practical activation of this type of programme has only taken place in a few large cities (in Turin since 1985, in Genoa since 1992 and in Milan since 1993) [13].

Social care sector

As far as the social care sector is concerned, we will distinguish for analytical purposes between formal and informal supply of care. The former - discussed in the chapter - concerns monetary transfer by the State to supplement the income of the cared-for person as well as the supply of services provided at a local level, in ad hoc structures or at the elderly person's home, by publicly or privately paid personnel. Informal care - which will be discussed in chapter 3 - concerns the interventions provided by the elderly person's informal network of support, made up of family members, neighbours and volunteers.

Monetary transfers by the state

Depending on the type and degree of disability which has been assessed by the Medical Commission of the local ASL, the non self-sufficient person in Italy is entitled to receive, thanks to a special fund provided by the Ministry of Interior, the economic support listed in table 2. It shows that people who are *partially disabled* (i.e. with a reduction of their working capability of more than "¾" of the total) and have a yearly income lower than 6.2 million lire can apply for an allowance of about 5 million lire a year. The income requirement is much less rigid - as it increases to little less than 23 million lire a year - for people who are *partially blind or deaf and dumb*, who, in addition to their income, can apply for a further allowance which for the blind amounts to 1.1 million lire and to 3.7 million lire for deaf and dumb people. The latter amount can also be received by people affected by a mild form of blindness (between 1/10 and 1/20) but only if they are unemployed and have a yearly income of less than 9.5 million lire.

Table 2: Allowances granted by the Italian State to disabled persons, according to kind/degree of disability, income level and age

Health prerequisite	Maximum yearly individual income (x 1000 lire)	Other prerequisites	Yearly amount of the allowance (in thousands of lire)	Denomination of the allowance
1. disability (difficulty in performing the tasks and functions of one's age) or deafness (loss of hearing higher than 60 decibels)	6.240	- 0-17 years old - attending schools, courses or undergoing treatments - not being a patient in a hospital - not receiving any special (cfr. n. 4) or communication (cfr. n. 5) allowance	5.000	attendance allowance
2. partial disability (higher than 74%)*	6.240	18 - 64 years old	5.000	payment
3. partial blindness (sight between 1/20 and 1/10)	9.500	unemployed	3.700	payment
4. partial blindness (sight worse than 1/20)	• not means tested • 22.800	- -	1.100 5.000	special allowance pension
5. deafness and dumbness*	• not means tested • 22.800	- • 18 - 64 years old	3.700** 5.400	communication payment pension
6. disability or total blindness (100%)*	• 22.800 • not means tested	• 18 - 64years old (or older than 18)' • not being a patient in a hospital free of charge	5.000 (o 5.400)' 9.400 (o 12.300)'**	pension companion payment

*: when they are 65, disabled people affected by this kind of disability receive the so called "assegno sociale" (social allowance, about 6,6 million lire) which is supplied by the Italian National Pension Scheme (INPS) and no longer by the Ministry of Interiors.
**: the same person can receive both allowances
': in case of blindness

Sources: - [36-40]

In case of *total blindness or total disability*, the amount of the allowance remains the same, but it is granted only if the income is lower than 22.8 million lire. Besides - which is the most relevant economic datum - these people can also apply for the so called "companion payment", which is not income-tested and amounts to 9 million lire a year (12.3 million lire in case of total blindness), provided the disabled person does not enjoy free institutionalization.

In short, the amount of State benefits envisaged in case of disability can vary from a minimum of 1,000,000 lire a year in the case of a partially blind person with a yearly income higher than £ 22.8 million lire, to £ 17.7 million lire in the case of a totally blind person unable to walk without the permanent help of a companion with an income less than 22.8 million lire, who can thus be beneficiary of both the "companion payment" (12.3 million lire a year) and of the disability pension (5.4 million lire). In order to gain an idea of the purchasing power of these amounts it should be remembered that, in 1995, the average yearly expense of one elderly person living alone was about 17.6 million lire [37] which leads to the conclusion that only the allowance envisaged for total blindness (pension plus companion payment) could ensure - excluding other forms of income - a consumption level equal to the average.

Table 3 illustrates how susbtantial the increase in the number of these allowances has been over the years, especially that of disability allowances and, within them, of those granted to the over 65 year old elderly, whose number has more than tripled between 1984 and 1995, reaching 6.7% of the corresponding age group. It must be underlined that - due partly to the phenomenon of local favouritisms, which has actually transformed these allowances into a hidden form of income integration allocated irrespective of the existence or not of any disability in the individual [41] - the distribution of such allowances throughout the country is very irregular. In some Central and Southern regions (Umbria, Abruzzo and Sardinia), for example, in 1994 the percentage of civil disabled people (32-34%) was almost double than in Piedmont, Lombardy and Veneto (16-17%), in the North of the country [37].

Table 3: Number of allowances according to type of disability, 1984-1997
(thousands, last column in percentage values)

Year	"Deaf-mute"	"Blind"	"Disabled" Total	of which over-65 years old with an accompanying allowance Absolute number	% on total over-65 population
1984	16,0	107,5	249,5	198,8	2.7
1987	14,7	110,6	773,0	214,3	3.0
1991	37,3	115,8	1.092,0	428,3	5.0
1995	40,0	120,2	1.264,3	610,1	6.7
1996	40,4	119,5	1.263,5	609,9	6.2
1997	40,4	117,2	1.229,0	590,0	5.9*

*: our estimate
Source: [38-40]

Recently, however, there has been an increase in the controls aimed at limiting such misuse of funds, with the result that, from a sample of 150,000 disability pensions controlled between 1997 and 1998 some 34,500 (23%!) have been revoked owing to the lack of the necessary prerequisites [42]. As a consequence, there has been a turnabout not only for disability pensions but also for companion payments to people over 65, the number of which has shown a substantial decrease in number.

In the last few years, apart from State allowances, local forms of contribution have been provided by several regional and municipal administrations in Central Italy (e.g. Trentino-Alto-Adige, Emilia-Romagna and Tuscany), which are distributed to families who care for non self sufficient elderly in their own home [43,44]. These contributions - which usually add up to no more than 600,000 lire per month - are mostly meant to be used to cover expenses for home help and, unlike the state accompanying allowance, are means-tested. In some cases - as in Tuscany - it is also possible to use this regional economic support to cover the care provided by persons (such as friends or neighbours) who do not belong to the family of the cared-for person.

The municipal social services

Due to the above mentioned division of the social care functions (see paragraph 1.2), it is the Communes, through their social services - even if coordinated by the Provinces and guided by the guidelines of the Regions - which have the task of assessing the care needs of the elderly and their families, and of deciding which steps should be taken in favour of the cared for elderly people. This statement is generally true, but it should be remembered that, owing to the partial enactment of the law concerning a social assistance national scheme, in Italy there exists a significantly high level of variability from region to region both in the level of expenditure and in types of intervention [37]. This variability refers both to the absolute level of per capita current expenditure borne by local Authorities for social care - in Northern Italy (138,000 lire a year) almost double than in the South (70,000) - and the relative weight of such expenditure on the total expenditure operated by the Commune (which in Valle d'Aosta and Friuli Venezia-Giulia reaches about 20%, almost three times higher than the 7% of Molise, Campania, Basilicata and Calabria).

In some regions, as it has previously been pointed out, the enforcement of ad hoc regional provisions has allowed the social services offered by the Communes to be integrated with those supplied by the ASLs. In the field of the care of elderly people, this coordination between the two sectors has brought about the creation of the above mentioned multidisciplinary Units of Geriatric Assessment (UVGs) made up of municipal and medical staff to facilitate a full assessment of the health and socio-economic needs of the elderly, and therefore to anticipate and formulate a plan for integrated care. As a matter of fact, the systematic diffusion of these UVGs all over the country is one of the priority actions stated in the National Health Scheme for the three years from 1998 to 2000 [45].

In many areas, however, the management of social care for the non self-sufficient elderly is still separate from health care, and the tasks of the Commune (coordinated by the Region) are therefore mainly concentrated on the provision of socio-economic care, in some cases integrated with social and health care interventions. Among the most common in Italy the following should be mentioned [28,29]:

- *economic assistance allowances* (temporary or permanent) to increase the personal independence of the recipient with household bills, medical care not provided for by SSN, etc;
- *social and health home care services* (Servizi di Assistenza domiciliare socio assistenziale, SAD) i.e. services of family/domestic nature (housework, bathing and

toiletting, feeding, laundry, accompanying etc) to allow the non self-sufficient person, whether elderly or not, to keep his/her own habits in the home environment;
- *hospitality in nursing homes*;
- *preventive socialization services* (for self-sufficient and partially non self sufficient persons): holiday breaks and recreational centres.

The nursing home

The traditional Italian nursing home has historically always been intended for indigent people who were unable to lead independent lives [46]. Even if these homes often took in chronically weak, sick and old people, in addition to the poor ,the economic conditions of the person remained more important than the physical ones in determining who could be taken in and who could not, which was reflected in the partial self-sufficiency of most of the in-patients. Table 4 shows how today instead - for reasons partially due to the introduction of the principles of managed competition and market economy in the Italian National Health System [47], making less convenient for a hospital to accept elderly patients, who usually require relatively long hospital stays [17] - nursing homes tend to admit, to a much greater extent than in the past, very old, seriously disabled elderly, who have care and health needs requiring the intervention of qualified personnel and care standards which differ greatly from those destined for independent persons [48].

The lack of modernization of most nursing homes means that the increasing demand for care facilities for severely disabled elderly remains mostly unmet. This is reflected by the low admission rate to nursing homes, which presently house about 2-3% of over 65 year olds [49], meaning that - as in most Mediterranean countries - it is a much rarer solution than in North-European countries [50]. In 1994, the total number of nursing homes for elderly in Italy was 4,836, with an estimated 287.500 beds, most of which (83%) are in medium-sized homes (with between 11 and 100 beds) [51].

Table 4: Disability degree of the elderly living in nursing homes in the Marche Region, 1979-1991 (percentage data)

		ASL n. 10 (N = 400)		Regione Marche (N = 4.152)
Disability degree	1979	1984	1991	1991
Self sufficient	61.9	48.0	33.5	52.8
Partially disable	18.4	9.0	8.9	8.2
Totally disable	19.7	33.0	57.6	39.0

Source: [48].

This low tendency to use nursing homes, especially in the South of the country, seems to reflect a generalised attitude among most elderly people, who declare that they would like "to die at home" [52], not to leave the place they live in and absolutely refuse to be transferred to institutions which are not their own [53]. These data are corroborated by hospital mortality rates, which show that in Italy only one elderly person in three (34%) dies in hospital, compared to much higher rates (between 50 and 80%) in countries like United

States, Canada or France [54]. All this should be interpreted in the light of the still traditionally strong support - though rapidly diminishing, for reasons that will be addressed further on - provided by other family members, rather than as a consequence of the introduction of alternative solutions which, as illustrated in the next paragraph, still remain relatively scarce.

New trends in the field of supports to the carers

There are not many legislative measures in Italy in favour of those who carry out caregiving tasks, and those which do exist have only recently been adopted. Recently the availability of part-time work was improved for public employees (law no. 662 of 1996), while many private employers are still very reluctant to agree to it "because of economic disincentives resulting from the structure of social security" [55]. To the employee who has to look after an elderly on a full-time basis - and cannot therefore profit by working part-time - the Social Security Reform law n. 335 of 1995 does allow a period of paid leave, but only if the dependent family member co-habits with the older person and, perhaps the greatest restriction of this measure, only up to a maximum of 25 days per year and 24 months in the whole working life [56]. For those who have to dedicate themselves to periods of continuous full-time caregiving - and this is the burden the family usually faces when having to care for a totally disabled elderly person - the only alternative presently available is to quit work for a period of "unpaid leave", generally limited to one year or less (even if a legislative decree currently discussed in Parliament extends that period to two years) [57]. It should though be underlined that this opportunity is only available to civil servants, as in the private sector the recourse to it is much less realistic, and often represents an "easy way to lose one's job" [58].

An idea of the difficulties which are currently faced in Italy by those who try to reconcile work in the labour market with informal family tasks can be deduced from the results of a survey carried out in some Milanese firms with a high percentage of female employement [59]. Thanks to the pressure exerted by female employees working night shifts - deemed as dangerous by industrial medicine and permitted by Italian law only if agreed through the collective negotiation (see law n. 903 of 1997, art. 5) - the trade unions of these companies were in fact able to obtain in 1989 exemption from night shift for women with children under six years of age or having to care for elderly or handicapped family members. When this request was extended to all female workers, the companies responded by closing the factories, and only after long negotiations, in 1994, did they permit a limited number of exemptions, established by a joint commission after examination of individual requests. The case shows clearly once again how the needs and difficulties of women are often very different from those of men, as work shifts are considered by the latter as mainly an opportunity to increase their income, while the former complain above all about the lack of time resulting from these [60].

This brief overview can be concluded with the preliminary results of a survey currently being carried out by I.N.R.C.A. (Italian National Research Centre on Ageing), based on structured interviews to 69 caregivers of non self-sufficient over 75 year olds, of whom 78% are women, 23% still working (in 4 out of 5 cases full-time), 41% retired and 35% housewives [61]. *Among those who are still working*, most (62%) do not appear to suffer in any way from being both carer and worker. Over a third (38%), however, complained of problems of excessive inflexibility at work - in terms of time schedules, leave of absence and holidays - as well as of lost career opportunities, in terms of more gratifying and/or better paid work, which would have meant moving or working full-time and therefore had to be turned down. *Among the non-employed caregivers* - housewives and pensioners - the percentage of those who state they have problems in their professional work due to caregiving activities drops to circa 20%, for reasons which are mostly linked to early retirement (among those who left work) and to "it did not allow me to work" (among the housewives). An interesting aspect which emerges from this study, in terms of formulation of suggestions, is represented by the high number of those - about 50% - who state *that the solution that would most help to reconcile work and caregiving* is "economic support to make it possible to better organise caregiving", a solution which among those who work is combined with a request for external personnel to supplement family care.

Roles of Family Carers of Older People Living at Home

The traditional role of the Italian family

As has already been seen, in Italy most elderly people have up to now found the necessary help within their own family, "primary group of kinship", whether they continue to live in their own home or go to live with other family members [62]. As a matter of fact many elderly, though not cohabiting with other family members, have a so-called "intimacy at a distance" relationship with them, as can be seen by the fact that 59% of elderly who live alone see their offspring once a day, 20% more than once a week and only 13% less frequently (Istat 1995b: 110-111), confirming that Italian elderly people, compared to their peers in other countries, have more frequent contacts with other family members [55].

This situation contributes to keep the rate of recourse to formal care services by elderly people relatively low - as already seen with respect to nursing homes (see 2.2.3) - making instead informal family care a widespread phenomenon. Cautious estimates indicate in fact that about 75-80% of elderly care - including all kinds of support intervention for the disabled, from economic support to physical care and psychological and relational support - is provided within the informal network of the enlarged family [55,63,64]. This confirms the role of the family as a "productive organization" which - widely speaking - produces goods and supplies services according to the needs of its members [65,66]: to improve or alleviate the economic condition of the poor elderly person [67]; to prevent dependency and progressive chronicity when the elderly person is admitted into an institution [68,69]; and to integrate possible home care services at a local level, thus improving their functioning.

Support from other sources, which are here only shortly summarised, is much less substantial. The enlarged network of relatives, active above all in rural communities, can sometimes represent a simultaneous care support for the elderly and a physical-psychological help to the caregiver [70]. Collaboration from neighbours - which can range from carrying out certain errands to keeping the old person company, or just keeping an eye on him/her, in order to give the family carer a short break - is a reality which seems to concern the minority of the elderly population [71]. Though often limited to urban areas and concentrated in institutes and hospitals, volunteers also play their part - in 1996 1,280 volunteer organisations were working in the elderly care sector, involving almost 70,000 volunteers [72] often providing support and counselling in place of the formal services [73,74] sometimes integrated by conscientious objectors (young men who, having chosen to do civil rather than military service, have recently become a growing reference point for care services supplied by Municipalities and Health Autorities) [75]. These non-familial support sources tend though in Italy to be sporadic, thus often ending up as a very bland kind of support to the role traditionally played by the Italian family. A recent survey carried out by the Italian Academy of Family Physicians confirms these results: (see Figure 2): based on a sample of 2,148 over 65 year olds contacted by 102 general practitioners throughout the country, at home, in nursing homes and in G.P. surgeries, the survey shows that the great majority (70-80%) of them receive help for the ADL and IADL from the family. In two cases - for the use of the toilet and the lifting out of and putting into bed of the elderly - the help of paid personnel is also frequently requested (30-40% of cases), while the role of public services and volunteers remains always very incidental, if not totally absent. This situation is made even worse by the lack of coordination among the different institutions [30].

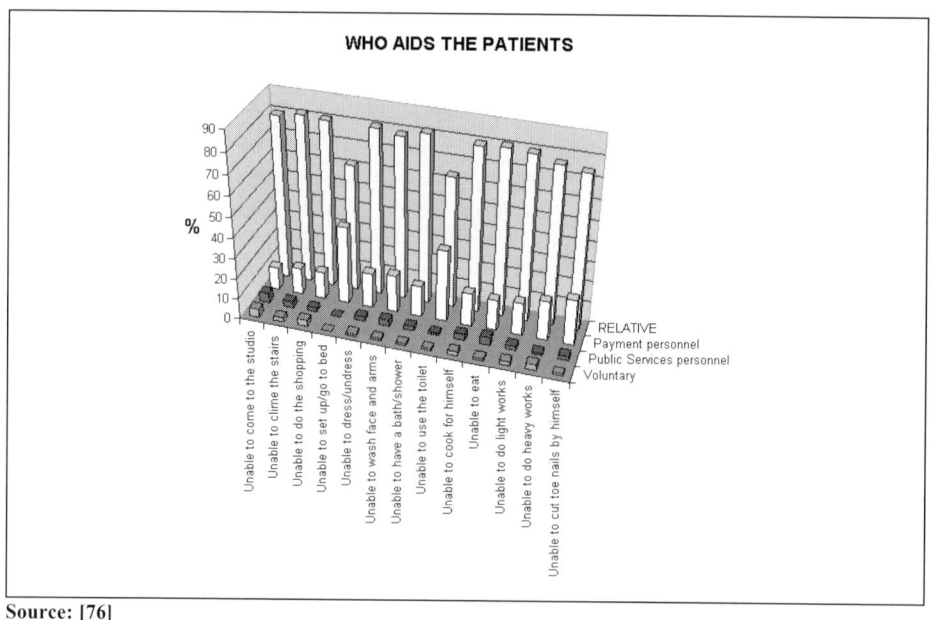

WHO AIDS THE PATIENTS

Source: [76]

Figure 2: Percentage of help provided to disabled elderly by the family as well as by private, public and volunteer personnel according to different ADL and IADL

The impact of demographic and socio-economic change

The family, therefore, finds itself today often alone in facing the increased care needs of the elderly population, just at a time when, on the contrary, the support which the family structure is able to provide is on the decrease. From a demographic point of view, in fact, the observed drop in the fertility rate on the one hand, and the reduction in the average family size, on the other hand (cfr. Table 5), contribute to a shrinking of the network of informal care which can be supplied within the intra-family structure, thus increasing the dependency of the single elderly person upon the community.

The reduction of potential support from the family is also a consequence of socio-economic factors, particularly the growing presence of women in the labour market, with obvious repercussions in the decreasing number of "pure" housewives and of people traditionally "delegated" to caregiving. Elderly care is ,in fact, in Italy no different from that in other countries [77,78], being supplied mainly by the female members of the family [79]. The above mentioned study carried out by I.N.R.C.A. in the Region of Marche (Central Italy) shows that, in a random sample of 171 caregivers of over 75 year old disabled people, circa four out of five care-givers (80,7% of the total) are women [80]. Data from one of the most industrialised areas of the country, the Region of Lombardy in Northern Italy, reveals furthermore that caregiving affects the majority of "middle-aged" women (between 45 and

65 years old), since 56% of them state that they have provided some kind of domestic work or nursing care to their parents in the last six months [79].

Table 5: Average household size in Italy, 1951-2024

	historical series 1951-1994					projections 2009-2039		
	1951-52	1960-61	1970-71	1980-81	1994	2009-10	2024	2039
Fertility rate	2,3	2,4	2,4	1,6	1,2	1,5	...	...
Average number of members per household	4,0	3,6	3,3	3,0	2,7	2,3	2,1	2,0

Sources: - [2,81,82]

Caregiving: a task "for the woman"

The diffusion of female caregiving in the whole country is, however, likely to be even broader than the latter percentage seems to suggest, since it does not take into account at least two phenomena: that there exist also women who, as spouses, care for their disabled husbands; and that in less industrialised areas the persistence of traditional habits are linked with higher rates of family - i.e. female - support. As a matter of fact, wives seem to be those who, in Italy, are "morally and factually obliged" to care for a disabled elderly person; in her absence or inability, the daughters must take over, followed by the daughters-in-law [62,83]. Talking of family care becomes therefore a euphemism, as most of the caring tasks are performed by women, also due to the frequent absence of cooperation by the sons [84,85]. It is emblematic that the daughters, even if they live further away from the parents than the sons, visit their parents more often and have much greater contact with them [86,87].

Furthermore, a woman often has to combine her caring tasks nowadays with her role as a grandmother, a figure which today is more and more involved in looking after the children of daughters and daughters-in law, who often have just become mothers - due to the increased mean age at first birth - and are involved in external working activities themselves [43,54,65,88]. This plurality of roles - daughter, wife, mother, grandmother, working woman - is certainly a contributary factor to the fact that middle-aged women, especially if "full-time" carers, are subject to a relatively high risk of depression and stress [89]. Aspects such as the loss of friends, of leisure time, as well as of the "right to have holiday" [90] should not be underestimated, since they are consequences which, in some cases, fall paradoxically on the figure of the daughter-in-law who cares for her mother-in-law, rather than on the husband/son. It can therefore be stated that it is mainly women who continue to bear the weight of the inadequacies of the Italian Welfare State, characterised - and not only in the elderly care sector - by a lack of services which has taken advantage of, and in turn generated, downright exploitation and lack of recognition of unpaid family work carried out by mothers, wives and daughters [91].

Even when immigrants are involved in caregiving, often living with the elderly they care for - a phenomenon which is rapidly growing in Italy, especially in urban areas, according to a pattern which has been already observed in other industrialized countries [92] - this support generally comes from women, who seem to have, due to traditions prevalent in their original countries - Philippines, South American as well as Balkan countries - a more accustomed and daily relationship with disease, suffering and death than Italian women [93-95].

Table 6 shows the increase in female participation in the labour market - compared to the fall of male participation - which has occurred in Italy over the past three decades. The importance of this phenomenon, which has been accompanied by demands for equal treatment for men and women in terms of career and professional opportunity [78], gives an idea of how urgently the challenge of reconciling work outside the home, housework and caregiving needs solutions in the form of reforms of the Italian Welfare System. In fact, the present growing burden of caregiving tasks involving elderly family members is in conflict with the greater participation in the labour market by women, a situation which for many women means that they keep on having to find work characterised by marginality, seasonality and discontinuity [96]. Data show in fact that in 1995 only 2.8% of men worked part-time in Italy, compared with 12.3% of the women, so that 70% of part-time employees were female, mainly employed in the services sector, where there is more flexibility [97,98].

Table 6: Activity rate by sex, 1960-1995

Year	Males	Females
1960	62,5	26,4
1965	59,3	22,8
1970	56,6	21,8
1975	54,6	22,4
1980	54,4	26,0
1985	54,7	28,2
1990	54,8	30,6
1995	51,7	29,2

Sources: [99-101]

Thus we can speak not only of a "double presence" of women, in the family and in the labour market [84,102,103], but even of "triple presence", when the number of tasks, already significant in their own family, is incremented by caring for one's own elderly parents or parents-in-law [104]. It is therefore not surprising that sometimes women who are overburdened on more than one front make the decision - just how voluntarily should be more deeply investigated - to give up paid work: a choice with consequences which are not limited to a loss of immediate income, but are also long-term, as they lead to a loss of pension benefits [105].

The crisis of traditional elderly caregiving patterns provided by the Italian family and its female members is confirmed, though indirectly, by recent research results. In particular, a survey carried out in 1993-94 among the 223 elderly recipients of the Municipal Home Care provided by the city of Ancona (Central Adriatic Coast) shows that, while 65% of them stated that they receive visits from their family members, only 47% confirmed getting concrete support from them, and 35% of the interviewed people admitted having to resort to private paid services [71]. From another study conducted in 1994 on an elderly population living in a mountain area of Central Italy [105-107] it emerged that 89% of the 139 over 65 year olds interviewed stated that they received help from their family; the latter consisted though mainly of friendship and company, and much less of effective help in personal care and housework. The same survey brought also to light - by comparing data collected in a similar study carried out in the same community in 1980 - that the elderly nowadays show a greater acceptance (or a reduced aversion), of nursing homes than previously.

These results, rather than questioning the traditional and primary role of the Italian family in caregiving, actually underline the "growing difficulty in combining this task with other daily activities, such as work, looking after children and other members of the family" [108]. They represent therefore a clear example of how the family increasingly needs support itself, if it wants to be able to care for its weaker members without having to supplement rhem, at their own expense, with the duties and roles of the State and the public care services. Otherwise the danger is that it might end up covering a double role: on the one hand it protects and defends the disabled elderly as an "active caring subject"; on the other hand, it very slowly becomes the "subject of demand" and the "object of intervention" [109]: demanding help, relief, and protection, but at the same time trying to prevent possible "caregiving pathologies", a symptom of a caregiving burden which is difficult to sustain and is linked to a conflict between the needs of the cared-for elderly person and the carer's personal exigencies [63], often results in anxiety, depression, insomnia, frustration, nervous breakdown or even the use of drugs [83].

Assessment

In Italy, assessment of the health condition of the elderly population and of the effectiveness of the intervention adopted to improve it, has traditionally made little use of standardized instruments. This is due in part to the lack of clear legislation on this matter,but also depends on the conscience or the whim of the individual practitioner concerned. Only in the last few years have there been signs of a cultural change, shown by a general reappraisal of the value that the quality of services has attained in the eyes of Italian society not only in the field of health. The legislative Decree n. 502 of 1992 has in fact started a series of legislative measures pointing out the quality factors that must be observed and respected by the health care services - defined by the Legislative Decree n. 517 of 1993 and the Decrees by the Ministry of Health of 24th July 1995 and of 15th October 1996.

All this legislation - including the National Health Scheme 1998-2000, at present under discussion in the Italian Parliament - has gone no further than theoretical formulations, apart from very rare exceptions at local level [110], fixing a series of indicators mainly centered on the reality of hospitalization, without defining precise assessment measures of effectivenes and quality in the context of primary care of the elderly.

In the customery practice, therefore, the standardized instruments adopted in Italy by the respective responsible for the care of elderly people and of their families are not numerous [30], and are probably used mostly by those practitioners who, apart from their clinical activities, also carry out research and scientific writing. Among the most common standardized instruments - beginning with those used to assess the health condition of the elderly person - the following should be mentioned:

For the multidimensional evaluation:
- AGED (Assessment of Geriatric Disability): computer aided procedure used to collect and evaluate information concerning the degree of self-sufficiency of the elderly and the correlated time of nursing and social care [30,111].

- B.I.N.A. (Breve Indice di Non Autoufficienza): this has been adopted as the official assessment means in the allocation of A.D.I. in Emilia Romagna [12] and for the certification of the condition of non self-sufficiency of elderly people in Nursing Homes in Friuli Venezia Giulia (L.R. no.67 of 1983 and L.R. no.49 of 1993) [16].
- C.T.M.S.P.: based on the model used by the Ministry of Health of Quebec (Canada), it was first employed in Italy in 1993 in order to determine the allocation of A.D.I. in some ASLs in Milan [112].
- G.E.F.I. (Global Evaluation Functional Index): a simple index for the total functional evaluation of the elderly person [30,113-115].
- S.V.A.D. (Sistema Valutativo dell'Anziano a Domicilio): Italian adaptation of the form used by the Ministry of Health of British of Columbia (Canada), it is used to assess the health of the elderly residing at home [30,116].
- V.A.O.R.-A.D.I.: the Italian adaptation of the U.S. Resident Assessment Instrument is used to assess elderly people who live in nursing homes [117].
- V.A.L.G.R.A.F.: instrument of functional evaluation based on graphic images used to assess elderly people who are residents in nursing homes or hospitals for long hospitalization [118].

For functional evaluation [115,116,119]:
- Scale of Activities of Daily Living (ADL): Italian adaptation of Katz's scale
- Scale of Instrumental Activities of Daily Living (IADL): Italian adptation of Lawton's scale
- Barthel Index: mainly used in the rehabilitation field [120].

For the evaluation of mental deterioration:
- Mini Mental State Examination: very rapid, it is among the most widely used and recognized [120,121].
- Short Portable Mental Status Questionnaire: very rapid, in the Italian version a question about about the President's name has been replaced by a question about the Pope's name [116,120].

For the evaluation of depression [122]:
- Geriatric Depression Scale (G.D.S.): it is among the most commonly used [117,123]
- Philadelphia Geriatric Center Morale Scale
- Measurement of Morale in the Elderly
- Geriatric Scale of Hopelessness
- Beck's Depression Inventory [120,124],

and, specific for demented elderly people:
- Cornell Scale for Depression in Dementia
- Depressive Signs Scale (DSS)
- Dementia Modd Assessment Scale
- Camberra Interview for the Elderly

As for the assessment of the state of health of the carer, the Relative's Stress Scale by Greene [125] is no doubt the most commonly used assessment instrument, given its extreme rapidity of administration, and it is used not only in hospitals or ambulatorial settings [120,126-128], but also for field research [90].

Apart from this instrument, in Italy the state of health of the carer is generally assessed by non specific and even non-standardized techniques. Among the rare exception is the previously mentioned survey conducted by INRCA in cooperation with CNR about "the role of women in the family care of the elderly" [90]. During this research, which is still being carried out, the following standardized measures were used: the Montgomery Caregiver Burden Measures [129], together with a series of non specific standardized instruments, such as the Norbeck Social Support Questionnaire [130], the Italian adaptations of Zung Self-rating Anxiety Scale and of Zung Self-rating Depression Scale [131] as well as the Life Satisfaction Index - A [132].

The need for suitable instruments of diagnosis and evaluation in this field, instruments which should also be sensitive to differences of gender, is affirmed by several authors and supported by research. Among these studies in the psychological field, is the work by Leonardi, who has produced a special paper "for the analysis of women's daily life" [133,134], as well as, in the field of sociological studies and discourse analysis, the work by Paoletti [135,136].

Case studies

Case 1

Female, aged 76, with osthoearthritis of the hips and knees, poor vision due to macular degeneration, and hypertension. Mobile with a frame within her home except for the stairs. Needs help with mobility outside, shopping cooking and housework.

Social circumstances (A): Older person living alone in an isolated farmhouse. Widowed. Little money. Daughter and son-in-law unemployed with four children, aged 9 months to 7 years, and live 5 kilometres away. Two other children of the older person live over 100 kilometres away.

In this situation, the first step would probably be to assess whether housing conditions would allow the mother to move in with one of her three children (starting with the closest female child) or whether the daughter living closest to her mother could move into her mother's house with her. Even if the daughter didn't move, she would be the one more "naturally" bound to look after her mother, going to her home to carry out the household chores her mother can no longer perform.

Social care: given the elderly woman's age and the fact that her daughter has got a large family and her two other children live far away, she should probably apply for help from the municipal social services. If she or her children have not already applied, she will be assisted in writing and sending the application to get suitable benefits (civil disability and partial blindness, since she is not in such condition as to be entitled to a companion payment) and also a social pension (if her income is below the amount stated by the law). If the economic conditions of the two children who live far away are not good, the Commune might decide to put her name on the list for a low rent Council house in order to avoid her having to live alone in the farmhouse. There will be a later assessment to determine whether to allocate financial aid - or to integrate State benefits or the SAD for help at home (but only in the Communes where the service has been activated).

Health care: the MMG is likely to propose the activation of a bimonthly ADP to keep the woman's health conditions under control - the ASL supplies, upon request, the necessary equipment for mobility . Since she is over 65, she does not have to pay for any health care.

The needs of the daughter/caregiver are not directly evaluated but they will be dealt with in the report written by the social workers to support the elderly woman's application for economic benefit: If the mother and the daughter decided to live together, integrated help measures would be likely to be taken which would better take into account the caregiver's needs. Only a few Regions give a monthly stipend to the caregiver for her work, but then only in cases of average or low incomes (below 50 million lire a year for two people, below 80 million lire for 5 or more people).

Social circumstances (B): Older person living alone in a ground floor flat in town. Widowed. Daughter and son-in-law are both teachers in full-time employment, with two children aged 7 and 1, and live within 1 kilometre in the same town.

In this case the most likely solution is the mother moving in with her daughter if the house is large enough. Otherwise, the daughter pays her mother daily visits helping her with some tasks (shopping, transport) and keeping her company as often as her family and work commitments allow. For the heavier chores, such as house cleaning, a charwoman helps and she is partly paid by the daughter. The daughter, overcoming resistance on the part of the mother, may resort to the help of a foreign live-in domestic, who will manage the house, thus assuring daytime companionship and night supervision.

Social care: Being in a favourable economic situation, the mother cannot expect to receive help from the Commune social services. She could apply for a special benefit for her partial blindness - since this benefit is not income tested - and a pension for her partial blindness (but only if her individual income is not higher than 22,8 million lire a year).

Health care: the MMG's visits and housecalls are free and guaranteed. If the elderly person's income does not exceed 70 million lire a year, she will not have to pay for any medical care.

Any needs of a medical nature (depression, stress, etc) which the carer may have will be evaluated only if communicated to her MMG or specialist.

Social circumstances (C): Older person living with spouse in 2-storey house. Retired with savings. Spouse is fit and well. No children. Bedroom, bathroom and toilet are upstairs.

The woman's spouse takes her downstairs daily, by himself or with the help of neighbours or external personnel (see answer 2) and helps her with the documents and bureaucratic papers (applying for and cashing pensions, drug prescriptions, payment of bills etc). External personnel is employed for housework, toileting and meals (see answer 2).

Social care: through the Municipal Social Service the old couple will probably be able to take advantage of the SAD, though they will have to pay for the carrying out of the tasks the husband can not cope with (owing to their income situation).

Health care: the MMG will probably propose a bimonthly ADP service.

The carer's practical needs could be assessed and partly satisfied by SAD, while eventual health problems (depression, stress etc) would be addressed by the MMG or specialists' visits. In cases where the household yearly income is less than 70 million lire, the carer will also be allowed to benefit from the health care fee exemption, since he is over 65.

Case 2

Male, aged 80, facing discharge from hospital following a stroke. Expected to be confined to bed or chair for several weeks with gradual recovery of mobility. Needs the help of one person for transfers, toileting, bathing and dressing.

Social circumstances (A): see case 1-A. In this case we can point out the following differences from case 1-A.

After trying to keep her father in hospital for as long as possible, the nearest daughter might decide to move temporarily to her father's home to help during the most difficult phase before his condition improves. Besides, she would probably apply to the municipal social services and ASL to receive some form of immediate help (see answer 2).

Social care: The municipal social services oblige him to obtain the benefits due for partial disability as well as the social pension, and supply the elderly person, at least temporarily, with SAD. If the incomes of the two children living farther away are not high, access to municipal economic facilities might be allowed to pay for the high temporary costs of care during the recovery phase. The same applies for the assessment of the availability of a council house.

Health care: ADI (Integrated Home Assistance) (provided it has been implemented in the patient's Commune) or a home nursing/rehabilitation service could be activated. If the daughter can guarantee a certain continuity of care, but this solution is viable only in Turin, Genoa, and Milan, a Home Hospitalization service could be activated. If these services are not available, the MMG can in any case suggest the activation of ADP (Programmed Home Care), firstly every four months, later on at longer intervals. The ASL supplies, upon request, the necessary health and sanitary equipment (hospital bed, wheel chair, etc). When able, the elderly person will apply, free of charge, to a certified rehabilitation centre to get appropriate recovery therapy. In his case all health care is free.

Social circumstances (B): see case 1-B. In this case we can point out the following differences from case 1-B.

Given her family and professional engagements, the daughter can be of help only for a short time and only for the lightest duties (shopping and payment of bills). She will pay external personnel for the heaviest duties.

Social care: Owing to their high income, the elderly man and his daughter will pay for home help. After discharge from hospital, they will probably need external personnel to guarantee night assistance, a problem which is often solved only through the services of foreign immigrants.

Health care: ADI (Integrated Home Assistence) could be activated where available or home nursing/rehabilitation services. If the family can assure a certain continuity of relationship - but this solution is viable only in Turin, Genoa and Milan - a Home Hospitalization service could be activated. If these services are not available, the MMG can suggest the activation of ADP (Programmed Home Care) firstly every four months, later on at longer intervals - the ASL supplies, upon request, the necessary health and sanitary equipment (hospital bed, wheelchair etc). The Health care is free of charge only if the yearly household income is less than 70 million lire.

Social circumstances (C): see case 1-C. The following differences from case 1-C can be pointed out.

The elderly woman's spouse will probably try to do the lightest housework asking for help from external personnel for the heavier tasks.

Social care: the elderly woman could be eligible for payment from municipal SAD, combined if necessary with help from external personnel.

Health care: provided it has been implemented in the elderly person's Commune, ADI (Integrated Home Assistance) or a home nursing/rehabilitation service could be activated. If the husband can guarantee a certain continuity of care, but this solution is only viable in Turin, Genoa and Milan, a Home Hospitalization service could be activated. If these services are not available, the MMG can suggest the activation of ADP (Programmed home care) firstly every four months, later on at longer intervals. The ASL supplies, upon request, the necessary health and sanitary equipment (hospital bed, wheelchair etc). All health care is free of charge provided the yearly household income is less than 70 million lire.

Besides what has already been said, for case 1-C, it must be added that in Turin, Genoa and Milan, Home Hospitalization could help to assess any suffering on the part of the carer more quickly and systematically, suggesting ad hoc support therapy.

Case 3

Female, aged 86, suffering from dementia. Frequent wandering by day and night. Frequent falls. Incontinent of urine and faeces.

Social circumstances (A): see case 1-A. Since the elderly person is not in a condition to look after herself and since none of her three children can accept her in his/her family for a long time, the most likely hypothesis is that the woman, after several attempts of staying with her children, will be institutionalized. In such a hypothesis the caregiver's role will be reduced to a financial contribution to meet expenses - which are very high - for residential care, apart from visiting the institutionalized mother.

Social care: The Municipal Social Services will help with the documents to get the following benefits: assessment of the mental state and subsequently the appointment of a Tutelary judge, access to State allowances for total disability, including companion payment; the choice of a nursing home; the actual admission to hospital; the Commune will also keep in touch with her 3 children to ask them for a financial contribution to cover the costs of the nursing home should the mother's income be insufficient until her personal possessions and estate have been sold.

Health care: A part of the above mentioned costs for residential care is reimbursed by the SSN to cover the costs related to various forms of health care. The elderly patient, once her disability has been assessed, will probably be exempt from payment of health care fees. Health care will be assured by the medical staff of the nursing home (according to ad hoc agreements) or, if there are no internal medical staff, by the MMG.

Since the mother has been institutionalized, the role of family carers would exist only if one of the children should pay frequent visits to the mother. In this case the carer's eventual needs would be assessed and valued only randomly by the staff of the nursing home. Otherwise the same situation as in case 1-A would be appliable.

Social circumstances (B): see case 1-B. Two hypotheses are possible: either the elderly woman will be institutionalized (in which case the situation is the same as in case 2-A), or she will stay in her home if somebody is willing to live with her. This possibility - much more likely in an urban context and if there are (which however is quite rare) daily centres for demented patients - would probably mean the appointment of a foreign female immigrant (whose work could possibly be shared with somebody else's during the day) with a view to assuring day and night assistance in exchange for reasonable pay. In this case the main tasks of the daughter carer would be to select a suitable person, probably with the help of associations working in the field of home help, to help her, to make her mother accept the new help especially during the first weeks, and to pay her should the mother's income be too low . The daughter/carer could however continue toileting her mother and looking after her, shifting the heavier tasks onto the paid staff.

Social care: If the daughter decided to look for paid staff to live at home with the elderly woman, the only possible help from of the Commune would be a list of reliable people who could be contacted for the job. In many cases, however, this service is offered by voluntary associations usually of Catholic background. Should institutionalization be the option, the Commune could help with the bureaucracy involved (see also 3-A), for instance to obtain a total disability pension (only if the personal income is less than 22.8 million lire a year) and the companion payment (which is not means tested).

Health care: In the case of admission to a nursing home, the situation is the same as for 3-A. If the elderly woman stays at her home with live-in staff, she will not have to pay any health care fees (which for this kind of pathology is not means tested) and she might take advantage - if available - of ADI (Integrated Home Care). Otherwise the MMG could suggest the activation of an ADP service. The ASL supplies, upon request, incontinence pads. If the patient lives in one of the few Communes where there is a daily centre for demented persons, she could spend some hours there with the assistance of specialized staff.

The eventual care needs of the daughter carer would not be assessed systematically and specifically, unless her mother frequents a daily centre for demented persons where assessment of the carers' care needs are often routine. In general the hardships and difficulties linked to the task of being a carer will be considered only if the carer herself takes the initiative and asks her MMG to assess her health condition. It is to be stressed that the involvement of the carer - though less heavy - would continue both in the case of the patient's institutionalization and if the patient should continue to live at home with the help of external staff who would be paid by the carer. Some help might come from joining one of the voluntary associations which have been created in Italy in the last few years to better protect the interests of demented patients.

Social circumstances (C): see case 1-C. The only differences with reference to case 1-C are the following:

Her spouse will try to best cope with the situation accepting any help that may come from outside the family (see Answer 2). His tasks will mainly be to watch over and to protect his partner, helping her with dressing and toileting and entrusting external staff with the other duties.

Social care: The Municipal Social services allow the couple to take advantage of SAD - though on payment - and help them to obtain any possible financial assistance to which they are entitled (disability pension - which is means tested -and companion payment). The woman's husband will probably use his savings to employ external personnel for night care and for the housework. Extra help might come from voluntary associations and self-help associations - if there are any in the area - which offer home care or assistance in daily centres through the activity of volunteers.

Health care: Where available, ADI could be activated. Otherwise, the MMG can propose the activation of ADP. The ASL supplies, upon request, incontinence pads. Health care is free only if the yearly household income does not exceed 70 million lire. If there is a daily centre for demented elderly, the husband could entrust them with his wife for some hours a day, so that his wife could be looked after by specialized staff.

Since the husband lives with his wife, his difficulties and problems could be assessed, more easily than in case A and B, by the staff of the social services of the Commune, by SAD operators, by the MMG and also by the personnel of the daily centres and voluntary associations which could give assistance to him according to the regulations described above.

Future Developments

Recent trends

The illustrated data and experiences have shown that formal care solutions destined to the frail elderly in Italy are still insufficient and only partially updated with respect to the changing needs of the users. The polarization of the existing alternatives, which are still prevalently restricted to the dichotomy between "home" and the "nursing home" - a definition which often indicates the traditional institution for poor elderly, rather than centres making available to their own guests integrated medical and social care - is a very clear indicator of this situation. Even less conspicuous and diverse is the supply of services to the caregivers, whether in monetary terms or in the form of counselling and specific health monitoring.

There are, at present, some indications that the situation is changing. First of all the Italian government has given its approval within the National Health Scheme for the three years 1998-2000 - which must be discussed by Parliament - a special section devoted to the elderly which clearly sets up as its main objective "to adopt policies of support to families with elderly people in need of home care (also with a view to safeguarding the health of women who are, in most cases, the main responsible for the assistance)" [45].

A new trend which has been taking place in Italy in the last few years - along the lines of a process already started in other countries [137] - is the setting up of "special units" for demented elderly people within settings used by non self-sufficient elderly people. For example, in 1995 the Lombardy Region (Northern Italy) began a three year experimental project, called "Alzheimer project", which created, inside already existing rehabilitation centres, 9 regional Alzheimer centres for research and care, with 20 beds each, which were followed by 60 more Alzheimer centres of the same size but only devoted to care. These centres were activated between 1995 and 1996 inside the RSAs existing in the region [138]. This example has spread to other regions incorporating, in some cases, not only residential care, but also daily centres and outdoor areas (the so called "Alzheimer gardens") for patients affected by wandering behaviour [126,139].

Another of the various initiatives undertaken for the reform of the Italian welfare system is the proposal for the setting up of a "Fund for non self-sufficient people" [140]. The proposal - suggested by a special commission nominated by the Prime Minister with the purpose of analysing the "macroeconomic compatibility of social expenditure" in Italy - envisages the creation of a national fund "to ensure that all citizens have access to financial assistance and medical care whenever the situation of non self-sufficiency occurs". The fund - following the Germany example [141] - should be financed through contributions paid by the workers as well as the employers, and it should supply an economic reward - even if delayed in time, by granting pension benefits - to caregivers (whether family members or not) who provide assistance to non self-sufficient elderly or, should home care not be possible, an adequate allowance to the elderly for institutionalization. Reaction to this project has been varied. Some are strongly in favour, while others insist on the need to keep expenses concerning the assistance of non self-sufficient people in a health care ambit, without transferring them to the social assistance or to a new "Social Safety Department", in compliance with the suggestions of the Commissions. In addition the proposal of providences for institutionalization has been criticized, as they have been considered a sort of indirect push towards the institutionalization of non self-sufficient elderly people [140].

Another recent initiative is the Bill proposed by the Minister of Social Solidarity concerning a series of "Norms to make working time, family time and care time compatible". The aim of this proposal, currently under scrutiny in Parliament, is to favour a

better coordination between work and family life including assistance, through the integration and the rationalization of the existing laws.The main measures which have been proposed are three:
- long unpaid leave from work (but calculated for pension purposes and career seniority), to assist one's spouse or relative (up to the third level of kinship) needing assistance;
- the supply of funds to cope with the expenses faced in such circumstances in the form of advances on future pay;
- incentives to the employers who allow part-time work, giving priority to the employees who assist relatives.

The costs for these provisions should be covered through the creation of a "National Fund for Flexibility" consisting of 130 billion lire in the first year and 170 billion lire in the following two years. The proposal, which could be favourably considered for its contents - despite some contradictions concerning the worker's non-payment during the periods devoted to assistance - appears to be rather too ambitious for the present Italian situation, which is characterized by a myriad of regulations concerning flexibility, but which is, paradoxically, too rigid when it envisages only periods of temporary discharge and not of horizontal or vertical part-time work on the same basis .

On the whole, however, the new proposals appear to be still too cautious and too modest for a health system mainly based on hospitalization, rather than on the safeguard and protection of people's health. This is demonstrated by the extremely low levels of public expenditure assigned in Italy to prevention, rehabilitation and primary assistance in general, while almost two thirds of the financial resources are absorbed by hospital care expenses [31]. It is worth noting that the level of health expenses contained in the Italian GDP (5.4% in 1995) is lower than that of other OCSE countries [142], but these resources are not well allocated. In this period of generalized cuts to public expenditure, the risk is that of "expelling" people affected by chronic pathologies from the system of health care, with a subsequent increase not only in problems in the sector of social assistance - notoriously weaker from an organizational and financial point of view - but also in the burden of assistance to be borne by the families [31].

Open Challenges

Formal home and residential care

In the light of the above mentioned current trends, the main resistance which the social and health policies for the elderly will have to face in Italy can be summarized as follows. With respect to formal care, two directions seem to represent a priority for the future political agenda. The first is centred on the strengthening of community care, through the quantitative and qualitative improvement of integrated social, medical, nursing and rehabilitative home care, in order to keep the elderly person's home as "the central point" of an "enlarged household" [143]. The professional qualification of practitioners and formal home carers should also be better aimed so as to allow them to respond more effectively to the needs of the dependent elderly person, for instance through the design and implementation of ad hoc preparation courses for "caregivers of disabled elderly people", who in Italy do not yet have a well-established juridical-professional relevance.

The improvement of residential care for the frail elderly is the second priority, to be made possible by the adoption of more quality- and user-oriented management formulas, in order to adequately care for highly disabled users. This means a radical change in the content of the care services provided by existing structures - whether these have kept their traditional denomination as "Casa di Riposo" or have changed (but often only by name) into Health Care Residences - in order to develop towards the model of a "Service Centre" [108]. The latter - intended as a service provider which has direct and continual contact with the users in its own area, in close collaboration with other social and medical support structures (general practitioners, day centres, hospitals, community services) - should coordinate and supply, to both in-patients (even temporary ones) and external users in the neighbourhood, care services such as laundry, hot meals, rehabilitation, in suitably personalised forms.

Recourse to residential structures - a solution which in Italy has so far meant almost always a definitive institutionalisation - could become, thanks to the coordination of a Service Centre, a sort of respite service, making it possible for families to have a break, albeit temporary and short term but nevertheless useful, and offering qualified services which can periodically substitute the help provided by family members, thus favouring their mental and physical recovery. The philosophy behind this kind of solution can be compared to the one which has inspired the "Integrated Home Care Services" implemented at the end of the 80s in Denmark, where an explicit purpose of the reform was the try to involve, on the one hand, staff of nursing facilities in the home care services and, on the other hand, home care workers in the nursing facilities [144]. The main purpose remains the development of a series of alternatives for the users, who can adjust and mix the different services according to their own needs situation, to delay as long as possible permanent institutionalisation, and to avoid overburdening the family of the cared-for person by providing suitable support to the necessary caregiving activities.

Family and caregivers support

Within this sector a more systematic and institutional collaboration between the family and external formal supports is urgently needed. A first way to achieve this is the widespread organisation of training-information courses on theory and practice for informal caregivers, like those already tried out by some Italian municipalities [75] and, on a national scale, by countries such as Germany. Parallel to this, it is necessary to potentiate (quantitatively as well as qualitatively) the supply of personnel capable of providing qualified counselling to elderly people in need of care and to their families [135], to improve the recourse of the users to existing support services, which in some cases at present is difficult [145].

Fundamental in this sense is the activity of the general practitioner, who can provide concrete support, advice and medical education to the family caregivers [83], but still too often works uncoordinated with the 'performers' in the care of the elderly, especially the municipal support services. First signs of a more decisive change of mentality in this field are, however, taking place on a local level, where integrated health and social elderly care services are now being implemented by some municipalities [146].

The heart of the matter is that the "subjective right of the family caregiver to respite measures" should be recognised, through a reconsideration of caregiving activities as an "intra-domestic work", and as such deserving to be safeguarded [147]. To this purpose, a decisive impulse could be provided by an appropriate reorganisation of the Health Care Residences into short-term respite services, but is also feasible, for instance, through solutions similar to Great Britain's "family placement scheme" [144], according to which, in order to provide respite to family caregivers, the cared for person is hosted temporarily by a so called "placement family", often middle-aged women with a residential home or nursing background, paid by the local authority. A better recognition of caregiving activities might also come from the provision of economic incentives - in addition to the existing companion payment - consisting of both tax relief and (partially even means-tested) benefits to those who care for the elderly disabled [83]. A further desirable measure - which has actually already been included in the proposals made by the above mentioned Ministerial Commission on the "macroeconomic compatibilities of social expenditure" - would be to recognise, for pension purposes, those periods of time which family members - or other informal figures - dedicate to caregiving tasks [43].

A better coordination should be achieved with regard to the variety of family, social and professional roles in which Italian carers - i.e. Italian women - are today absorbed. As far as the *labour market* is concerned, there is an urgent need for support measures which recognize, for instance, the right to periods of "children leave" to allow them to care for the own parents, a provision which various political parties and trade unions have long been asking for [56]. Besides developing part-time work, other measures which could ease the present rigidity of labour activity and conciliate it better with elderly caregiving are an increase in paid leave - similar to what is already happening for instance in Sweden [144] - as well as flexibility in time schedules [43]. In general, what is needed is a philosophy of "organised flexibility" which, using an integrated approach towards the individual - and not being limited to only identifying single aspects, such as the individual role of worker, parent, or caregiver, but all of them concurrently - can create solutions which take into account the requirements of working hours, service hours, times of family life, and of their possible reciprocal influence on social life [148]. As already shown by some surveys carried out abroad, the advantages and satisfaction which can be achieved by playing a variety of different roles - as is the case of the carer and worker, besides that of spouse and mother - can often ward off the stress which sometimes results from caregiving [149], making it possible to carry out the latter in a coordinated manner with other tasks. In these circumstances, it is likely that paid work will provide the caregiver with a mental-physical "break" and any potential resentment towards caregiving will be offset by positive effects which are usually obtained only using external "respite services" [150-152].

With respect to this area, too, it can be observed that concrete proposals are already available - see the above mentioned proposal regarding the "Norms to make working time, family time and care time compatible" - although it is hard to tell if and when they might become reality. In conclusion, a global approach towards the care of the frail elderly is desirable, through the promotion of services which - without saddling the caregiver with further tasks which he or she does not have the means necessary to accomplish and without relinquishing the need to respect the needs of the cared for elderly person - are able to ensure to both parties a proper and flexible support, with the help of qualified and personalized counselling and supervision [103]. The worry of medical expenditure, the short length of governments, and the actual tendency, highlighted by the mass media, to focus on longer lifespan and "successful ageing" rather than the problems of the non self-sufficient elderly and their carers, have so far prevented in Italy the initiation of systematic reforms able to make the most out of public and private resources in a "Welfare mix" perspective [153,154]. It is to be hoped that the more sensitive attention which has been paid to the problem recently in the country will rapidly find actual realisation.

---

[1]Unless otherwise indicated, this is the age limit which will be used in the text to indicate that a person or a population is "elderly".

References

[1] U.S. Bureau of Census Global Ageing into the 21st Century. Wallchart. Washington D.C.: U.S. Government Printing Office, 1997.
[2] Eurostat, Demographic statistics 1997. Luxembourg: Office for Official Publications of the European Communities, 1997.
[3] Istat, *Indagine Multiscopo sulle famiglie - Volume 11: I disabili.* Roma, 1995.
[4] Istat, *Anziani in Italia.* Bologna: Il Mulino 1997.
[5] C. Giammarchi and M. Mengani, M. Aspetti quantitativi della disabilità nella popolazione anziana. *Rassegna Geriatrica Gerontechnology* **32(1/2)** (1996) 67-76.
[6] R.L. Kane et al, Using ADLs to establish eligibility for long-term care among the cognitively impaired. *Gerontologist*, **31(1)** (1991) 60-66.
[7] M. Mengani et al, L'aiuto assistenziale della famiglia agli anziani non autosufficienti residenti a domicilio: situazione attuale e prospettive future. *Difesa Sociale*, **75(4)** (1996) 139-148.
[8] Istituto per la Ricerca Sociale, Coordinamento e integrazione dei servizi socio-assistenziali con i servizi sanitari. Roma: Ministero dell'Interno, 1984.
[9] Disegno di Legge del Governo "Disposizioni per la realizzazione del sistema integrato di interventi e servizi sociali". Prospettive Assistenziali, **30(122)** (1998) 33-40.
[10] M. Paci, Disuguaglianza, esclusione e nuova domanda di welfare state. Alcune riflessioni. In: E. Bartocci (ed.), Disuguaglianza e stato sociale. Roma: Donzelli Editore, 1996.
[11] G. Di Pasqua, L'importanza dell'ente locale per una nuova politica dei servizi sociali, in Oggidomanianziani, **8(4)** (1995) 5-11.
[12] Giunta della Regione Emilia-Romagna, Deliberazione n. 5105 del 12/10/1994, Direttiva su criteri, modalità e procedure per la contribuzione alle famiglie disponibili a mantenere l'anziano non autosufficiente nel proprio contesto. Bologna, 1994.
[13] CENSIS, *Home care per anziani. La mappa dell'offerta.* Milano: Franco Angeli, 1996.
[14] L. Colombini, anni di legislazione a favore degli anziani, in Oggidomanianziani **8(4)** (1995) 15-62.
[15] M. Dogliotti, La posizione dei parenti e dei pubblici poteri, in M. Dogliotti et al, (eds.), I malati di Alzheimer: esigenze e diritti. Torino: UTET Libreria, 1994.
[16] Ministero della Sanità - Centro Studi Tutela della salute degli anziani: materiali e indirizzi per l'attuazione del progetto-obiettivo. Roma: Istituto Poligrafico e Zecca dello Stato, 1995.
[17] M. Lucchetti and G. Lamura, G. Le politiche per la salute degli anziani in Italia, in R. Colantonio et al (eds.), Environment and Ageing: the state of research in Germany and Italy, proceedings of the 5th Meeting of the Italian Association of the "Alexander-von-Humboldt" Foundation Fellows held in Urbino on 23-24 May 1997, Milano: Guerini Editore 1998, (in press).
[18] C. Hanau, La razionalità nella scelta dell'assistenza domiciliare. *L'Assistenza Sociale,* **48(1)** (1994) 55-116.
[19] F. FabrisL'ospedalizzazione a domicilio (O.D.). *Geriatria* **9(1)** (1997) 13-18.
[20] C. Facchini, Le donne nelle solidarietà familiari. In: G. Lazzarini (ed.), Anziani e generazioni. Milano: Franco Angeli, 1994 329-341.
[21] G. Nervo, Prendersi cura degli anziani malati. *Géron*, **3(4/5)** (1993) 13-18.
[22] F. Santanera et al, Anziani malati cronici: i diritti negati. Torino: Utet Libreria, 1994.
[23] E. Abruzzese, La casa di riposo. Un caso limite di non comunicazione. In: G. Lazzarini (ed.), Anziani e generazioni. Milano: Franco Angeli: 397-411.
[24] C Scarafiotti et al, Caring activities for non self-reliant old aged and support to the families within the framework of a local geriatric assistance pattern, in Proceedings of the European Conference "What kind of legal and social protection for frail older persons? The ageing society and personal rights", held in Rome on 19-22 June. Rome, Fondazione Finney - Commission of the European Union, 1996: 296-299.
[25] A. Venchiarutti, The legal protection of disabled old people, in Proceedings of the European Conference "What kind of legal and social protection for frail older persons? The ageing society and personal rights", held in Rome 19-22 June 1996. Rome: Fondazione Finney - Commission of the European Union, 1996.
[26] F. Palmisano, "Interdiction" and "incapacitation" - The public guardian, in Proceedings of the European Conference "What kind of legal and social protection for frail older persons? The ageing society and personal rights", held in Rome 19-22 June 1996. Rome: Fondazione Finney - Commission of the European Union: 104-109.
[27] F. Corezzi, Il ridisegno della spesa sociale. Studi sul *welfare* italiano - 1° Rapporto: la previdenza. Roma: Liberetà, 1997
[28] Labos, Quartà età e non autosufficienza. Roma, Edizioni T.E.R, 1988.

[29] Comune di Ancona - Servizio Servizi Sociali ed Educativi, Normativa Socio-Assistenziale Anno 1997. Delibera Consiliare N. 176 del 17.03.1997 (unpublished manuscript).
[30] G. Abate et al, Assistenza Domiciliare Integrata (A.D.I.). Indagine conoscitiva sulla situazione nazionale. Roma: Consiglio Nazionale delle Ricerche (Progetto Finalizzato Invecchiamento) 1995.
[31] A. Banchero, L'offerta di servizi: dall'asssitenza primaria alla long-term care. In: M. Trabucchi and F. Vanara (eds.), Rapporto Sanità '98. Priorità e finanziamento del Servizio sanitario nazionale: le fragilità. Bologna: Il Mulino, 1998 315-343.
[32] P.U. Carbonin et al, Il ricorso ai servizi sanitari: risultati dello studio del Gruppo Italiano di Farmacoepidemiologia nell'Anziano (GIFA) sulle caratteristiche dell'ospedalizzazione nelle divisioni di Geriatria e di Medicina Interna in Italia, in La salute degli anziani in Italia. Atti del Convegno tenuto a Roma il 21-22 marzo 1995. Roma: CNR-Istituto di Ricerche sulla Popolazione: 1997 91-110.
[33] Redazione, La drammatica esperienza del figlio di una anziana malata cronica non autosufficiente, Prospettive Assistenziali, 119 (1997) 20-23.
[34] F. Santanera, Sancito dalla legge 4 agosto 1955 n. 692 il diritto degli anziani cronici non autosufficienti alle cure sanitarie, comprese quelle ospedaliere. Prospettive Assistenziali, 1997 119: 5-7.
[35] Redazione, La Corte di Cassazione conferma il diritto dei malati cronici alle cure sanitarie. Prospettive Assistenziali, **117** (1998) 32-34.
[36] G. Ferraro, Provvidenze legislative a favore dei mutilati ed invalidi civili, ciechi e sordomuti. Compendio informativo-statistico 1991. Roma: Ministero dell'Interno, Direzione Generale dei Servizi Civili, 1992.
[37] S. Adamo et al, Il ridisegno della spesa sociale. Studi sul *welfare* italiano. 3° rapporto: L'assistenza. Roma, Editrice Liberetà, 1997.
[38] Ministero degli Interni, Provvidenze legislative a favore dei mutilati ed invalidi civili, ciechi e sordomuti. Roma, Ministero dell'Interno, Direzione Generale dei Servizi Civili, 1988, 1991 (as well as unpublished data for following years).
[39] Ministero degli Interni, Provvidenze legislative a favore dei mutilati ed invalidi civili, ciechi e sordomuti. Roma, Ministero dell'Interno, Direzione Generale dei Servizi Civili, 1988, 1991 (as well as unpublished data for following years).
[40] Ministero degli Interni, Provvidenze legislative a favore dei mutilati ed invalidi civili, ciechi e sordomuti. Roma, Ministero dell'Interno, Direzione Generale dei Servizi Civili 1998 (unpublished data).
[41] M. Paci, La sfida della cittadinanza sociale. Roma: Edizioni Lavoro, 1990.
[42] S. Carli, Falso 1 invalido su 4: il Nord eguaglia il sud, *La Repubblica*, 25 July, 1998.
[43] E. Credendino, La società degli anziani e i diritti della persona - La relazione tra carer e anziano non autosufficiente. L'anziano come risorsa per la comunità. *La Rivista di Servizio Sociale*, **37(1)** (1997) 65-77.
[44] M. Sabbatini, Per gli anziani affido, sicuro. Il Comune **4** (1998) 32.
[45] ASI (Agenzia Sanitaria Italiana), Il testo del Piano sanitario nazionale per il triennio 1998-2000. Inserto Speciale **6(20)** (1998) I-XXIII.
[46] G. Cosmacini and C. Cenedella, *I vecchi e la cura. Storia del Pio Albergo Trivulzio*. Bari: Editori Laterza,1994.
[47] P. Vineis and E. Paci, Epidemiology and the Italian national health service. *Journal of Epidemiology and Community Health* **49** (1995) 559-562.
[48] M. Mengani, Il grado di autosufficienza degli anziani nelle Case di Riposo della Regione Marche. *Prisma* **11(32)** (1993) 1-76.
[49] C. Facchini, Gli anziani e la solidarietà tra generazioni. In: M. Barbagli and C. Saraceno (eds.), Lo stato della famiglia in Italia. Bologna: Il Mulino, (1997) 281-290.
[50] C. Glendinning and E. McLaughlin, Paying for Care: Lessons from Europe. London: Social Security Advisory Committee, HMSO, 1993.
[51] C. Renzi et al, Registro Nazionale delle Case di Riposo. *Quaderni di Volontariato* **6** (1994) 31-135.
[52] A. Bavazzano and P.G. Taiti, L'assistenza alla persona anziana non autosufficiente. *Anziani oggi* **8(1)** (1996) 11-24.
[53] L. Cataldi and R. Pace, Integrazione tra assistenza domiciliare e reti familiari per la cura degli anziani. *Giornale di Gerontologia* **45(5)** (1997) 323-332.
[54] V. Buratta and R. Crialesi, Le famiglie dei disabili: profilo socio-demografico e relazionale. *Rassegna Italiana di Sociologia* **37(3)** (1996) 477-499.
[55] J. Ditch et al, A synthesis of national family policies 1994. Heslington: European Observatory on National Family Policies (University of York), 1995.
[56] L. De Santis, Increasing the rights of carers: an initiative of the Italian Pensioners' Unions, in Proceedings of the European Conference "What kind of legal and social protection for frail older

persons? The ageing society and personal rights", held in Rome 19-22 June. Rome, Fondazione Finney - Commission of the European Union: (1996) 263-269.
[57] G. Cinque and S. Fucile, Non solo madri. *Liber&tà*, **3** (1998) 12-15.
[58] G. Lamura, Rapporto sui risultati dello studio pilota INRCA-CNR "Il ruolo della donna nell'assistenza famigliare all'anziano non autosufficiente". Ancona: INRCA (unpublished manuscript) 1997.
[59] M. Bergamaschi *et al*, Un benessere insopportabile. Identità femminile tra lavoro produttivo e lavoro di cura. Milano: Franco Angeli, 1995.
[60] R. Fontana and P. Schifano, Soggetti sociali non identificati: le turniste. *Studi Organizzativi* 18(2) (1987) 79-109.
[61] G. Lamura *et al*, (eds.), Il ruolo della donna nell'assistenza famigliare all'anziano. Rapporto di sintesi sullo studio condotto presso 69 famiglie residenti nel Comune di Senigallia (An) nel periodo novembre-dicembre 1997. Ancona: I.N.R.C.A. 1998 (in press).
[62] J. Horl, Il ruolo delle reti informali e delle organizzazioni formali nel sostegno sociale. *La ricerca sociale*, 37: 68-92.
[63] Pernigotti, L. (1994) L'anziano ammalato e la sua famiglia, in G. Lazzarini (ed) *Anziani e generazioni*. Milano: Franco Angeli, (1988) 379-395.
[64] F. Dell'Orto Garzonio and P. Taccani, *Conoscere la vecchiaia*. Roma: NIS, 1990.
[65] G. Vicarelli, Introduzione, in G. Vicarelli (ed) Familia mirabilis. Ruoli femminili e reti familiari nelle Marche degli anni Novanta. Ancona: Transeuropa, (1994) 7-16.
[66] P. David and G. Vicarelli, (eds.), *L'azienda famiglia*. Bari: Laterza, 1983.
[67] A. Florea, Vita familiare e relazionale, in ISTISSS (ed) La famiglia anziana: terza e quarta età a confronto. Roma: Ministero dell'Interno, (1994) 47-86.
[68] E. Scabini (ed.), *Famiglia e salute*. Milano: Vita e Pensiero, 1989.
[69] D. Sau, Contributo dell'operatore all'adattamento ambientale dell'anziano istituzionalizzato ed alla conservazione dei rapporti con la famiglia, In: G. Lazzarini (ed.), Anziani e generazioni, Milano: Franco Angeli, (1994) 441-446.
[70] R. Serini, Invecchiare in provincia: differenze di genere e rapporti fra generazioni. In: G. Lazzarini (ed.), Anziani e generazioni, Milano: Franco Angeli, (1994) 447-454.
[71] M. Mengani, Il servizio di assistenza domiciliare. Ancona: Il Lavoro Editoriale, 1995.
[72] N. Manzi, Volunteering and frail older persons, in Proceedings of the European Conference "What kind of legal and social protection for frail older persons? The ageing society and personal rights", held in Rome 19-22 June 1996. Rome, Fondazione Finney - Commission of the European Union: 41-51.
[73] C. Pettenati *et al*, Vademecum Alzheimer. Milano: Associazione Italiana Malattia di Alzheimer, 1997.
[74] P. Spadin, Problema della famiglia e del carico assistenziale. In: F. Marcellini *et al*, Conoscere il malato di Alzheimer. Ancona: I.N.R.C.A., 1998 25-29.
[75] P, Taccani *et al*, Gli anziani nelle strutture residenziali. Roma: Nuova Italia Scientifica, 1997.
[76] Accademia Italiana dei Medici di Famiglia - Dipartimento Italiano Medici di Famiglia - Cenacoli di Ippocrate Indagine sullo stato di salute e sul supporto ricevuto da anziani ultrasessantacinquenni. Unpublished data, 1998.
[77] C. Estes *et al*, The long term crisis. Elders trapped in the no-care zone. Newbury Park: Sage Publications, 1997.
[78] G. Giumelli, Informal caregivers e persone anziane: alcune riflessioni. *Senectus* 1(3) (1994) 9-19.
[79] C. Facchini, Women and the network of family solidarities: the Italian case. In: P. Pitaud and R. Vercauteren (eds.), Vieillir dans les villes de l'Europe du sud. Ramonville: Edition Érès, 1994 105-116.
[80] G. Lamura et al, The role of women in the family care of disabled elderly. In G.R. Andrews *et al*, (eds.), XVI World Congress of Gerontology - Book of Abstracts. Adelaide: International Association of Gerontology, 1997 599.
[81] A. Golini *et al*, scenari per il possibile sviluppo della popolazione delle regioni italiane al 2044. Roma: CNR-IRP, 1995.
[82] Istat, *Sommario storico di statistiche sulla popolazione 1951-1987*. Roma, 1990.
[83] G. Baldassarre, Il ruolo della famiglia nell'assistenza all'anziano non autosufficiente: problemi, risorse, proposte. *Giornale di Gerontologia*, **(43)6** (1995) 303-311.
[84] L. Boccacin, Gli anziani e la salute. Il sostegno delle reti familiari. *La ricerca sociale*, **43/44** (1990) 113-129.
[85] M.A. Aveni Casucci *et al*, Lavoro femminile e invecchiamento. *Giornale di Gerontologia*, **43(12)** (1995) 771-776.
[86] Istat, Famiglia, abitazioni, servizi di pubblica utilità. Indagini Multiscopo sulle famiglie. Anni 1993-1994. Roma, 1994

[87] N. Negri, Genitori e figli: egoismo, altruismo e senso del dovere in G. Lazzarini (ed) *Anziani e generazioni*. Milano: Franco Angeli, 1994, 315-328.
[88] M.G. Melchiorre and G. Vicarelli, I tempi di un centro urbano. Famiglie e servizi a Chiaravalle Chiaravalle: Amministrazione Comunale, 1995.
[89] V. Cigoli and G. Gilli, L'incontro tra famiglia e servizi. In: V. Cigoli (ed.), Il corpo famigliare. L'anziano, la malattia, l'intreccio generazionale. Milano: Franco Angeli, 1992, 235-252.
[90] M. Mengani and G. Lamura, Attività di supporto, stile di vita e salute degli assistenti informali di anziani non autosufficienti: un'analisi qualitativa. Poster presented at the 42° National Congress of the Italian Society of Geriatrics and Gerontology. Roma (book of abstracts in press) 1997.
[91] G.B. Sgritta, Famiglie e solidarietà intergenerazionale: transizione demografica o crisi politica? *Difesa Sociale*, **175(5)** (1996) 15-34.
[92] S.M. Neysmith and J. Aronson, Working conditions in home care: negotiating race and class boundaries in gendered work. *International Journal of Health Services*, **27(3)** (1997) 479-499.
[93] M.G. Melchiorre, Lavorare dove e perché. In: G. Vicarelli (ed.), Di qua e di là dal mondo. Donne straniere nelle Marche. Ancona: Istituto Gramsci, 1994 47-74.
[94] M.G. Melchiorre, Le donne immigrate. In: E. Moretti and G. Vicarelli (ed.), Una regione al bivio. Immigrati e mercato del lavoro nella Regione Marche. Ancona: Osservatorio Regionale del Mercato del Lavoro, 1997 85-151.
[95] L. Ziglio, Nuove tendenze dell'immigrazione femminile. In Proceedings of the Symposium "Le mille e una donna". Milano: Amministrazione Comunale, 1990 59-67.
[96] P. Vinay et al, Women of the South in European Integration: Problems and Prospects. Brussels: DIOTIMA, Centre for Research on Women's Issues, Commission of the European Communities, Equal Opportunities Unit, 1991.
[97] G. Barile, G. Lavoro femminile e condizione familiare. *IRER Notizie*, **36** (1990) 7-18.
[98] Istat, Rilevazione delle forze di lavoro – *Media*, Roma, 1995.
[99] Istat, Annuario Statistico Italiano, Roma, 1997.
[100] Istat, Statistiche del lavoro. Volume 26. Roma, 1986.
[101] Istat, Introducing Italy (bilingual Italian-English edition). Roma, 1995.
[102] L. Balbo, La doppia presenza. *Inchiesta*, n. 32 (monographic issue), 1978.
[103] C. Saraceno, (ed.), Il lavoro mal diviso. Bari: De Donato Editore, 1978.
[104] F. Bimbi, Gender, "gift relationship" and the welfare state cultures in Italy. In: J. Lewis (ed.), Women and Social Policies in Europe. Work, Family and the State. London, Edward Elgar Pub, 1993.
[105] G. Lamura et al, Social change and care needs in an elderly mountain rural population in Central Italy. In: G.R. Andrews et al, (eds.), XVI World Congress of Gerontology - Book of Abstracts. Adelaide: International Association of Gerontology, 1997 527-528.
[106] M. Mengani (ed.), Gli anziani in un contesto montano. Ancona: INRCA, 1995.
[107] G. Lamura et al, Disability, family support and care services: two case studies in Central Italy. In: G.R. Andrews et al, (eds.), XVI World Congress of Gerontology - Book of Abstracts. Adelaide: International Association of Gerontology, 1997 298.
[108] M. Mengani et al, Family care for the disabled elderly residing at home present and future. In: Proceedings of the European Conference "What kind of legal and social protection for frail older persons? The ageing society and personal rights", held in Rome on 19-22 June. Rome: Fondazione Finney - Commission of the European Union, 1996.
[109] R. Scortegagna, What kind of social and legal protection? In: Proceedings of the European Conference "What kind of legal and social protection for frail older persons? The ageing society and personal rights", held in Rome on 19-22 June. Rome, Fondazione Finney - Commission of the European Union, 1996 300-305.
[110] Legge Regionale n. 19 del 12 maggio, Istituzione dei Comitati consultivi misti per il controllo di qualità dal lato degli utenti, presso i presidi ospedalieri e le più rilevanti strutture sanitarie non ospedaliere. Bologna: Consiglio Regionale della Regione Emilia-Romagna, 1994.
[111] S. Lucarini et alValutazione del fabbisogno di nursing infermieristico e tutelare in residenza protetta mediante la scala A.GE.D. (Assessment of Geriatric Disability). *Giornale di gerontologia*, **45(3/4)** (1996) 246.
[112] C. Hanau and E. Pipitone, Analisi della domanda di cure domiciliari in tre U.S.S.L. di Milano. Quaderni di Cure Paliiative, (4) (in press), 1998.
[113] D. Cucinotta et al, Proposta e validazione di un semplice indice per la valutazione funzionale globale dell'anziano, il G.E.F.I. Giornale di Gerontologia, **37(1)** (1989) 31-36.
[114] S. French et al, Assistenza Domiciliare Integrata nel Sanvitese: confronto per sesso secondo il grado e il tipo di autonomia. *Epidemiologia & Prevenzione*, **20(2-3)** (1996) 263-264.

[115] D. Cucinotta et al, La valutazione multidimensionale geriatrica. *Giornale di Gerontologia*, **45(10)** (1997) 641-644.
[116] g. Abate, Trial clinico controllato su efficacia ed utilità dell'Assistenza Domicialiare Integrata (A.D.I.). Mauale di istruzione. Chieti: Università degli Studi, 1993.
[117] F. Lattanzio et al, Valutazione multidimensionale. Strumenti di seconda generazione. Anziani Oggi, **9(1)** (1997) 11-32.
[118] P. Morosini et al, VALGRAF: una nuova soluzione grafica per la valutazione longitudinale dello stato funzionale degli anziani ricoverati in rreparti per lungodegenti e in case protette. Giornale di Gerontologia, **40(4)** (1992) 111-118.
[119] L. Ferrucci et al, Dagli studi epidemiologici alla messa a punto degli strumenti di valutazione. In: Comune di Dicomano (ed.), Gli anziani a casa: uno studio a Dicomano. Firenze: Alpha Libri, 1993 79-96.
[120] F. Fabris et al, La cartella clinica geriatrica. Una proposta di valutazione funzionale multidimensionale. *Minerva Medica*, **80** (Suppl. 1 to n. 12) (1989) 1-56.
[121] O. Zanetti et al, Depressione e stress in 103 caregiver di pazienti affetti da malattia di Alzheimer. *Giornale di Gerontologia*, **45(3/4)** (1997) 294.
[122] R. Rozzini and M. Trabucchi, Epidemioogia della depressione nell'anziano. Giornale di Gerontologia, **44(2)** (1996) 103-110.
[123] E. Antonini et al, La scala di depressione geriatrica. In: Comune di Dicomano (ed.), Gli anziani a casa: uno studio a Dicomano. Firenze: *Alpha Libri*, 1993 79-96.
[124] A. Vespa et al, Relazione tra depressione, senso di solitudine, fattori sociali e malattia negli anziani. *Geriatria*, **8(3)** (1996) 213-218.
[125] J.G. Greene, Measuring behavioural disturbance of elderly demented patients in the community and its effects on relatives: a factor analytic study. *Age and Ageing*, **11** (1982) 121-126.
[126] L. Bartorelli, L'assistenza all'anziano demente. *Giornale di Gerontologia*, **45(9)** (1997) 599-604.
[127] R. Fabrello et al, Stress del caregiver nell'assistenza del soggetto anziano non autosufficiente di sesso femminile, a domicilio. *Giornale di Gerontologia*, **45(3/4)** (1997) 296.
[128] R. Girardello et al, Implicazioni psicologiche nell'assistenza a domicilio di anziane non autosufficienti: correlazione con il numero di figli. *Giornale di Gerontologia*, **45(3/4)** (1997) 266.
[129] R.J.V. Montgomery et al, Caregiving and the experience of subjective and objective burden. *Family Relations*, **34** (1985) 19-26.
[130] J.S. Norbeck et al, The development of an instrument to measure social support, *Nursing Research*, **30** (1981) 264-269.
[131] C. Conti, Le scale di valutazione in psichiatria. Caratteristiche generali. Torino: UTET Libreria, 1995.
[132] J. Liang, Dimensions of the Life Satisfaction Index A: A structural formulation. *Journal of Gerontology*, **39** (1984) 613-622.
[133] P. Leonardi (ed.), Curare nella differenza. Psicoterapie del disagio femminile. Milano: Franco Angeli, 1995.
[134] P. Leonardi, Depressione e differenze di genere: interventi al femminile. *Epidemilogia & Prevenzione*, **20**(2-3) (1996) 255-257.
[135] I. Paoletti, Caring for older people: a gendered practice. Paper presented at the International Sociological Association (ISA) Conference, Montreal, 27 July- 3rd August, 1998.
[136] I. Paoletti, A half life: Women caregivers of older disabled relatives. *Journal of Women and Ageing*, (in press) 1999.
[137] M.G. Ory, International perspectives on the establishment aqnd evaluation of dementia special care units (SCUs). In: G.R. Andrews et al, (eds.), XVI World Congress of Gerontology - Book of Abstracts. Adelaide: International Association of Gerontology, 1997.
[138] R. Rozzini, L'assistenza alle persone affette da demenza. *Giornale di Gerontologia*, **44**(10/11) (1996) 705-710.
[139] Centro Alzheimer Per non dimenticare. Ancona: Centro Disturbi della Memoria e Malattia di Alzheimer INRCA (brochure), 1998.
[140] Redazione, La relazione conclusiva della Commissione Onofri su previdenza, sanità e assistenza. Prospettive Assistenziali, **118** (1997) 24-31.
[141] G. Lamura and M. Mengani, M. La nuova "assicurazione sociale dell'assistenza" tedesca. *La Rivista di Servizio Sociale*, **35**(3) (1995) 33-47.
[142] B. Grossi, I cambiamenti in atto nel Servizio Sanitario Nazionale. In: M. Trabucchi and F. Vanara (eds.) ,Rapporto Sanità '98. Priorità e finanziamento del Servizio sanitario nazionale: le fragilità. Bologna: Il Mulino, 1998 25-81.
[143] I. Gennaro, Definition for a "Home without walls", in Proceedings of the European Conference "What kind of legal and social protection for frail older persons? The ageing society and personal rights", held

in Rome 19-22 June 1996. Rome, Fondazione Finney - Commission of the European Union:, 1996 258-262.
[144] B.J. Coleman, European models of long-term care in the home and community. *International Journal of Health Services,* **25(3)** (1995) 455-474.
[145] B. Barbero AvanziniFamiglia e servizi sociali. Milano: Franco Angeli, 1994.
[146] F. Piangerelli, Assistenza domiciliare, si cambia. *Corriere Adriatico*, 2 September, 1998.
[147] A. Florea and E. Credendino, Old aged families and carers. Support services and protection programs: the project of Fondazione Finney, in Proceedings of the European Conference "What kind of legal and social protection for frail older persons? The ageing society and personal rights", held in Rome 19-22 June 1996.
[148] P. Vinay, Mutamento e continuità: i caratteri di una regione. In: G. Vicarelli (ed.) Famiglia mirabilis. Ruoli femminili e reti familiari nelle Marche degli anni Novanta. Ancona: Transeuropa/Saggi, 1994. 17-41.
[149] C.L. Jenkins, Women, Work, and Caregiving: How Do These Roles Affect Women's Well-Being? *Journal of Women and Ageing*, **9(3)** (1997) 27-45.
[150] M.G. Secchi and G. Andreini, Servizi presenti, servizi possibili. In: P. Taccani (ed.), Dentro la cura. Famiglie e anziani non autosufficienti. Milano: Franco Angeli, 1994 217-246.
[151] L. Dennerstein, Mental Health, Work, and Gender. *International Journal of Health Services,* **3** (1995) 503-509.
[152] B. Murphey *et al*, Women with Multiple Roles: The Emotional Impact of Caring for Ageing Parents. *Ageing and Society*, **17(3)** (1997) 277-291.
[153] A. L. Fadiga Zanatta and M.L. Mirabile Demografia, Famiglia e Società. Come cambiano le donne. Roma: Ediesse Editrice, 1993.
[154] P.U. Carbonin *et al*, Gli insuccessi delle politiche sanitarie per l'anziano e la crisi della Sanità nei Paesi Sviluppati. *Difesa Sociale*, **73(2)** (1994) 135-162. Rome, Fondazione Finney - Commission of the European Union: 231-235.

Chapter 6

The Netherlands
(February 2000)

Susan G.M. Adam
Nivel – Netherlands Institute of Primary Care
P O Box 1568
3500 BN Utrecht
The Netherlands

Jack B.F. Hutten
Nivel – Netherlands Institute of Primary Care
P O Box 1568
3500 BN Utrecht
The Netherlands

Introduction

Like most other Western European countries, the Netherlands has been confronted with a steady increase of the number of older people in its population. The percentage of inhabitants aged at least 65 grew from 12.8 in 1990 to 13.5% in 1999[1]. Compared to other countries, this development started relatively late: most member states of the European Union already passed this last percentage in 1990 [2]. According to De Boer [3] this implicates that Dutch health care and social services have been less markedly confronted with a sharp rise in demand from older people. Therefore services have remained of high quality, covering a broad range of facilities. Vollering [4] and Giarchi [5] also concluded that the availability of services for the elderly is rather complete and comprehensive in the Netherlands compared to a lot of other European Countries. However, the demographic differences mentioned above will be reduced in the coming decades. Therefore, the structure and availability of services for older people in the Netherlands are currently discussed and reconsidered.

This section provides a rough outline of the position of older people and their family carers in Dutch society. The emphasis is mainly laid on the general policies towards these groups.

Background

In general an ageing society has important implications for the amount and types of health and social services needed, e.g. because of an increase of morbidity, especially chronic conditions and co-morbidity [6]. Furthermore, the potential of informal care providers, such as family members and friends, has decreased in the Netherlands during the last years [7,8]. Smaller families, a higher participation of women on the labour market, an increasing number of single elderly and changing attitudes on living conditions, family relations and privacy are the main causes. As a consequence the appeal to professional services will rise.

Besides a quantitative growth of the demand for health and social services, the type of care that is needed is also expected to change [9]. On the one hand, because of an ageing population a shift is taken place from more medical technical curative services towards more social and care-oriented services such as personal assistance with, e.g. bathing and dressing, cooking and other housekeeping activities, and social activities. This means that a broader range of services is required: a mixture of social and health care services provided at home or within the community. On the other hand, more specialised technical nursing activities are required, e.g. for specific groups of chronically ill and pain-relief for terminal ill patients (palliative care). This last development is enforced by the introduction of new technologies which can be used in a home care setting and as a consequence more severe cases can be cared for at home.

Simultaneously with a strong increase of their number, the social position of older people is changing. In the near future most older people will have a higher level of education and their personal financial resources will improve. This means that a larger group of relatively affluent older people will be able to arrange their own care and services. Furthermore, there is a growing recognition of the government and politicians of the need to give voice to service users such as disabled and older people [10]. The empowerment of these groups, e.g. by the foundation of users' organisations, is an important tendency in the Dutch society. They demand a high quality of care which imposes a greater burden on all (professionals) caregivers.

In sum, we can say that in Dutch policies a shift is taken place from 'a service-oriented' approach towards a 'person-centred' approach. This means that not the availability of services but the demands of patients or clients steer the care that is provided [11]. In this way services need to change and care must be tailored to the individual needs of each patient taken into account their personal circumstances, lifestyle and financial situation. Also De Boer [3] identified the policy aspiration to provide a 'tailored service delivery' for older people. This can be reached by further privatisation, decentralisation and separation of housing and care.

Policy and practice towards older people and their family carers

Services for older people in the Netherlands are mainly provided by private non-profit organisations and, to a lesser extent, by some public organisations. They operate within the legal and policy framework that is developed by the government.

Since the late 1970s the policy makers have been focussed on the goal to let older people live as long as possible in their own houses or social environment. However some difficulties occurred to reach this goal. In 1994 the advisory commission on the modernisation of the care for older people (*Commissie Modernisering Ouderenzorg*) published their report *Ouderenzorg met toekomst* (Care for older people with future). Central in this report were the problems concerning the relation between living and care facilities and the necessity to cut back the costs of residential services for the elderly (mainly the old people's homes). The commission listed the most important bottle necks in the care for older people. Firstly, although there are possibilities to reduce some expenditures, people have to be aware that, because of the increasing number of elderly in the Dutch population, an increase in the public expenditure for care is necessary.

Secondly, there are severe problems and obstacles in maintaining elderly people as long as possible in their own houses or social environment: houses are often not adapted for the special needs of the elderly and there are some serious (financial) problems to provide the amount of home care that is required.

Furthermore, the commission stressed that, though most elderly want to stay in their own home as long as possible, they will not do that at any price. At least a part of the elderly will, also in future, choose to live in an old people's home when necessary. It is predicted that the percentage of older people living in those homes will not change in the future. Finally, because of the large amount of care providers, care is fragmented which can affect the efficiency, quality and continuity of care.

The commission's recommendations are elaborated in two policy documents which are recently published: *Zicht op Zorg* (View on Care) and *Zorgnota 2000*. In these documents the government proposes some radical changes in the organisation and financing of care for older people. As mentioned the main policy goal is to give the clients or patients the central position in the care system. This is expressed in the four principals:

- The main starting-point is the self-determination of clients: older people themselves are basically responsible for their own situation. Therefore they have to be taken seriously by professional care providers, their independence and privacy have to be respected, and the older people themselves should decide what kind of service they need. If an old person is unable to make these decisions, an agent should take over to defence the interest of that person. If possible, this should be the informal carer who is most involved in the daily care of the old person.

- Professional services need to be focussed on the support of the older people in his/her own existence. Professional care providers should not take over the responsibilities but should start at the abilities of an individual which are still available.
- The care system must take into account the individual diversity: all people are different and live in different conditions. This means that the available services also should be divers and flexible.
- A justified allocation of available resources is required. Therefore support and care should be provided regardless the person's position or, e.g. income.

To reach these objectives, the Dutch care system needs to be modernised in many respects.

Decentralisation and regionalisation

The government realises that needs of older people can only be met by a further decentralisation of responsibilities and authorities. At a regional level, services can be planned more adequately and they can more easily be confronted with the needs of the elderly population. Concretely, the Netherlands is recently divided into a number of regions and in each region a so called *Zorgkantoor* (Care Office)[1] is situated. The idea is that each Care Office will become responsible for all the care in its region that is financed through the AWBZ[2]. The Care Offices must negotiate with and contract professional care providers. The government expects that this will have a positive influence on the cost containment and the quality of the care that is provided.

Co-operation and co-ordination

Extended coherence in the social and health care system needs to be facilitated by a further financial integration of different services and the promotion of co-operation, communication and co-ordination in the provision of care. Although the process of harmonisation of the financing and organisation of services in the Netherlands is developing more quickly compared to other European countries, still a number of financial and organisational boundaries between services need to be broken down. A concrete policy measure is, e.g. that from 2001 all old people's homes will be financed through the AWBZ-act in the same way as nursing homes and home care services. Another important development in this respect is the formation of so-called *Zorgketens* (Chains of Care). These are regional co-operations of different care providing organisations which work together on formalised or institutionalised basis.

The policy goals mentioned above not only affect the organisational and financing structure of the care system but have also significant consequences for the kind of care that is provided. The shift from institutional forms of care towards cheaper home or community based services and 'informal care' (voluntary care as well as family care) will be continued.

Financing

A justified allocation of the available resources implies policy measures regarding cost containment and a stronger call for efficiency in the provision of services. The Dutch government wants to change the current situation where 'money follows the provision of care' into a situation where 'care follows the money'. In this respect two radical developments in the financing system can be mentioned. Firstly, the traditional 'lump sum' - financing system, in which care organisations received a fixed budget based on characteristics of their catchment area, will be replaced by an 'output' -financed system, in the year 2001. Secondly, the Personal Budget-scheme that is introduced in 1996 will be extended. In this scheme clients receive a personal budget instead of actual care. With this budget the clients themselves are able to buy the care they need and choose their own care provider.

Since the beginning of the 1990s, attempts are made to introduce market strategies, such as competition, in health care to improve flexibility and efficiency in the provision of services. It is mainly implemented in the Dutch home care system where several new commercial or for-profit agencies entered the 'market'. However, some questionable effects on the accessibility and quality of the services appeared. The competition between the new agencies and the traditional home care services was considered as unfair. Commercial organisations were not obliged to provide the whole broad package of services and could select their own clients. Furthermore, there were important differences in personnel management (e.g. with regard to salaries and training) and the involvement of the organisations in quality assurance activities. As a consequence a complex market was established which did not improve but, more likely, threatened the independent position of the clients. Therefore, the Dutch government was forced to interfere. In 1998 the entrance of new home care organisations was temporarily frozen. All existing organisations must meet the same criteria regarding the accessibility and quality of care. This means that the opportunities for competition in the provision of home care are strongly reduced.

Reducing waiting lists

An important problem in the implementation of the new policy towards older people in the Netherlands are the available resources. Nowadays long waiting lists exist for most of the services. They are caused by budget problems and shortage of staff. The financial resources are already too low and do not fully take into account the increasing demands. Qualified personnel is difficult to find because of the relatively bad image of the sector (low status, poorly paid) and the increasing number of people who want to work on a part-time basis.

Recently, some clients on a waiting list for home help services took the matter to court. The independent judge decided that they have a legal right to these services and that the responsible organisations, in this case the Care Offices, are obliged to arrange these services. The Dutch government has given high priority to the reduction of waiting lists. This can be reached by expanding the amount of services, improving the efficiency in the provision of care and providing more adequate information about waiting lists to the clients. Furthermore, it is essential that the problem should be solved at a regional level.

Assessment

Another policy tool to strengthen the position of older people in the care system and to allocate the available resources is the new assessment system which is introduced in 1998. In this new system the assessment of the needs of older people is, in general, no longer the responsibility of the professional care providers as it was before. Nowadays there are 85 *RIO's (regionale indicatieorganen*: Regional Assessment Organisations) in the Netherlands which assess the needs of people with regard to all caring facilities such as home care, old people's homes and nursing homes. An important difference with the old situation is that the assessment may not be steered by the availability of services. It should be an objective, comprehensive and independent judgement of the actual needs of older people.

Informal care

As mentioned the Dutch government recognises the importance of informal or family carers, especially for the care of frail elderly with chronic conditions and physical or mental restrictions. 'Informal care' facilitates the autonomy of older people: they can stay in their own house and will be less independent on professional health and social services. It has also important financial consequences. The ministry of health [11] stated that the public expenditure on care for the elderly is limited because most care is provided by people in the direct social environment of older people. It is important to mention that children do not have a formal obligation to take care of their parents as in some other European countries. Therefore, special attention must be given to the strengthening and support of family carers.

In the next section the most important available professional services supporting older people will be described. The third section gives more information about the position, problems and supporting facilities of family carers. An accurate assessment of actual needs of older people and their family carers is an important condition to provide care and support. In section four the new assessment system will be presented. In the fifth section the actual provision of care to older people and their family carers be more explicit by the description of three standardised cases. Finally, in the last section the future developments will be discussed.

Health and Social Care for Older People: Structures and Functions

The Netherlands has established a complete and comprehensive system of health and social services for its population of older people. It contains a wide range of 'community-based' as well as institutional or residential services and facilities. Because of the process of substitution of care, emphasis is laid on the further development of services situated in the direct social environment of older people. More tasks have moved from institutions to care providers situated in the community. Furthermore, there is an ongoing process of integration, co-ordination, and co-operation between services. This process occurs within the health and social care systems separately as well as between these two systems. As a consequence, the structure and functions of the services are likely to change.

In this section information will be presented about the most important health and social services for old people: primary health care (general practice and home care), institutional services, day care facilities and social support.

Primary health care

The Netherlands has a well developed system of primary health care with two core services: general practice and home care. These two services are separately organised and financed. But General Practitioners (GPs) and e.g. community nurses co-operate in daily practice.

Furthermore, some allied health services are part of the primary health care system such as physiotherapists and dieticians. Moreover, mental health care for older people is mainly the responsibility of mental health advisory services (RIAGG). GPs can refer their clients to them if they need help.

General practice

One of the main characteristics of the Dutch health care system is the strong central position of GPs. Almost all inhabitants are registered at a general practice, the so-called list system, and specialist or hospital care is only accessible after a referral by a GP. The position of Dutch GPs can be compared with those in the UK and Denmark: gatekeeper, fixed lists, working in independent practice (no fixed salary). The average list size in the Netherlands is 2300.

About less than half of the GPs work in single handed practice, 10% work in multidisciplinary health cares and the remaining in partnerships or group practices. The number of GPs in single handed practice is expected to drop in the near future.

Because of GPs' central role in the Dutch health care system, they are the most important physician providing health care to older people. The GP is responsible for those who are living in their own houses as well as those living in old people's homes. Only older people in nursing homes (almost 3% of the people aged 65 or more, in 1998) are not the responsibility of the GP but of special nursing home doctors.

Because patients have to be referred to specialist care by a GP, he or she can co-ordinate, guide and monitor the care for a specific patient. The Dutch Association of General Practitioners (LHV) stresses the importance of the GP for the older population. According to them, common chronic conditions such as Diabetes type II, COPD and Rheumatism must to be treated and monitored in general practice. The Dutch College of General Practitioners (NHG) has developed a number of standards of care. In these standards guidelines for good treatment and practice are formulated. There are standards which are especially relevant for elderly people. It is, however, very difficult to meet these standards in the daily practice, e.g. due to the high workload of Dutch GPs. A possible solution for this problem is the recent introduction of practice nurses[3] in general practice. Their main task will be to perform periodical checks of people with chronic conditions.

In principle GPs could play an important role in the support of the family carers of older people. Because of their co-ordinating function, GPs could gain a general overview of the particular needs of family carers. However, there is no empirical data available to verify to what extent they are actually involved in these matters.

Home care

Home care is a very important part of the care for older people. In the Netherlands the term Home care is used for all professional types of care, help and support delivered by nurses or home helps to sick, disabled, frail and/or older people in their own homes or those of relatives. In its essence it contains nursing, caring and housekeeping activities.

In 1998 almost 600.000 people received some kind of home care: most of them (80%) were aged 65 or over. On average they received almost 3.5 hours of care per [11].

Since the beginning of the 1990s the structures and functions of these services have changed strongly. In nearly all regions in the Netherlands, the former regional home nursing or cross association and the regional organisation for home help services merged into one regional home care organisation. However the relation and co-operation between home nursing and home help services still varies between regions. Some home care organisations already operate so called integrated teams which provide integrated care (health and social care) to avoid overlap between the services of home nurses and home helps. Others only merged at an organisational level but operate two separate departments for the two kinds of services. As mentioned in section 1, new private agencies entered the 'market' and started to provide certain home care services.

Consequently, there is now a variety of organisations providing home care in the Netherlands. Most, but certainly not all, belong to one of the two umbrella organisations that exist: the National Association for Home Care (LVT) and the Branch-organisation for Home Care in the Netherlands (BTN). The first consists of traditional public home care organisations, while the new (non)profit organisations are mainly members of the latter. The umbrella organisations promote the interests of its members in e.g. collective bargaining with government and insurance companies, and play a crucial role in the implementation of quality assurance activities in the sector.

Home nursing care

Legally all residents of the Netherlands are entitled to receive home nursing care which can be reached 24-hours-a-day and care can be delivered in the evenings, nights and weekends if necessary. Patients are entitled to a maximum amount of nursing care at home: 2.5 hours a day or three visits a day, for an unlimited period of time. Patients who need more intensive home nursing for a limited period of time, mostly terminal care or patients who are waiting for admission to a nursing home, can make an appeal to additional home care.

In general, three types of nurses work in home care [12]. Community nurses (*Wijkverpleegkundigen*) have had either four years of higher vocational training or 3.5 years in-service training in a hospital with another two years of intermediate vocational training. Nurses in the community (*Verpleegkundigen in de wijk*) have had 3.5 years in-service training in a hospital to become a registered nurse but did not have additional training in community nursing. And, finally, auxiliary community nurses (*Wijkziekenverzorgenden*) who either had two years in-service training in a hospital or nursing home and a six-month course in community nursing or three years intermediate vocational training in nursing. Community nurses are considered as first level nurses and nurses in the community and auxiliary community nurses as second level nurses. Community nurses can perform a wide range of tasks such as hygienic and other personal care (e.g. bathing, help with lavatory, help with activities of daily living), routine technical nursing procedures (such as injections, dressings, stoma care, bladder washout), more complicated technical nursing (e.g. epidural anaesthesia, handling respirator, catheterisation), patient education, psychosocial activities, and involvement in the evaluation of care. Auxiliary nurses are also qualified to perform most of these tasks, except more complicated technical nursing procedures and the evaluation of care. In addition, auxiliaries more often provide hygiene care and give less often psychosocial support. Furthermore, all types of nurses are involved in the support and stimulation of care provided by the partner, other family members or informal carers.

Home help services

The home help service is officially defined as "help of a domestic and caring nature, occasionally supplemented by help of a personal and supporting nature, offered to all inhabitants of the Netherlands who need at least help of a domestic nature related to illness, recovery, old age, handicap, death, psychosocial, and personal problems that threaten the maintenance of the household". Its objectives are to support families and individuals in need and enable them to live as independently as possible [13].

Home help services are performed by home helps with a variety of qualifications and, therefore, a wide range of different tasks and responsibilities [12,14].

Officially, unqualified home helps (*ongediplomeerd helpenden*) are only allowed to do the housework like cleaning the home, washing dishes, washing and ironing. Qualified home helps (*gediplomeerd helpenden*) do the housekeeping and some caring tasks as far as they can not be done by the members of the household, like bathing, help with lavatory, and providing general and family support like shopping, take for a walk, administrative support (filling in forms). Qualified home carers (*gediplomeerd verzorgenden*) mainly carry out hygiene and personal care, some housekeeping activities, they organise the household and they provide support in case of psychosocial problems. Finally, specialised home carers (*gespecialiseerde gezinsverzorgenden*) support households with multiple complex problems. Also the support and stimulation of the informal carers of an older person is considered as an important part of the work of specialised or qualified home helps or carers.

Residential services and housing facilities

Dutch residential services and institutional care are considered as one of the best in Europe [5]. There is a wide variety of residential services such as: nursing homes, old people's homes, sheltered housing and service flats. There is a long tradition in these kinds of services and therefore, the number of older people living in residential services was, for a long period of time, one of the highest in Europe. The next table shows that the percentage of older people living in an old people's home has dropped dramatically in the past years, especially in the age group 65-79.

Table 1. Percentage of people aged 65 or more living in an old people's home in the Netherlands

Age Group	1985	1990	1995	1997	1998
65-69 yrs	0.6	0.4	0.3	0.3	0.2
70-74	2.3	1.5	1.1	1.0	0.9
74-79	7.1	5.2	3.8	3.3	3.0
80-84	18.0	14.6	11.4	10.5	9.8
85-89	32.4	29.8	25.1	23.2	22.2
90-94		44.7	40.9	38.1	37.1
95+		49.6	51.6	50.6	50.4
Total	**7.7**	**6.7**	**5.7**	**5.3**	**5.1**

These figures show that especially people in the oldest age groups live in an old people's home.

Furthermore, although the percentage of older people with chronic diseases and co-morbidity is increasing, the percentage living in nursing homes remained constant over the last ten years (between 2.5% and 3.0%) [11].

As a result, institutional services are more focussed on the care of real frail older people instead of relatively healthy old people as they did some years [15].

Most people in residential services are older than 75 years. About half of the people aged 90 or more, live in a nursing home or old people's home [11].

Old people's homes

As mentioned the number of old people's homes has decreased and they more or less lost their original functions. They are mainly run by private foundations. The inhabitants have their own private (small) rooms and there are a lot of common facilities such as small shops, a hairdresser, pedicure and a wide range of recreational activities.

Many homes have special accommodation on the premises for self-reliant older people who need help occasionally [12]. The number of these so-called *aanleunwoningen* has increased markedly during the past decade. The elderly living in this type of sheltered housing run an independent household, but are able to use certain facilities and services provided by the old people's homes [16].

Nursing homes

Nursing homes (*Verpleeghuizen*) have an important position in the health care system in the Netherlands [17]. They provide long-term intensive care for somatic and psycho-geriatric older people with multiple pathology, disabilities and handicaps. There are three types of nursing homes: those for somatic patients, those for psycho-geriatric patients, and combined type with separate wards for both categories. The latter is most common and its number is expected to increase in the near future [18]. More than 95% of the nursing homes are private non-profit organisations; the remaining 5% is owned and run by municipalities.

Medical care is provided by specialised nursing home physicians with an average ratio of one full-time doctor per 100 beds. Nursing staff consist mainly (85%) of so called level B auxiliary nurses. Furthermore some allied health professionals are employed such as physiotherapists, occupational therapists, speech therapists, activity or recreational therapists, psychologists, dieticians, and social workers [17]. There are also volunteers working in nursing homes, mainly involved in social care and activities [18].

Nursing homes provide care in a clinical as well as an ambulatory setting. In 1997, 77% of the nursing homes also delivered day care [19]. Other relatively new provisions that can be mentioned are night admissions, weekend and day treatment, respite care, crisis intervention and the consultative task of the nursing home doctor towards old people's homes and primary health care staff.

The focus on the self-determination of older people stresses the need to improve the privacy of people living in nursing homes. The number of patients per room dropped in the last years, but still a large majority of patients have to share their room with at least two other people.

The original purpose of old people's homes was to offer an adequate living environment to those among the older people who can only manage on their own with difficulty. Because of the stricter admission criteria of old people's homes and also because of the fact that residents require more intensive care, the difference between the populations of both types of organisations is fading. Therefore, they are now in a transformation process to merge into a new type of organisation.

Day care facilities

Like in most of the other countries, day care facilities for the elderly in the Netherlands have increased during the past decade. There are organisations or centres which are focussed on leisure activities. Day care for frail elderly is provided in nursing homes, old people's homes and specific facilities, e.g. for demented elderly.

Social services

Community or social care such as meals-on-wheels, special transport services, leisure activities and all kinds of other support facilities, is mainly the responsibility of the local authorities. However, the actual provision of these kinds of services is mainly done by voluntary organisations. A lot of the social services are provided through neighbourhood centres (*wijk- en buurtcentra*) which are mostly part of the general social and community work: e.g. providing meals, leisure activities etc. In some areas these services are provided by the old people's homes in so called '*huiskamer-projecten*' (living room-projects). Furthermore, there are organisations related to church which are also active in areas of the general care for the elderly. They are mainly financed through governmental subsidies and private contributions.

Roles of Family Carers of Older People Living at Home

Introduction

As mentioned in the first section, demographic developments will alter the amount and type of care that old people need. Furthermore, it is concluded that the role of informal care will become of great importance in the near future. Informal care can be divided in family care and care provided by voluntary workers. Family care includes help and support to sick, disabled, frail and/or older people by family members, neighbours and other people of their social network. In contrast, voluntary help is help provided by people who did not have a social relationship with the dependent person [20]. In this section more insight will be given in the role, problems and supporting facilities of family carers. This means that the other forms of informal care are left aside.

Family care in historical perspective

Social support has always been very important in Dutch society. After the second world war a period of reconstruction followed. Policy was concentrated on income and housing. The population was increasing very fast and there was also a housing shortage. In those years, the first residential homes for older people were built. Elderly were stimulated to go to live in a home for the elderly, partly to make room for families with young children (during the general housing shortage). There was quickly a steep increase in the number of older people being accommodated in those homes.

The 1970s was the decade when economic decline set in. The welfare agenda changed from a supply system with an open-ended budget to a cost-oriented system. Policy was oriented on a decrease of the growth of the number of residential homes. Social services were decentralised and the substitution of institutional care for community care increased efficiency [15,21].

Since the middle of the 1970s, as a consequence of the increasing number of elderly and financial problems for the Dutch government, informal care became very important [19]. Before that time, no special attention was paid to informal care, like family care. However, the government realised that the number of older people would increase very fast and very strong in the near future, with financial consequences. Therefore, government policies were more and more focussed on home care and informal care instead of institutional care. Cheaper alternatives of professional care were developed and special attention was and is still given to enforce and support informal care. Since the middle of the 1980s informal care is fully accepted and is generally established [22].

However, although the need for informal care was increasing, there were important changes in society that affected the availability of family care such as the reduction in the average family size, the growth of the number of single older people, and the development that family members and friends live at larger distances from each other [23-25]. Furthermore, more women are participating on the labour market. In 1995, 49% of women between 20 and 64 years of age had a job outside their homes. It is estimated that this percentage will raise between 63 and 73% in 2020 [26]. It is also expected that the wishes of older people are changing. They prefer to stay independently as long as possible and do not want any interference with their private lives or cause someone inconvenience.

In sum, it can be concluded that on the one hand family care will have a more important role in the care for older people. On the other hand the potential of family care is expected to decline in the near future.

The next part of this section describes who receive family care, who the family carers are, the kind of care they provide and the problems they experience. Furthermore it describes possible solutions and developments for the future.

Who receive family care?

It is estimated that 11% of the Dutch population older than 6 years (1.5 million people) have problems with regard to personal and/or domestic care. This does not mean that they are all in need of care or support. About 500.000 persons have a severe disability and as a consequence they do need care. This group of dependent, frail people includes relatively more women and older persons. However approximately 25% of the people who need care are younger than 44 years (De Boer et al., 1994). Persons with a more severe disability more often receive professional care. In addition, the role of family carers remains of great importance (De Boer et al., 1994).

Of the people needing help at home, 80% receives informal help [5]. More than 50% of them only receive informal help [23].

The chance to receive care from a family carer is highly related to the living conditions of the older person. People who live with a spouse or their children are more likely to be supported by a family carer than people who live alone. The next table presents figures about the living conditions of older people in 1998.

Table 2. Living conditions of older people in the Netherlands, in 1998 (in percentages)*

Living	
Alone	44%
With spouse, without children	51%
With spouse and children	2%
With children, without spouse	3%

* Own calculation based on CBS [27].

What kind of care is provided?

Family care can be divided in three types of care, namely emotional care, personal care and domestic care. Examples of emotional care are keeping someone company and showing interest in someone. Personal care is related to activities which include physical intimacy like washing and dressing and helping someone to go to the toilet. Domestic care includes housekeeping activities like cleaning, cooking, washing and shopping.

In the Netherlands, personal care and domestic care are the types of care which are most often provided by family carers [23,28]. Exact allocation between services is not clear. On the one hand research showed that approximately 66% of family care consists of domestic care and 33% (also) consists of personal care [23]. On the other hand research [29] showed that carers most often provide emotional support (41%). Domestic care was given in 18% of the cases and personal care was given less often (2%).

Who provides family care?

The number of people who provide family care is high. Approximately 1,3 million people (11% of the adults) regularly provide family care to sick, disabled, frail and/or older people [28,30,31]. Family care is given by family members like spouses, children (in law), brothers/sisters and other family members, neighbours, friends and acquaintances. Although family carers are a heterogeneous group, most care is provided by spouses and children [25,32].

The various carers provide different kinds of care. Roughly a distinction can be made between partners, children and other people who provide care. Furthermore men and women provide different kinds of care.

Most of the caring tasks are still performed by women [28]. Of all family carers about 70% is female [29]. 15% of all women older than 16 years of age provides family care. The percentage of men in this age group who provide care is lower, namely 7%. From this we can conclude that about twice as much women compared to men provide family care. An explanation for this may be the traditional role pattern in which women are carers and men are breadwinners. Furthermore most women (68%) in the Netherlands have part-time jobs [33]. However, research showed that people who work part-time not always provide more often family care than people who work full-time [23]. Men who care for their spouse provide all kinds of care. However, other men (mostly sons) more often provide domestic care, like doing the shopping, and administrative tasks such as filling in forms. In general, those activities are more often provided by men than by women [25].

As mentioned there are not only differences between men and women in providing family care but also between the various types of carers, like partners, children and other people.

Family care internal to the home is most often provided by partners and care external to the home is primarily provided by daughters (children): 44% of the family carers are daughters (in-law) and 24% are partners [31].

Care which is provided by partners is equally provided by women and men [34]. They are mostly the primary caregiver and provide all kinds of care: personal, emotional and domestic care. Mostly they do not experience giving care as family care. They take it for granted [32,34] and they consider it is a part of their lives to care for their spouse [24]. In general, they provide intensive care and they receive less help or support from others [34].

Research showed that 70% of the partners experience the care they provide as heavily. The care which is provided by them is more difficult than the care provided by daughters or other carers. Furthermore, partners often suffer from a poor health themselves because they are often at an advanced age. For those people it is not always easy to provide (intensive) care.

Domestic care is most often provided by children, mainly by daughters and daughters-in-law [22,32]. Daughters often feel obliged to care for their parents (mostly their mother) [34].

Other family carers like brothers and sisters of the older person provide personal, emotional and domestic care [31]. Almost 75% of these carers are female [34].

Problems of family carers

As mentioned many older dependent people receive help on a structural base. They often need extensive care. Therefore, many carers are under considerable stress; psychological, physical and/or financial [24,25]. Research by Van der Lyke [22] showed that a part of the family carers feel depressed, have a poor health, are chronically tired and/or live in social isolation [22]. Several factors are responsible for the extent of stress, like the health status of the caregiver and the relationship between the dependent person and the caregiver. Providing care may also lead to extra financial costs which can be caused by for example travelling expenses and extra heating when the one who needs care lives in with the caregiver [25].

Furthermore, Janssen [35] distinguished three types of stress; care stress, relation stress and network stress. In his research in 80% of the situations there was care stress, in 50% relation stress and in 19% network stress. Care stress is stress which is related to the care itself, for example physical disorders/symptoms like difficulties with lifting, tiredness and sleeplessness. Many carers also complained about being housebound. They have to stay at home all the time because they cannot leave the dependent person alone for little while. Relation stress is caused by the attitude of the dependent person towards the family carer. Carers complained about the demanding nature of the dependent person, the orders which were given and the lack of appreciation. The third type, network stress is not caused by the behaviour of the dependent person but by the behaviour of other family members. In some cases the family carers are not practically or emotionally supported by their family members like their brothers and sisters [35]. Family carers expect support and loyalty from them, but the other family members are often uninterested [32]. Disappointment is the result of this. Furthermore, family carers have the feeling that they are solely responsible and that leads to stress [35,36].

Family care is also most often provided by people who have children themselves. So, family carers who have children living at home [29] may experience double stress, because they take care of someone external to the home and they have to run their own house. This may lead to a stressed relationship both with the one who receives care and their spouse or children [32].

It is generally known that family carers only then stop providing care when they are under considerable stress. Because of this, it is of great importance to support those carers in the interest of both the dependent people as the carers themselves, because burnout of family carers could lead to negative consequences for both of them.

The family carer will need care from the professional health and social care system. This leads to extra costs. The family carers need to take care of themselves and will not be able to care for the dependent person like they did before. Other people need to take care of the dependent person and it is not always easy to arrange this.

Support activities for family carers

As the importance of family care grows and the fact that family care may also lead to negative consequences, as mentioned above, it is important to support family carers. In the Netherlands, a lot of support activities have been developed in the last decade. The aims of the activities can be divided in three types, namely to give the family carer emotional, practical or financial support.

Emotional support is given by for example interest groups, contact offices and support groups. Practical support is provided by professional care and by activities like courses and education meetings. Furthermore the career leave, the emergency leave and the persons-bound budget may give financial support.

Emotional support

Since 1993 there is an interest group for family carers, the 'Landelijke Organisatie Thuisverzorgers (LOT)' (National Organisation Family Carers). This organisation promotes the interests of family carers and supports family carers and institutions who want to establish regional contact offices.

Contact offices have been established all over the country. Those contact offices organise support groups. The aim of support groups is to bring family carers, who are in comparable situations and have more or less the same problems, together. Discussing with other people who have similar experiences gives the participants support and courage to go on. Often only to talk about it results in a great relief. Mostly the support groups are classified according to the disease of the person for whom they care. For example there are support groups for carers of dementing people and for carers of patients with cancer. There are also discussion groups in which both the family carer and the one they care for can participate. The supporting groups vary in content and set-up, like the number of meetings and the group size. Patients' association, the consumers' organisation or a professional organisation are often the initiators and have the supervision. Professional organisations provide facilities for support groups to organise meetings.

Practical support

As mentioned above practical care can be divided in: professional care, respite care, courses and education meetings.

Firstly, professional care is mostly given as a supplement of family care. Research by De Boer [3] showed that elderly who receive family care more often also use home care (help) than those who do not receive family care. Probably family carers are the intermediary between people who need care and the professional caregiver, like home help [3].

Stress of family carers is often the result of insufficient cooperation between professional and family care. It is important that vulnerability of family carers is recognised in an early stage and that the carers receive support when necessary. It is important that family carers are supported by professional caregivers in order to be able to continue giving care. This is a part of the work of community nurses and home help.

Second, respite care is professional care which is provided to give family carers a break from caring [37]. Types of respite care are reception at home or reception external to the home, like day treatment and day care (dag opvang) but also other types of temporary care by another person than the family carer. Aim of respite care is to relieve family carers of their task temporary and to give them the opportunity to go window-shopping one afternoon, to go on holiday or to visit someone. Respite care is important because without it activities like shopping are not possible for some family carers, because they can not leave the care dependent person alone [38].

Thirdly, courses are also activities which provide practical support. Professionals give those courses. The aim of courses is to carry over information about diseases and to practice skills. Exchange of experiences and emotions is not the purpose of these meetings. Also the courses are divided according to the diseases of the care demanders. An example of an available course is a reanimation course for family carers of cardiac patients. Initiators of courses are home nursing services, home care organisations, hospitals and patients' associations [38].

The central idea of education meetings is the exchange of information. Other initiatives to support family carers are the development of brochures to carry over information and the possibility for family carers to call a certain telephone number to ask for information or to relieve one's feeling. However most of the telephone numbers are meant for patients and not for the family carer [38].

Financial support

In the Netherlands also financial support activities have been developed to stimulate and support family carers to provide care. Those activities are two types of leaves, the personal budget and financial compensation.

Recently, in the Netherlands two types of leaves were introduced: the career leave and the emergency leave. Since 1 October 1998, the career leave gives employees the possibility to take a leave of 2-6 months for caring or educational reasons. The benefit is related to last earnings but makes up a maximum of NLG 960 a month. [15].

The emergency leave means leave for care of a sick relative. There is no statutory scheme for this leave but this form of leave is beginning to appear in collective labour agreements. The emergency leave does neither entitle the employee to any specific amounts of days off nor wage compensation. The employee has to negotiate this with the employer. In some collective agreements, employees receive their normal wage during the emergency leave. The use of the emergency leave is not registered, but approximately 2-3% of employees use the leave during the year.

In the Netherlands, care dependent persons are eligible for a personal budget for care. The budgets are founded on a regular basis at 1995. A personal budget can be defined as cash payments given to care dependent persons with which they can buy their own care. Care dependent people may also use the personal budget to hire and pay their family carers. The personal budget is for some family carers the perfect invention. They receive money for the care they provide and in addition they are entitled to social insurance as premiums are being paid for them. Particularly, payments are a solution when family carers have to give up their job in order to be able to provide care [37].

Another possibility to stimulate giving family care is to found a financial or material compensation, for example direct financial compensation, as mentioned above or taxational (taxwise) compensation. However, some family carers do not want to receive money for the care provided. They feel it is natural to provide care to their relatives. They think that payment of family care will hamper the relationship between the family care and the care dependent [37].

Furthermore research [39] showed that in general a financial allowance does not increase the willingness to provide family care. In fact for activities with little effort the willingness to provide care decreased [39]. In the Netherlands, the general opinion is that providing or receiving family care does not need to be related to a financial [32].

From this section it can be concluded that nowadays, there are a lot of support activities for family carers in the Netherlands. Unfortunately, it is not clear who make use of those activities and who do not. At the same time, hardly no research has been done on the effects of the activities.

Assessment

The main goal of the Dutch health and social system is to provide 'tailored services' to support older people and their family carers. The first step towards this goal is to identify and define the real needs of those target groups. Therefore, an accurate assessment procedure is required. This section presents more information about the new system which is recently introduced in the Netherlands.

Before 1998 the needs of older people were assessed by professional care providers, mostly social workers or community nurses. They assessed the amount and type of care which was required. The result was that the provided care was more supply-oriented than demand-oriented. This means that the available care was taken into account by deciding which type and amount of care had to be provided. In January 1998 RIO's (Regionaal Indicatie Orgaan: Regional Assessment Organisation) were introduced. Nowadays there are 85 RIO's in the Netherlands [40]. RIO's are financed by the municipalities and they cover an area of on average seven municipalities and 250.000 inhabitants [41].

One of the tasks of RIO's is to assess the needs of older people with regard to home care, old people's homes and nursing homes. Furthermore some RIO's also carry out assessments for e.g. facilities for disabled people (transport and wheel chairs), for social facilities (meals on wheels) and for housing adaptations and technical aides.

The original of RIO's is to provide objective, independent and integral assessments [11,40-42]. This means that the assessment is based on general, objective criteria without being influenced by other factors (like the supply of care and the costs) and includes the complete package of care and services [41]. Therefore, a common protocol of the BIO (Breed Indicatie Overleg: Broad Indication Consultation) is developed [42,43].

Basically all applications for care are dealt with in the same way. However to handle cases efficiently, three different types of procedures have been developed: direct consultation, emergency consultation and the standard procedure.

Generally the procedure is as follows. The assessment procedure starts with the registration of all relevant personal information. After that the physical condition of the dependent person is observed. Diseases (e.g. heart problems), disorders (e.g. breathing) and/or limitations (e.g. limited freedom of movement and stair-climbing) are registered. At the same time environmental factors are taken into account like the presence of a partner who is able to provide some care (family carer) or the availability of a supporting devices. Subsequently the assessor and the applicant determine the aim of the care. Then the assessor considers whether the care which is required is also available [41,43]. When that type of care is available, the financier (health insurance fund or municipality) carries out a 'rightfulness test' and finally care is provided [41].

As mentioned above there are three types of procedures. When there is a demand of care, it firstly has to be decided which procedure needs to be followed. This depends on the demand of the client, the kind of problem, the situation of the client and the information which is available about the client or has to be asked for and the expertise which is needed for an adequate problem analysis and an appropriate choice of care [43].

The three types of procedures are direct consultation, emergency consultation and the standard procedure. Some demand of care can be dealt with directly by telephone or at the desk of the RIO. For some acute services, like administration of medicine and wound care, it is possible to decide directly what kind of care needs to be provided. The emergency consultation is for urgent care demand. In crisis situations for example when the partner of a demented elderly dies the emergency procedure may be followed. The assessment procedure will be finished within 24 hours or care is available directly and the indication follows afterwards.

In all other situations the standard procedure is followed. The standard procedure includes three different variants: the shortened standard procedure, the normal standard procedure and the extensive standard procedure.

In case of the shortened standard procedure the assessor does not visit the care demander at home. The assessment is based on a telephone call. This is mostly the case in situations in which already sufficient information about the client is available or when it concerns a demand of care for which there are standard arrangements. For a normal standard procedure assessment is formed by a telephone call and/or a house visit and if necessary by consulting dossiers. A long-lasting intensive care at home or a lengthy stay in an institution is always discussed multidisciplinary. The extensive standard procedure is needed when a specialist consult is needed additional to the information collection by the assessor. For a specialist consult you may think of a consultation by an ergotherapist or a situation in which a complicated adaptation of the house is required [43].

The effectiveness of the assessment as it is carried out by the RIO's has not been evaluated till now because the RIO's were introduced only two years ago in January 1998.

At the end of 1999 some evaluation studies were started. The Dutch government will receive the first results at the beginning of 2001 [11].

The protocol of the BIO also includes an optional section to roughly assess the vulnerability and needs of the primary informal carer. Firstly, it is indicated what type and amount of care is provided by the informal carer. There is a list of 17 activities, including e.g. bathing, dressing, eating, social activities and emotional support. The assessor asks the informal carer about the frequency of the activities. Furthermore, the number of hours of informal care is asked. Finally, the list is presented to the family carer to indicate which kind of support might be required. However, it is not clear whether this is done in all assessments by all RIO's.

Case Studies

In this section the actual provision of care to older people and their family carers will be made more explicit by the description of three standardised cases. These cases vary in the nature of the illness and disabilities of the older person. Furthermore per case there are three variations in the social circumstances of the older person and those of the family carers. For each case, three questions will be answered:

- What role(s) would the family carer typically occupy on caring for the older person?
- What services would typically be provided to support the older person?
- How would the family carer's needs typically be assessed and what support would typically be provided for the carer?

In reality the provision of care is determined by many aspects which are not mentioned in the case descriptions. Therefore it is only possible to describe the situation at a general level. This means that e.g. specific personal circumstances (such as the quality of the family relations) and differences between regions and communities can not be taken into account.

Case 1

Female, aged 76 with osteoarthritis of hips and knees, poor vision due to macular degeneration, and hypertension. Mobile with a frame within her home except for the stairs, Needs help with mobility outside, shopping, cooking and housework.

Social circumstances (A): Older person living alone in an isolated farmhouse. Widowed. Little money. Daughter and son-in-law unemployed with four children, aged 9 months to 7 years, and live 5 kilometres away. Two other children of the older person live over 100 kilometres away.

The role of family carers If the older person wants to stay in her own home, the daughter living close by will probably be the most important carer. Especially in rural areas family relations are often very close and children are more or less socially obligated to take care of their parents. The fact that the daughter and son-in-law are unemployed will even increase this social pressure. The daughter will mainly be involved in the practical acute daily support of the woman consisting of e.g. housekeeping activities, shopping and cooking. Also more incidental activities such as a visit to a doctor or hospital are mostly likely the responsibility of the daughter. This means that she visits her mother each day to see how she is doing and what kind of help she needs. The daughter will be responsible to arrange the required support (e.g. by asking other people such as her partner, neighbours or other family members), but most of the times she will provide it herself.

Because of the distance, the two other children will not be involved in the daily support. They sometimes take over the care for the older person in the weekends or help with some incidental tasks which can be planned ahead. Maybe, depending on their own financial situation, they could support their mother and sister financially. This is, however, not very common in the Netherlands because of the available social security system which provides money to the older person and to the unemployed daughter and son-in-law.

Professional services Given the severity of the physical condition of the older person, she has at least applied for home help services. The assessment procedure will be done by the RIO (Regional Assessment Organisation) which estimates the needs of the older person. Probably the older person will receive a limited number of hours of home help support by an unqualified home help. The home help will visit the older person once or twice a week to do some regular housekeeping activities such as cleaning the house, washing and ironing. The Netherlands is a densely populated country and therefore, home help services are also available in most of the rural areas. The home help will frequently communicate with the daughter living close by to gear their supporting activities.

Furthermore, a General Practitioner (GP) will regularly visit the older person to check her hypertension and other physical impairments. In some cases this could be done by a community nurse. Also a treatment by a physiotherapist might be needed. The municipality will also provide some supporting services. Because of the restricted mobility outside, transport services will be arranged. There are e.g. special taxi's (*deeltaxi*) available which enables older or disabled people to travel without making an appeal to informal carers.

Assessment and support of family carers In the situation as described above, the GP will probably keep an eye on things and can, if necessary, offer more information about the available supporting activities for family carers. It is however questionable whether these services exist in small rural areas. The home help might also support the family carer, but she is not trained to do so. Probably most support will be received by members of the social community such as neighbours and friends.

Social circumstances (B): Older person lives alone in a ground floor flat in town. Widowed. Daughter and son-in-law are both teachers in full-time employment, with 2 children aged 7 and 11, and live 1 kilometre in the same town.

The role of family carers The daughter and son-in-law have limited opportunities to provide help and support with daily activities, due to their full-time jobs and caring responsibilities for their own two children. They will mainly provide incidental support and emotional care, if necessary. Furthermore, they will take care in the weekends. Given the age of the grandchildren and the fact that they live near their grandmother, the grandchildren might be involved in some activities such as shopping. However, the largest part of the practical support is expected to come from neighbours who will most likely also be older persons.

Professional services It is most likely that the older person will apply for home help services. As in situation A, the assessment procedure will be done by the RIO. However, it is expected that this woman will receive more hours of home help support because of the restricted opportunities of her children to provide care. An unqualified home help will probably visit this woman on a daily basis (except the weekends) to help her with most housekeeping tasks. The problems related to cooking are most likely to be solved by calling in the 'meals-on-wheels' -services which are available in most urban areas. Other community services which can be used are e.g. transport services and leisure activities. The

GP and, if necessary, a community nurse are mainly responsible for the medical care provision.

Assessment and support of family carers In this situation family carers only play a minor role, so assessment and support is not really required.

Social circumstances (C): Older person lives with spouse in 2-storey house. Retired with savings. Spouse is fit and well. No children. Bedroom, bathroom and toilet are upstairs.

The role of family carers The main difference between this case and the other two cases is the fact that the old person lives with her spouse. Obviously, he is the main family carer and he provides most support and help with daily activities, especially because he is fit and in good health.

Professional services The couple will receive home help services. The amount and type of professional services depend on the abilities of the spouse to do housekeeping tasks. In general, an unqualified home help will visit the couple a few times a week to help with the housekeeping tasks. Furthermore the couple can make use of the available social and medical services as mentioned above. In this case, some adaptations in the couple's house seem to be necessary. If possible, a bedroom, bathroom and toilet can be built down stairs or technical aides such as a stair elevator can be installed. The couple has to apply for these facilities at the RIO or a special department of the municipality.

Assessment and support of family carers It is very important in this case that the professional caregivers (the GP and, to a lesser extent, the home help) are aware of the vulnerability of the spouse. They have to realise that he takes care of his wife 24 hours a day and 7 days a week. Therefore there is a real chance that he will become overloaded, especially because there are no children to fall back on. These professionals have no validated and reliable instrument to assess the needs of the family carer in a systematic way. They can also do some kind of assessment by observation and during a visit they can ask the spouse or his wife how things are going on. The home help will support the husband and wife with housekeeping tasks and emotional support, although this is officially not a task of an unqualified home help. Further social support, e.g. leisure activities or courses, will be provided by neighbourhood centres or other community services, if necessary. It is unlikely that the spouse will ask for respite care because those services are mostly used for family carers of psycho geriatric patients. Besides, the female in this situation can stay in their own home independently, if her husband needs or wants to go out.

Case 2

Male, aged 80, facing discharge from hospital following a stroke. Expected to be confined to bed or chair for several weeks with gradual recovery of morbidity. Needs the help of one person for transfers, toileting, bathing and dressing.

Social circumstances (A): Older person living alone in an isolated farmhouse. Widowed. Little money. Daughter and son-in-law unemployed with four children, aged 9 months to 7 years, and live 5 kilometres away. Two other children of the older person live over 100 kilometres away.

The role of family carers Firstly it has to be decided whether it is possible to take care of the man in his own home or whether it is preferable to transport him to a nursing home to recover. All family members will be involved in this decision. Many Dutch hospitals employ liaison nurses who guide and arrange the discharge from the hospital to the home situation. She will also assess the social circumstances of the patient. If the older person receives care at home, the daughter who lives close by will probably be involved in the daily housekeeping activities such as cooking, washing and cleaning. It is also likely that she will help with personal care such as bathing and dressing.

Professional care The liaison nurse will arrange the home care facilities which are needed. This can be technical (nursing) aides, home help services and home nursing care. Furthermore, she will inform the GP of the older person about his return and the kind of medical care that the patient needs. The RIO (Regional Assessment Organisation) will perform a direct assessment to define the needs and required professional services. Most likely a (auxiliary) community nurse will visit the patient each day to provide hygiene and personal care. She will do some routine nursing procedures and keep in touch with the GP who is medically responsible. Next, at least in the first period, the patient will also get some extra support in housekeeping activities by an unqualified home help. After a while there is a real possibility that a qualified home help will take over because she carries out hygiene and personal care, some housekeeping activities, she organises the household and provides support in case of psychosocial problems. Furthermore, the care dependent person will get a tele-alarm system for emergency calls.

Assessment and support of family carers A sort of assessment of the abilities of the family carers to perform caring activities is done before the hospital discharge. The liaison nurse might inform the family carers about possible supporting services or give them advice about the treatment and care of the patient.

Social circumstances (B): Older person lives alone in a ground floor flat in town. Widowed. Daughter and son-in-law are both teachers in full-time employment, with 2 children aged 7 and 11, and live 1 kilometre in the same town.

The role of family carers In these circumstances, the family carers are unable to provide or help significantly with housekeeping activities and personal care. Therefore it is more likely, compared to the former situation, that the patient will be temporarily admitted in a nursing home. Theoretically it is possible that the daughter applies for an emergency leave to take care of her father. But, as mentioned in section 3, this is still very uncommon in the Netherlands.

If the patient goes directly to his own house, the liaison nurse of the hospital will arrange the home care facilities which are needed.

Professional care The situation is nearly the same as described in social circumstances (A). The main differences are the number of hours of home help care that are required because of the inability of the family carers to contribute to the care provision. A (auxiliary) community nurse will visit the patient several times a day to help with e.g. bathing and dressing and housekeeping activities. Furthermore, a tele-alarm system will be installed for emergency calls of the patient.

Assessment and support of family carers In this situation family carers only play a minor role, so assessment and support is not really required.

Social circumstances (C): Older person lives with spouse in 2-storey house. Retired with savings. Spouse is fit and well. No children. Bedroom, bathroom and toilet are upstairs.

The role of family carers If the older person stays at home and receives care at home, his wife will be the primary family carer, especially because she is in good health. Maybe some neighbours or friends will help her with practical tasks such as shopping. Besides her own routine housekeeping activities, the wife will help her husband with hygiene and personal care like dressing, bathing and going to the toilet.

Professional care As in the two other situations, the RIO will perform a direct assessment to define the needs and required professional services. Assuming that the woman will do her own housekeeping activities no unqualified home help services will be provided. Some additional assistance is required by a (auxiliary) community nurse, namely routine technical nursing procedures, some help with personal care (but definitely less than in the circumstances A as described above) and keep in touch with the GP. Furthermore some technical aides for e.g. bathing will be available, if necessary.

Assessment and support of family carers A sort of assessment of the abilities of the wife to perform caring activities is done before the hospital discharge. The liaison nurse might inform the wife about possible supporting services or gives her advice about the treatment and care of the patient. Furthermore the GP and (auxiliary) community will keep an eye on things, but the needs of the wife will not be assessed systematically. It is possible that she will call a voluntary organisation which provides additional services.

Case 3

Female, aged 86, suffering from dementia. Frequent wandering by day and night. Frequent falls. Incontinent of urine and faeces.

Social circumstances (A): Older person living alone in an isolated farmhouse. Widowed. Little money. Daughter and son-in-law unemployed with four children, aged 9 months to 7 years, and live 5 kilometres away. Two other children of the older person live over 100 kilometres away.

The role of family carers It is obvious that the woman needs someone to care for her 24 hours a day, 7 days a week. The family carers will be unable to provide this care. Therefore it is most likely that the woman will be admitted in a nursing home. In the Netherlands, it is uncommon that older people live with their children. However, because of the long waiting list for an admission in a nursing home, this might be a temporary solution. When the woman stays in a nursing home, her children will come for a visit or take her out for some leisure activities.

Professional care The RIO (Regional Assessment Organisation) will perform a comprehensive assessment procedure and probably decide that the woman must be admitted in a nursing home. Given the severity of the situation an emergency consultation is required. In the nursing home nurses will take care of the woman. The medical care is not any longer the responsibility of her own GP but is taken over by the nursing home physician. If the woman has to wait for a place in a nursing home, she might visit a day care facility and spend the night with her daughter who lives close by.

Assessment and support of family carers Because the woman stays in a nursing home, this is not longer required in these circumstances.

Social circumstances (B): Older person lives alone in a ground floor flat in town. Widowed. Daughter and son-in-law are both teachers in full-time employment, with 2 children aged 7 and 11, and live 1 kilometre in the same town.

Because of the severe condition of the woman, this situation is comparable with the former one. The daughter and son-in-law can not offer permanent assistance to the woman. Therefore it is most likely that she will be admitted in a nursing home.

Social circumstances (C): Older person lives with spouse in 2-storey house. Retired with savings. Spouse is fit and well. No children. Bedroom, bathroom and toilet are upstairs.

The role of family carers In this situation, it is less sure whether the woman will be admitted in a nursing home because her husband is still vital and could, basically, take care of her permanently. It is, however, not known how long he is able to do this. Taking care of a person with dementia is a heavy burden because it goes with all kinds of practical difficulties and (mostly) emotional problems. If the husband indicates that he can not copy anymore, the woman will be probably admitted in a nursing home.

Professional care As long as the woman is cared for by her husband, a wide range of professional care will be available for the couple. Probably, a home help will support them with housekeeping tasks and personal care. Given the severity of the woman's condition, most likely she will visit a day care centre during day time. All kinds of activities are organised for psycho geriatric patients. During the weekends, a community nurse might visit the couple to see how things are going. The GPs will still be responsible for the medical treatment.

Assessment and support of family carers As mentioned a section of the BIO protocol assesses the needs of informal carers. Probably this is used in this case by the RIO. Furthermore, all professional caregivers will keep an eye on him to see whether he still can handle the situation and will not be overloaded. Furthermore, the husband can fall back on several respite services from neighbourhood centres or voluntary organisations. Volunteers e.g. can look after his wife, when he needs or wants to go out. Maybe some neighbours or friends will help the husband with some practical tasks (e.g. housekeeping activities, shopping), assist with personal care (e.g. dressing) or temporarily take over the care for the woman (respite care). It is also possible that the husband participates in meetings with other partners of a person with dementia. At these meetings they receive a lot of information about the disease and the care that is needed. Contact with people who have similar experiences often provides emotional support. Often these kind of groups also organise leisure activities for the partners of the care dependent persons.

Future Developments

This section provides a rough overview of the social position of older people and their family carers and the available health and social services in the Netherlands. As mentioned, important changes will occur in the near future. Some changes are related to the formal care system, others to the role and position of informal or family carers.

The most important challenge is to transfer the Dutch care system from a 'service-oriented' to a more 'person-centred' system. Support and care need to be tailored to the individual needs of each patient taken into account his/her personal circumstances, lifestyle and financial situation. Therefore a number of important changes in the organisational and financing structure of the health and social services are or will be implemented. Firstly, a further decentralisation of responsibilities will be required. Planning of facilities will become the responsibility of regions. Secondly, the co-operation, communication and co-ordination between services will be improved. Thirdly, the introduction of personal budgets will be extended which enables older people to buy their own services. This gives them the opportunity to pay 'informal carers' (such as neighbours) for their support. Fourthly, a new assessment system was introduced to assess the real needs of older people objectively, comprehensively and independently.

In the Netherlands the network of family carers is changing. The potential of informal care provided by partners and close family members (mainly children) is expected to decrease in the near future. However, because of the increase of the number of older people in society, more attention will be given to so called intergenerational support [28]. Continuing the current policy to combine caring and working, stimulate the participation of elderly in giving family care (intra generational care). People grow older and they longer stay vital. Because of that elderly should care for elderly in the future [23].

An important conclusion of this section is that only limited information is available about Dutch family carers. It is interesting that a new assessment system is introduced to define the actual needs of the older people. Although this system also includes a small section about the needs of family carers, it is unknown whether this section is practically used and whether it provides valid and reliable information about the vulnerability of family carers. The further development of such a system is important because it may prevent that family carers will become overloaded and, consequently, will be unable to continue their caring activities. As mentioned in section three, a wide range of facilities are developed to support family carers. However it is difficult to reach those people who are mostly in need of these services in an early stage. Therefore, an early warning system is required to predict the vulnerability of family carers. This system has to be used by professional caregivers in all situations regardless the severity of the problems of the older person.

Notes

[1] The administration of the 'care offices' is carried out by the Health insurance fund with the largest number of insured persons in that particular region. Care offices are non-governmental organisations which work within the legal framework of the AWBZ determined by the government.

[2] General Act on Exceptional Medical Expenses. This social health insurance scheme covers the entire Dutch population and includes e.g. most services for older people such as nursing homes and home care.

[3] In the Netherlands, the term *Praktijkondersteuning* (Practice support) is used because the activities can also be performed by staff without a nursing background, but other relevant qualifications.

References

[1]   CBS. (Centraal Bureau voor de Statistiek. Maandstatistiek Bevolking, 48 (2000) 29-31.
[2]   J.B.F. Hutten and A. Kerkstra A (eds.), Home Care in Europe: a country-specific guide to its organisation and financing. Aldershot: Arena Publishers, 1996.
[3]   A.H. De Boer, Housing and care for older people: a macro-micro perspective (proefschrift). Utrecht: Universiteit Utrecht, 1999.
[4]   J.M.C. Vollering, Care services for the elderly in the Netherlands. Amsterdam: Tinbergen Institute, 1991.
[5]   G.G. Giarchi, Caring for older Europeans: comparative studies in 29 countries. Aldershot: Arena Publishers, 1996.
[6]   W.J. Nusselder, Compression or expansion of morbidity? A life-table approach (thesis). Rotterdam: Erasmus University Rotterdam, 1998.
[7]   OECD. Caring for frail elderly people: Policies in evolution. Social policy studies no. 19. Paris, OECD, 1996.
[8]   A. Walker *et al*, Older people in Europe: social and economic policies. Brussels: European Commission, 1997.
[9]   D.M. Modly, Home health care worldwide: an introduction to global issues. In: D. Modly *et al*, (eds), Home care nursing services: international lessons. New York: Springer Publishing Company, 1997.
[10] A. Walker, An overview of home and community care in Europe. In: A. Walker, (ed.), European home and community care 1998/99. The Official EACHH Reference Book. London: Campden Publishing Limited, 1998.
[11] Ministry of Health, Welfare and Sports (Ministerie van VWS). Zorgnota 2000. Den Haag, 1999.
[12] A. Kerkstra,. Home care in the Netherlands. In: J.B.F. Hutten and A. Kerkstra (eds.), Home care in

Europe: a country-specific guide to its organisation and financing. Aldershot: Arena, 1996.
[13]   W. Van den Heuvel and H. Gerritsen, Home-care services in the Netherlands. In: A. Jamieson (ed.), Home care for older people in Europe. A comparison of policies and practices. Oxford: Oxford University Press, 1991.
[14]   S. Arts et al, In de gezinsverzorging. Utrecht: Landelijk centrum verpleging en verzorging/NIVEL, 1997.
[15]   T. Rostgaard and T. Fridberg, Caring for children and older people: a comparison of European policies and practices. Copenhagen; the Danish National Institute of Social Research, 1998.
[16]   C. Tunissen and M. Knapen, The national context of social innovation: The Netherlands. In: R.J. Kraan and J. Baldock (eds.), Care for the elderly: significant innovations in three European countries. Frankfurt am Mein: Campus Verlag, 1991.
[17]   M.W. Ribbe, Care for the elderly: the role of the nursing home in the Dutch health care system. *International Psychogeriatrics*, **5(2)** (1993)213-222.
[18]   A. Meijer,. Nursing homes in Europe: a comparative study of the organization and financing of nursing homes in five European countries. Wageningen: LUW, 1998.
[19]   J.M. Spaan and L.P. Bartels, Verpleeghuiszorg. In: cijfers 1993-1997. Utrecht: Nederlandse Vereniging voor verpleeghuiszorg, 1999.
[20]   A. Hommel et al, Informele zorg; Een kritische reflectie; commentaar bij beleid. *Tijdschrift voor Gerontologie en Geriatrie*, **26(5)** (1995) 220-223.
[21]   B.J.M. Welling, Zelfstandigheid en ouderenzorg: een evaluatie-onderzoek in een wooncentrum voor ouderen. Nijmegen: ITS, 1998.
[22]   S. Van der Lyke, Mantelzorg maakt patienten. *Tijdschrift voor gezondheid en politiek*, **13(2)** (1995) 7-9.
[23]   RMO/RVZ. Zorgarbeid in de toekomst: advies over de gevolgen van demografische ontwikkeling van vraag en aanbod zorg(arbeid). Den Haag/Zoetermeer, 1999.
[24]   W.J.M.J. Cuijpers, De werking van ondersteuningsgroepen voor centrale verzorgers van dementerende ouderen. Nijmegen: KUN, 1993.
[25]   Steenvoorden MAGA. Mantelzorg voor ouderen in Nederland: de stand van zaken en mogelijke verbeteringen. *Tijdschrift voor Gerontologie en Geriatrie*, **24(2)** (1993) 66-69.
[26]   A. Van den Bergh Jeths, Economische en sociaal-culturele ontwikkelingen. In: Volksgezondheid Toekomst Verkenning 1997. VII Gezondheid en zorg in de toekomst. Bilthoven-Maarssen: RIVM-Elsevier/De Tijdstroom, 1997.
[27]   CBS. Statistisch Jaarboek 2000. Voorburg/Heerlen: CBS, 2000.
[28]   M.S.H. Duijnstee et al, Mantelzorg voor mensen met een chronische ziekte; een literatuurstudie naar de rol van mantelzorg voor mensen met een chronische ziekte op basis van Nederlandse studies gepunbliceerd in de periode 1980-1993. Utrecht: NIZW, 1994.
[29]   M.G.H. Dautzenberg et al, Vrouwen van een middengeneratie en informele zorg voor ouderen. *Tijdschrift voor Gerontologie en Geriatrie*, **27(4)** (1996)141-149.
[30]   F.L.J. Tjadens and M.S.H. Duijnstee, MSH. Visie op mantelzorg. Utrecht: NIZW, 1999.
[31]   A.H. De Boer et al, Informele zorg: een verkenning van huidige en toekomstige ontwikkelingen. Rijswijk: SCP, 1994.
[32]   G. Van den Brink, Een schaars goed: de betekenis van zorg in de hedendaagse levensloop. Utrecht: NIZW, 1999.
[33]   F.L.J. Tjadens and M.S.H. Duinstee MSH, Mantelzorgondersteuning in Nederland anno 1998: een stand van zaken. In: RMO/RVZ. Achtergrondstudies bij het advies Zorgarbeid in de toekomst. Den Haag/Zoetermeer, 1999.
[34]   T. Janssen and C. Woldringh, Centrale verzorgers van ouderen: verschillen en overeenkomsten tussen verzorgende partners, dochters en overige verzorgers. Nijmegen: ITS, 1993.
[35]   T. Janssen, De betekenis van de familie voor de centrale verzorg(st)er van hulpbehoevende oudere mensen. *Tijdschrift voor Gerontologie en Geriatrie*, **19** (1998) 185-191.
[36]   A.M. Pot, Caregivers' perspective: a longitudinal study on the psychological distress of informal caregivers of demented elderly. Amsterdam: VU, 1996.
[37]   S. Weekers and M. Pijl, Home care and care allowances in the European Union. Utrecht: NIZW, 1998.
[38]   G. Goudriaan et al, Mantelzorgers steunen, waarom en hoe? Utrecht: NIZW, 1995.
[39]   M. Van der Doef, Mantelzorg tegen betaling?: meningen van mensen uit Tilburg. *Medisch Contact*, **46(25)** (1991)798-800.
[40]   Stip, Indicatieorganen in Nederland: een wegwijzer. Enschede: Stip, 1999.
[41]   R. Huijsman and J. Degen, Rio's als schakel in een regionale keten: betrokken partijen zijn het spoor enigszins bijster. *Ouderenzorg*, **2(4)** (1999) 20-21.
[42]   C. Carbo, Luis in de pels. *Zorgvisie*, **8** (1999) 11-13.
[43]   Stip. De werkwijze van het indicatieorgaan. Informatiebulletin 1999b;2(4):1-10.

Chapter 7

Poland
(September 1998)

Barbara Bień
Department of Clinical and Social Gerontolgoy
The Medical Academy of Bialystok
15-230 Bialystok
Kilinski str. 1
Poland

Beata Wojszel
Department of Clinical and Social Gerontolgoy
The Medical Academy of Bialystok
15-230 Bialystok
Kilinski str. 1
Poland

Barbara Polityńska
University of Bialystok
Faculty of Pedagogy & Psychology
20 Swierkowa Str. 15
PL-15-328 Bialystok
Poland

Jolanta Wilmańska
Department of Clinical and Social Gerontolgoy
The Medical Academy of Bialystok
15-230 Bialystok
Kilinski str. 1
Poland

Introduction

Within the context of Europe, Poland belongs, in demographic terms, to those countries with intermediate levels of ageing. In 1996, the median age for women in the population was 36 years and for men 32.5 years. Poland crossed the threshold for old age in demographic terms as far back as in 1968, and in 1997: 16.2% of the population were aged 60 or more, and 11.7% were 65 years or more. There is substantial variation in the regional distribution of demographic ageing throughout Poland. Even greater variation in ageing is seen between urban areas, where they form 17.6% of the population (exceeding even 30% in some regions).

The previous, present, and projected distribution of the elderly population is shown in Table 1.

Table 1. Growth and structure of the elderly population in Poland by age groups (figures in percentages)

	1970	1996	2000*	2020**
People over 60 in the whole population	13.0%	16.1%	18.0%	22.4%
60-64	35.4	28.7	26.8	28.9
65-69	27.4	2637	25.0	26.7
70-74	19.0	20.9	21.9	19.8
of which 60-74	81.8	76.2	73.7	75.4
75-79	10.4	11.2	14.8	
80+	7.8	12.6	11.0	
of which 75+	18.2	23.8	25.8	24.6
	100.0	100.0	100.0	100.0

*according to the demographic prognosis produced by Rosset in 1970
**according to the Central Statistical Office, estimates produced in 1996

According to the demographic prognosis produced by Rosset in 1970, the proportion of the young elderly (60 to 74 years) is to fall by around 8% in relation to the number of older people in general during the next 30 years, whereas the proportion of very old people (aged 75 and over) is to increase from 19.0 to 26%. According to the demographic prognosis of the Central Statistical Office for 2020, the percentage of people over 60 years will reach 22.4% and those over 65 – 15.9% respectively.

Nowadays, in many industrialized countries, newborn girls can expect to live about 80 years and newborn boys about 75 years. The corresponding figures in Poland are 77.0 years and 68.5 years, respectively.

The present day situation in Poland makes the task of preparing a report on the system of care for older people a particularly difficult one. The political changes brought about in 1989 and the ongoing period of transformation of the state have brought about many changes in the existing organisational structures. The system of health care which is currently in the process of being created is not yet clearly defined because of the continuing transformation of the state and delays in legislative proceedings.

Among the many factors contributing to the lack of stability and gaps in the present system of care for older people, the following have a particularly strong influence:
1. The deep economic crisis which affected Poland at the time of the downfall of the communist system and the early period of transformation to a free market economy, had a fundamental effect in preventing the realisation of many social policies

2. The introduction of a free market economy together with protectionist activities concentrating on the social effects of these reforms (an increase in unemployment; taking early retirement)
3. Giving exaggerated priority to government social policies which were designed to protect the poorest groups in society, above all the unemployed and their families
4. Delays in introducing reforms to the social security and health care systems
5. The co-existence of many mutually uncoordinated acts of parliament dating back to the system of care provided during the period of so-called "real socialism" as well as legislative acts which as yet have not gained parliamentary approval
6. Psycho-social conditions and limitations in peoples' ability to adapt to the ongoing changes, especially in the case of older people, who were used to passively waiting for all services to be provided for them
7. Regional differences giving rise to an unequal provision of care facilities both from the public sector and from non-governmental sources

The majority of people in Poland received the political changes and the move towards democracy with enthusiasm. They led to evident successes in the area of democratisation of public life and state finances. Nevertheless, many election promises made by successive political parties as they came into power, relating to the social welfare responsibilities of the state, did not become widespread practice. As a result the existing welfare system is not fully effective, stabilised or cohesive. It is a mix of elements left over from the old system, combined with the new system of government.

The socialist welfare system was two dimensional in nature [1,2]. On the one hand it consisted of a dictated distribution and centrally controlled state sector, on the other hand mainly informal family assistance. These two sectors mutually complemented each other, though there was no room for co-operation between them. At first, it was the aim of the welfare policy of the state to take over all forms of provision of social security from the family and informal caregiving groups. The informal care sector, however, gradually gained increasing significance in compensating for the ever increasing ineffectiveness of state sector welfare provision. In the socialist society, to all intents and purposes, it is true to say that the private sector was not allowed to exist, and the voluntary sector was marginalised and effectively under state control [3]. There was no room for non-governmental, charitable or private organisations of any kind.

The classical welfare triangle during the period of socialism in Poland was largely distorted. A schematic representation is given in figure 1, from which it can be seen that the family was the basic and most important care provider, with support from state institutions, whereas the commercial and voluntary sectors *de facto* had a very small role to play in what was essentially a two dimensional model of welfare.

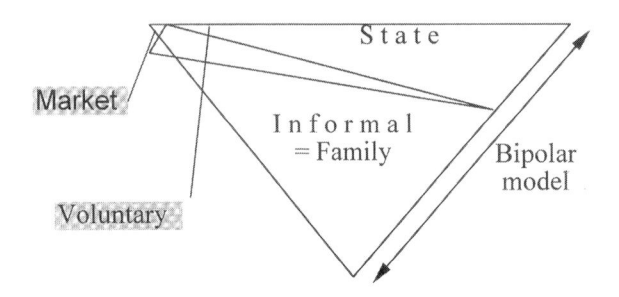

Figure 1. The welfare triangle in communist Poland

During the years of economic depression in Poland from the late nineteen eighties to the beginning of the nineteen nineties, this two dimensional model of care began to change. The reasons for this were, above all, the economic difficulties experienced by the state. Increasingly, the inability of the state to meet its welfare obligations led to greater demands being made on family carers to provide the services required by disabled members of their families. The currently preferred pluralistic model of health and social care (market services, voluntary and self-help organisations), although beginning to emerge, has still not reached any really significant level. Given this situation, sociologists warn of the risk of the emergence of a 'welfare gap' especially in relation to older people with disabilities [1].

Nevertheless, the social policies of recent years have encouraged the formation of non-governmental organisations of both a commercial and voluntary nature. Such developments would enable the creation of a multi-dimensional system of welfare, based on a pluralistic approach to the provision of care. The changes required to bring this about, above all necessitate a decentralisation of service provision and transference of responsibility for care provision from a very centralised system to provision of care at a local level. However, due to the large budget deficit of the state, this increase in responsibilities as far as local authorities are concerned has not been accompanied by the necessary funding subsidies. Moreover, the new local authorities, overwhelmed by the vastness of the task facing them, do not always fully appreciate the needs of older people, nor see them as a priority.

Society as a whole has suffered a decrease in the standard of living and as a result more people have turned to social services for help, leading to a relative decline in access to these services as far as older people are concerned. This statement cannot be fully supported owing to the lack of directly comparable research from all over Poland, but there is indirect evidence to support it from the work of Synak in the voivodeship (county) of Gdańsk [1]. His research findings show that the proportion of people receiving social security benefits of any kind in 1992 was more than double that of 1989. At the same time, however, in relation to older people, a similar increase was only seen in relation to those living in towns and cities (benefits related mainly to helping with rents for accommodation), whereas in rural areas there was even a small decline in those in receipt of benefits. In a longitudinal cohort study of the residents of a large city (Bialystok), the proportion of 75 year old respondents who had had at least one contact with a social worker during the past year rose from 5% in 1979 to 9% in 1994 [4].

Increased state financial support is directed predominantly at the poorest groups in society, mainly families affected by unemployment and homeless people, whereas the proportion of older people among those receiving welfare benefits has declined in relative terms. This is especially evident in certain rural areas, where the proportion of older people among those receiving benefits has fallen from 51.2% in 1989 to 22.5% in 1992 [1].

From research carried out in small communities it can be seen that financial support from the state nonetheless exceeds all other forms of aid, especially in the form of services [1]. The range of services and their availability has started to decrease, however. This is as a result of the introduction of fees for help in the form of services, at a rate determined according to the income per member of the household. Care services which are free of charge have been restricted only to those groups of people meeting certain criteria as far as income is concerned. In reality, decisions regarding the provision of social welfare facilities are considered only in respect of those people who actually apply for them. No records are kept detailing the needs of the population with regard to health and social welfare considerations, and the knowledge of older people with respect to these forms of assistance is at best extremely limited.

Health and social care services were for many years integrated under the jurisdiction of a single government ministry - the Ministry of Health and Social Welfare. In spite of the many disadvantages of a centralised system, co-operation between these services at the level of the provision of basic health care services, enabled the co-ordination of medical and social services to be carried out effectively.

In 1990, social services were separated from what became the Ministry of Health and were transferred to the jurisdiction of the Ministry of Employment and Social Policy. This brought about the disintegration of the co-operation which had previously existed to tackle the complex medical and social problems which in particular affected those in older people age groups [5]. It is true that the new Act of Parliament relating to social services allows extensive opportunities for compensatory provisions, not just in the form of financial assistance and provision of services, but also of social work and counselling [6], but widespread experience shows that its main effect has been to provide a formal statement of the rights of a potential user of the services to the limited financial resources of the local centres providing social welfare services [7]. The bill does not provide special privileges for older people as a potential client group, but defines certain criteria which are to grant the provision of state aid for certain issues, namely poverty, homelessness, chronic conditions, unemployment, drug addiction and alcoholism.

The new law regarding social services is based on the premise of pluralism in the provision of care, transferring responsibilities for care to a number of different organisations, as well as encouraging the active participation of those in receipt of the services. This is particularly difficult to bring about as a consequence of the helplessness and apathy in terms of actively responding to one's duties as a citizen, engendered by the previous system [8]. In relation to older people there is the additional problem of the lack of cultural models for this kind of behaviour, very often a failing state of health and technological considerations [2].

It is important to emphasise that in 1991, social services consumed 5.5% of the state budget, whereas in 1996 this had risen to a figure of 9.9% (the proportion consumed by health care fell over this period from 16.1% to 15.4%) [9]. In spite of the increased state support for those suffering the greatest levels of poverty in society, the category of people most severely affected were older people living in rural areas, where the problems of old age combine with poverty and disability to produce the greatest difficulties [10].

Health care policy in Poland is among the few state-run sectors which as yet has not been affected by the complex reforms accompanying the new political system. The bill relating to health care facilities passed in 1991 and the act of Parliament relating to health care and health insurance passed in 1997, have been introduced in a fragmentary and experimental way in a few primary health care facilities. It is estimated that the reformed types of primary health care, based on the family practitioner model, have been introduced in nearly 20% of primary health care services. These reforms will be introduced in full in 1999, following the administrative reforms for the country agreed by Parliament in recent weeks, which are to bring about the decentralisation of central government authority and finances. For the time being, the majority of primary health care provision still functions according to the principles of the old system, and is financed directly from the state budget.

The old-style system, which is ineffective both financially and in organisational terms, is strongly criticised by both patients and health care staff, as well as the managers themselves. However, the introduction of the complex reform of the health care system has been deferred up until now, because of the high costs associated with the introduction and establishing of the proposed new system, delays resulting from the training of the new family practitioners (the existing model of health care was *de facto* based on the provision of only specialist services) as well as resistance from some sectors of the medical profession themselves. This situation changing however, as Parliament has finally passed the necessary legislation to implement these reforms from the beginning of 1999.

Basic health care provision for older people is at present provided by general medical doctors based in community health clinics with a catchment area determined on a regional basis. In areas which have introduced the new reforms, primary care is the remit of family practitioners. As in the case of the provision of social care and social services, basic health care provision under the reformed system will not bring any special privileges for older people. No specialist services exist for older people and then are still to be treated under mainstream provisions. It is only at the level of specialist medical care that provision is made in the form of Specialist Geriatric Clinics, but these only exist in the larger cities and thus access to them is disproportionate.

In the area of hospital provisions, there is a high 'geriatrisation rate' of general medical wards. In the majority of hospital departments, the proportion of older patients exceeds 50% [11].

The number of rehabilitation facilities for older people suffering from chronic conditions is very small, which results in extended periods of hospitalisation in general hospitals and limitations as far as the process of rehabilitation itself is concerned. In 1994, as many as 33% of 75 year olds living in towns and cities considered that gaining access to hospital treatment was difficult (15 years earlier, 20% of those asked in this age group voiced the same opinion) [4].

In 1994 around 30% of older people considered that access to dental treatment was difficult, whereas in 1979 only around 6-7% of older people expressed this opinion [4]. It should be mentioned here that over the period concerned, many dental surgeries were privatised, which may have given rise to the expressed difficulties in gaining access to dental treatment under the state health care system.

The delays in introducing reforms to the health care system based on independent financial resources from health insurance (and not as to date from the state budget), in the context of very low rates of pay and the frustration experienced by the medical profession, have led to numerous protests from this professional body. This has been reflected in a worsening of the quality of medical services and the development of a "shadow market" in medical services, where patients unofficially pay for services they receive within the state health service [12]. This has led to inequalities in opportunities for services and the 'spontaneous commercialisation of health services' [13].

The realties of the existing system of welfare for older people in Poland during a period of transformation in the political system, which have been briefly presented here, lead to a number of somewhat sad reflections. One of them is the conclusion that public institutions do not meet their responsibilities in terms of tending satisfactorily to the care needs of older people who are sick or disabled. Given this situation, the greater majority of care tasks are left to the family, and supplement the state sector of care provision.

In the Polish tradition, the family is expected to fulfil all the basic care tasks in relation to its members [14]. In comparison to western countries, the family in Poland has remained close to a traditional picture. To a large extent this is as a result of the traditional model of a multi-generational model of living together and the consequent mutual connections that this brings about between the generations. In his research based on a nation-wide study conducted in 1967, Piotrowski [15] reports that 67% of people over the age of 65, who had children, lived with their children. This situation was true of the rural population to a greater extent (76%) and to a lesser extent (57%) of those living in urban areas. Between 1979 and 1994 the proportion of people aged 75 living with their children in a multi-generational family in the city of Bialystok fell from 41% to 34% among men and from 51% to 35% among women [5]. Similar figures have been reported in nation-wide research conducted by the Main Office of Statistics (GUS) in 1985 [16]. These figures indicate that there has been a gradual disintegration of multi-generational families in Poland.

In the past, and equally in the present day, living together in multi-generational families has rarely been a situation arising out of choice, but as a consequence of the difficulties in obtaining housing for young people. This is especially true for the category of people defined as the 'young old'. In the case of the 'old old', living together often signifies that help and care is being given by younger members of the family, who have often taken the older sick or disabled person in to their own home. On the basis of comparative research, Synak has formulated the hypothesis that over the past twenty years, the support and help of older parents directed towards their adult children has increased, whereas the help of children directed towards their elderly parents has been reduced [14,17]. Older people give assistance to their children, seeking to minimise the effects of the economic crisis, and are able, at the same time, to count on their help at times of illness or disability. Synak concludes that during times of crisis, the protective function of the family is even increased [1]. Data from 1985 show that 76% of people were helping their parents, whilst 73% were receiving help from them [16]. Children are the most important source of support for older people. The most common form of family help is nursing and care offered at times of illness. Symptomatic of this is the fact that during times of illness only 2% of people over the age of 60 reported that they expected help from a nurse, but 58% said that they counted on their children, whilst 54% said they expected it to come from their spouse (husband or wife) [16]. In her research, Kotlarska-Michalska reported that 87% of older people receive nursing care from their families, and only 13% from neighbours or institutions [18].

A fundamental role for the family in the welfare system for older people should be regarded as a positive phenomenon. However the resources of the family are limited and it is essential that it should receive support from the state. The possibility is even being considered that close family members, most frequently women who do not go out to work, should be paid for their services from state funding [1].

In contrast to the family, the role of the voluntary sector remains marginal. Voluntary organisations struggle with both financial and organisational difficulties. Self-help organisations are also emerging [19], but their development is limited because of financial difficulties, poor co-operation with local authorities and the lack of models and traditions to follow.

The weakest point in the pluralistic welfare system is the private sector, despite the removal of any legislation which formerly restricted such practice. It would seem that the development of this sector is, to a large extent, dependent on the economic situation of the country in general and on government policies in particular.

The aspects of the pluralistic system of welfare care which have been introduced in Poland in the 1990s as described here, are insufficient to confirm the presence of widespread reforms, and *de facto* the shape of the welfare triangle has changed but little. In practice the family carries out the functions of caring for older people both from the formal (legal) point of view and in reality, and is assisted by help from the state only in situations of extreme crisis. Typical examples would include situations of extreme poverty, or being left alone in conditions of severe pathology or disability. The lack of a family, or its inability to cope are reasons for being given high priority for institutional care run by the state social services, where places remain scarce and waiting lists extremely long. The waiting time to gain a place in institutional care varies from several weeks to several months or even years, depending on the region of the country.

In summary, one may be inclined to conclude that Poland is not developing any policies for the care of older people nor a multi-dimensional system of care for older people. The Polish parliament has ratified most of the international conventions relating to human rights, but these only minimally affect the legal status of older people. They give rights to all people, but the oldest in society are unable to ensure that they gain full benefits from them [20].

Health and Social Care for Older People: Structures and Functions

Health care

What is the place of older people in the existing system of health care? Older people have the same guarantee of the right to free health care as all other citizens of the Republic of Poland. This includes free access to all parts of the health service, as well as receiving prescribed drugs at rates subsidised by the state, irrespective of the age of the patient.

The basic structure of the health service did not change in any significant way after 1989 in comparison to the former period of socialist rule.

Basic activities connected with prophylactic care and treatment for the majority of the population are carried out by community health centres in towns or villages. These units serve the population of a defined area (e.g. in towns - specified streets and numbers of houses are defined as belonging to a given health centre). The community health centres form the central part of a network of institutions in a given region which together are called the District Health Administration. A network of these administrative authorities, in turn, covers the whole country. There are some exceptions to this organisation of basic health care facilities. In particular, they relate to those professional groups which have their own medical services organised directly by the Ministry responsible for them (professional soldiers, the police, employees of the state railways and their families) and employees of large industrial enterprises who have health care organised especially for their use.

In the local and rural health centres, services are offered in the area of four main medical specialities: general/internal medicine, paediatrics, obstetrics and gynaecology and dental services. Doctors work together with nurses (including community nurses), social workers and auxiliary staff (reception staff, dental assistants, administrative personnel). It is usual for health centres to have at their disposal basic diagnostic facilities (ECG, analytical laboratories, sometimes Ultrasonography). The larger health centres employ several general medical doctors, and patients may choose which doctor they wish to consult at any time. It is often the case, however, that the medical staff themselves decide to divide responsibility for the region they serve among themselves (this is especially true of home visits) and the patient's right to choose a doctor is not respected in practice.

Also at the level of primary care, but separate from the community health centres and under the direct supervision of the District Health Administration, there is a network of specialist clinics (e.g. neurological, rehabilitation, cardiology, diabetes) as well as hospital departments dealing with primary care specialities (usually - internal/general medicine, paediatrics, obstetrics and gynaecology and surgery). These departments are based in towns or peripheral regions of large cities. Access to specialist care or admission to hospital is subject to a referral by a doctor from the community health centre. It is often the case that the specialist clinics take over the responsibility for the care of patients within their specialist field. As a result, patients are often treated by a number of specialists at the same time.

At the next level in the hierarchical structure of the health service, is the voivode or county hospital which has specialist outpatient departments and institutions with which it closely co-operates. It is characterised by offering a range of specialist services and a high level of diagnostic and treatment services which are available to people from the whole of the county served by the hospital.

At the next level, that of the region, there are the highly specialised Teaching Hospitals of the University Medical Schools and Specialist Health Administration (e.g. regional oncology centres, dermatology units and units for the prevention and treatment of tuberculosis), which serve a region incorporating several voivodeships/counties. At the highest level there are national medical institutes for selected, narrow specialities, which, where necessary, are available to serve the citizens of the whole country.

What is the place of the older person in the system of health care in Poland described above? The fact that primary care is offered at the level of community health centres serving specified local areas is a large advantage for older people as it means that health care is provided on the patient's doorstep (this aspect of health care gained the support of experts from the World Bank [21]). Elderly people are the main clients of the community health centres. As a rule, they consider access to and the quality of care offered by these health centres to be of a high standard. In a longitudinal cohort study carried out in Bialystok from 1979 to 1994, only between 5% and 9% of older people reported difficulties in gaining access to a doctor either at the community health centre or in the form of a home visit [5].

The doctor is obliged to provide active counselling in the case of conditions which provide a significant risk from the epidemiological point of view (e.g. tuberculosis, venereal diseases, diabetes). Older people *per se* are not considered to be a group that is particularly at risk, and only come to the attention of the medical profession when they themselves actively seek treatment (spontaneous referral). There is no programme of prophylactic care for older people (with one or two rare exceptions [22], and at the point of retirement they cease to be included in the programme of prophylactic diagnostic tests which are required of all employees. The only exception to this are the screening tests which have been carried out in Poland for many years and which include older people, in relation to the early diagnosis of cervical cancer and radiological screening tests for tuberculosis, which have now been dropped owing to financial restrictions.

The doctor remains a central and dominant figure in the primary health care system. In relation to older people, this is seen in an increased frequency in the number of home visits made by doctors in comparison with nurses [5]. Home visits by community nurses are a rare form of care available to older people. This is one of the most striking and glaring gaps in the Polish health care system, particularly when compared to the countries of western Europe. The existing legislature does not provide a clear definition of the role and duties of a community nurse. There is little information with regard to what happens in this respect in practice nationwide. Nevertheless, from research at a community level carried out in a large urban area [23] it is apparent that the most frequent tasks carried out by community nurses in the care of older people are, in order of priority: injections and measurement of blood pressure, taking blood samples for diagnostic purposes and changing dressings. An important function of the nurse's role emphasised in this research is her psychotherapeutic role, however little importance is paid to her help in getting prescriptions or helping to maintain personal hygiene in those under her care.

Community health centres are open only on weekdays during specified hours (at the latest up to 19.00, where several doctors are employed). This lack of access to health centres, even on an emergency basis, out of normal working hours means that the accident and emergency hospital services are heavily used for one-off emergency interventions by older people. This form of intervention, which is extremely costly to the health service, is frequently over-used or even abused [21]. In 1994, in the city of Bialystok, as many as 18% of 75 year old people were attended by the accident and emergency services at least on one occasion during the year (5% used the service three times or more in that year). Accessibility of the accident and emergency services was considered to be the best in relation to all other aspects of the health service (fewer than 2% of respondents considered it to be difficult to gain access to these emergency services) [5].

Rehabilitation services are insufficiently developed and difficult for older people to gain access to, as they are focused, in the main, on dealing with injuries. Since 1995, priority of access has been given to people who are below the age of retirement, in an active drive to reduce the number of people gaining invalidity status and thus benefits. Institutions offering rehabilitation services and trained staff are very unevenly spread throughout the country. The lack of information concerning the needs of the population in terms of disability and economic restrictions have meant that rehabilitation services have not been brought closer to the prospective service users, as far as location is concerned. Many regions of the country lack the necessary facilities and specially trained personnel and as a result, access to these services is effectively limited to larger urban areas [24]. In the research carried out in Bialystok and referred to earlier, between 3.5% and 10.5% of the population (depending on their age and sex) had access to these services during the previous year. When the frequency of mobility problems in older population is considered, this reflects a relatively low level of access to rehabilitation services. It can safely be assumed that in rural areas this situation is even worse. In practice, there are no professional services for the rehabilitation of older people who are housebound.

Owing to a lack of hospital beds (especially as far as wards catering for chronic illnesses and geriatric rehabilitation are concerned) [21] ,older people, especially those of very advanced age, have difficulties in being admitted to hospital. This was confirmed by the community research in Bialystok. In 1989, as many as 55.2% of 70 year old people, and in 1994 - 33.3% of 75 year olds, reported difficulty in getting access to hospital treatment [5].

Geriatrics, as a medical speciality, has not yet found for itself a properly defined and respected role in the present system of health care. It is true that there do exist a few Specialist Health Centres for Geriatric Care in larger cities (mainly at the level of the voivodeship), but their activities are mainly restricted to providing medical consultations, very rarely are they able to offer rehabilitation services, community interventions or prophylactic care for older people.

In recent years there has been an increasing tendency for health services to become privatised (private doctors' and dentists' surgeries and to a much lesser extent, private hospitals). In 1996 more than a third of medical practitioners and nearly 90% of dentists were in private practice (for some, private practice was their only source of income, but most were also employed in the state sector) [21]. Owing to the lack of a system of private medical insurance, the costs of private treatment are not refundable, and thus are available only to a limited group of financially advantaged people. Nevertheless, older people take advantage of private medical services to the same extent (around 30%) as younger age groups [25]. The pressure on private medical services - in spite of the impoverishment of society - may be a sign of dissatisfaction with the services offered by the public health service, but equally offers a totally free choice of specialist, reduces the waiting time for the consultation, or diagnostic tests, as well as making access to hospital treatment frequently easier [21].

In 1991 the right to free prescriptions for retired people (with the exception of war veterans and their families as well as voluntary blood donors) was withdrawn [26]. The cost of medicines is partly refunded by the state, but at the same rate for all age groups. Since drug prices are no longer regulated and are open to the conditions of the free market, the costs of medicines are, in many cases, a substantial financial burden for older people, who are one of the main groups of consumers. In this respect, the situation for retired people and those in receipt of state invalidity benefits has declined significantly within the free-market system.

Older people, according to health service legislation, have, in theory, unlimited and free access to all medical services, both on an outpatient and inpatient basis and to community nursing services and equipment for the disabled etc. In practice, these services are not always available sufficiently, mainly for financial reasons. Regional differences have a great role to play here in terms of the resources available locally as far as health services are concerned, especially in relation to the patient's place of residence - urban versus rural areas [10].

Alongside the primary care structures described here, in recent years there have also been a number of experimental centres where family practitioners are based in certain areas of the country. In future, it is intended that they should replace the community health centres. The family doctor is to care for the whole family, starting from the pregnant woman and the newly born infant and ending with people in advanced old age. The new system of primary care is to be introduced in 1999 and will be based on funding provided by health insurance and not, as hitherto, from the state budget. Up to the present, however, the new health policies have not taken into consideration in any significant way the needs of older people. These needs are not reflected in any of the proposed principles of health care which are to be introduced.

Social services

Since 1990, a modern system of social services in Poland has been in the process of construction. This process was started as a result of the new Act of Parliament on social services passed on 29th November 1990 [27]. The main aim of social services became to help and facilitate individuals and families to survive difficult life situations, which they would not have been able to cope with using their own resources, possibilities and rights. The law divides the task of providing social services between local authorities and government administration. It also states that in organising social services, the local government and state administrative authorities set up for these purposes should co-operate with the various community organisations and individuals who are actively working in this area in their localities.

The first major organisational change was to set up, at the level of voivodeships, a Voivode/County Administration Unit for social services and, at the local level, centres for social services.

The Voivode Administration Unit for social services is responsible for performing the tasks laid down for it by the Voivode/Mayor. These include: drawing up an account of the needs and available resources for social services, organising and funding homes run by social services and dealing with referrals to residential homes, ensuring that commissioned work is carried out, organising training and professional courses for social services staff, and supporting the activities of non-governmental organisations.

The direct "hands-on" organisation of public social services for older people is the responsibility of community centres for social services. These are separate entities which have legal status and are funded by local government administration. The fundamental task for these centres is to provide community assistance for people living in their own homes. This includes: financial and material aid, care benefits and social work. The second aspect of the work of public social services is the placement of people in need of permanent care in residential homes run by social services.

Access to services provided by social services (financial aid and services) is determined on the basis of an administrative decision. This is made on the recommendation of one person - the director of the social services centre concerned, on the basis of an assessment of the client's social circumstances. It is required that clients should co-operate with the services to bring about an improvement in their own situation. Lack of the required co-operation or wasting existing resources may lead to assistance being limited or withdrawn entirely.

The right to financial assistance from social services is applicable to those older people who do not have any other sources of income, or to situations where the income per capita in the family does not exceed the lowest state pension and one of the following conditions pertain: poverty, homelessness, physical or mental disability, long-term illness, inability to cope with the care situation, alcoholism, drug addiction, and natural or ecological disasters. Entitlement to benefits depends on the financial and legal situation of the client, as well as recognised needs. They may be agreed on a permanent or temporary basis, or for specific purposes (such as for clothes, food, heating and rent subsidies).

Care services provided in the client's own home are available to people who are in need of the help of other people with regard to the activities of daily living, where the family is unable to provide this kind of help or the person concerned does not have a family. The services include help with meeting everyday needs, basic hygiene, nursing care which has been advised by a doctor and, as far as possible, ensuring that the person maintains contact with his environment. If the income per person in the family does not exceed the lowest rate for pensions, then these services are free of charge. In the remaining cases, the range of services provided is determined by the centre for social services according to need and the fee is established on the basis of the cared for person's income [28]. Since 1st January 1993, ensuring that a full range of care services is available is the responsibility of the local authority. These services are run by community centres for social services, which employ their own care staff or hire services from community organisations or private companies. In 1995, 93,662 people in Poland received this kind of help from social services, the majority of whom were older people. The providers of these services, apart from the staff of social services departments, were, to a significant extent, non-governmental institutions (33%) - such as the Polish Red Cross and the Polish Committee for social services, or other agencies, such as private care agencies [29].

Older people who remain in their own homes are, by law, entitled to social support (non-financial types of assistance), which includes help with arranging matters of an administrative nature, their financial affairs, and helping to ease difficulties with maintaining contacts with their surroundings and environment, as well as advisory services. Social services staff may, for example, represent their clients in court in matters concerning maintenance payments, they arrange matters connected with disability and pension benefits, and they are obliged to investigate the financial circumstances of people who are required to make maintenance payments. It is as a result of these activities that demands on the budget of the local authority are, to a large extent, limited, so that a greater number of people are able to benefit from the help of social services. Social services staff, within the context of their work activities, are also allowed to seek sponsors for their clients to ensure that they have sufficient basic food products, for example, clothes, shoes, and may apply to employers, institutions, organisations or schools, suggesting ways of providing help for those in need of assistance. Thus, apart from providing services of a financial nature (such as benefits), social services centres may employ a wide range of non-financial forms of assistance to help their clients.

Alongside some centres for social services there are also mental health clinics, alcohol advisory services or a confidential telephone advisory service. Social services also run day centres or care centres for older people. Depending on the needs of the person concerned, they may provide day care, food, basic care services, as well as meeting higher level needs, (such as providing a sense of security for older people, facilitating social contacts and helping to maintain self-esteem).

Meals are provided in their own homes for people with physical disabilities, Christmas and celebrations to mark other occasions, such as Senior Citizen's Day, are organised for people living alone, as are coach outings, rehabilitation courses, and services for washing clothes and linen as well as repairing household equipment. The fee for attending a day centre is determined according to the cost of the food provided. In 1985, there were 151 day centres throughout the country, which had at their disposal 5,616 places; by 1996 this figure had risen to 213 day centres with 11,368 places [9].

It should be said, that the services described here are those provided for by the new legislation, but in practice, provision is very variable and in some areas insufficient or even absent.

As mentioned above, social services centres (mainly in large towns and cities) work together with various other non-governmental community organisations, trying to solve problems that are the common task of both. The following organisations offer the widest range of services to older people:

The Polish Committee for social services (material and financial help, care services in the home, cultural and educational activities, legal assistance and help with food and meals)

The Polish Red Cross (material and financial assistance for people and families finding themselves in a difficult situation - collection and distribution of clothes, household equipment and furniture)

The Association of Friends of the Terminally Ill "Hospice" - help for people in the terminal stages of cancer, hospice teams providing home care and offering free medical (and other) services to people cared for in their own homes by their families, hospice facilities providing 24-hour care for people with no families and who do not have the right conditions to be cared for at home - a charge for these services is made on the same basis as in homes run by social services.

Institutional facilities are provided in the form of social services residential homes which may have a local or wider catchment area. These homes are run for different client groups (for older people, those with mental handicaps, people with long-term and psychiatric illnesses). Owing to greater investment in this area and the building of new homes, the waiting time for a place has, generally speaking, been reduced from a few years to a few months [30], though this does not apply to all regions of the country, and the number of places available still does not meet the needs of the community at large. In 1990, in Poland, there were 629 institutions providing 24-hour care which were run by social services (with a total of 68,020 places and a waiting list of 13,426), whereas in 1996, there were 872 (with 81,333 places and a waiting list of 11,974). Only a proportion of these places (20.4%) are earmarked for older people [9]. It is necessary to remember, however, that in the remaining homes, a significant proportion of the residents are within this elderly age group (over 50% of the residents of all the homes run by social services are people over the age of 60 years). In recent years, standards in these homes have improved, and rehabilitation and therapeutic services have been introduced to a significant extent. Very often, day centres have been set up alongside these homes, providing day services not only for the residents of the home, but for the community at large. Residential fees for social services homes for adults, run by local authorities, amount to double the lowest state pension, though individual residents are not required to pay more than 70% of their whole income for living there (in certain circumstances, residents may be partially or fully exempted from payment).

It should be emphasised that not all older people who qualify for the various forms of assistance from social services actually take them up. Some older people decide against this form of help for a variety of different reasons: pride prevents them from seeking help of this kind, financial considerations (they feel that the amount that they are required to pay for social services is too high) or as a result of a mistrust of unknown people. A proportion of older people simply do not have any access to contact with social services (they may not know where the centres are located, and they may have limited knowledge about the possibilities of receiving financial support, and material or care services). In a large city such as Bialystok, which is the administrative centre for the voivodeship, only 46.8% of people over the age of 60 were able to state where the centre for social services was to be found - in spite of the fact that in this particular case, its location was extremely 'user-friendly' (it was located in the same building as the community health centre) [19]. In addition, the new principles on which the social services administration is based require that older people should play an active role in solving their own problems, but at the same time, they ignore the realities which prevent them from doing so [2].

On the other hand, in the last number of years, the proportion of older people receiving help from social services has dropped, especially in rural areas. The groups which have received most help in the period of social, political and economic transformation which the country is going through at present are the unemployed and single mothers with dependent children. In 1995, families in which people were unemployed made up 50% of those receiving support from social services. Since 1993, 55-60% of the unemployed do not have the right to claim unemployment benefits, and almost half this number qualify for receiving the help of social services [30]. The law on social services makes the right to receiving benefits dependent (among other things) on the *per capita* income in the family, which may not exceed the lowest rate for state pensions. The consequence of this ruling is that a large proportion of older people are not entitled, as a result of the legislation, to take advantage of financial benefits. By far the majority of them have their own pensions or sickness and disability benefits which, as a rule, are at the level of, or just a little higher than, the cut-off defined by the means testing for entitlement to free social services.

A further problem is the limited funding at the disposal of the social services centres, especially against a background of ever increasing need. As a result, the services offered to clients do not always satisfy their expectations. It is often the case that resources are insufficient to meet even mandatory services (such as benefits for pregnant women and child benefits), to say nothing of meeting the costs of discretionary services (such as care services for older disabled people) [31].

The fact that the administrative buildings in which social services are housed are often unsatisfactory, combined with the large number of clients registered and the high caseload carried by social workers (on average 150 cases), leads to a situation in which contact with the client loses the personal and confidential character essential to its success and social workers frequently do not have time to focus on the individual needs of the client, which too are of the essence in work with older people. These are factors which have a very negative influence on the image of social services in the nineteen nineties [32].

A community team approach to primary care

The formal separation of the Ministry of Health from the Ministry of social services brought about a division in responsibilities and a deterioration in co-operation between health care and social services. It would seem, however, that the new legislation in the area of social services has brought about a general improvement in fulfilling their obligations. At the same time, however, co-operation between medical staff and social services has disintegrated at the primary care level, a claim that is supported by findings from a longitudinal cohort study carried out in a large town [5].

The community care team which, in the context of the health care system which has existed in Poland for many years, used to consist of the general medical doctor, a community nurse and a social worker was highly rated by those under its care, as well as by health care experts [21]. At present, team work between the health sector and social services sector has been weakened, which has led to a deterioration in the community team's ability to diagnose and intervene in the socio-medical problems of old age. In the day to day reality, first-line geriatric care at the primary care level is offered by the doctor and community nurse who, for obvious reasons, concentrate mainly on medical problems. In cases where, in the course of their routine assessment, they become aware of the unmet social or care needs of the individual, they inform the social worker, who then carries out an extensive assessment of the client's social circumstances and negotiates the different types of services available with the older person in need of care. Community nurses frequently voice the opinion that they are inadequately trained to work with older people, and their greatest difficulty arises from having to assess and plan the delivery of care independently, together with providing health education [33]. Care of older patients is but one of the many tasks of the community nurse. There have even been suggestions that community nurses should have courses in professional development to train them to deal with the principles of organising social care services for older people and their families, including specialist training in interpersonal communication which focuses on older client group under their care.

Since one of the characteristics of the pathology of old age is the mutual interdependency of health status and social conditions, it is reasonable to require that new forms of co-operation should be developed between health care and social services agencies, especially at the level of community care. These needs have not been addressed by any of the legislation passed to date, though at a local level there are spontaneous attempts to set up agencies which take both these aspects of care into account.

Roles of Family Carers of Older People Living at Home

The situation of the family carers of older, disabled people has never been the subject of research on a wide scale in Poland. It has usually been the case that the role of family carers has been seen from the point of view of older people themselves.

The fundamental role of the family in providing care for older people is mainly the result of the traditional model in which multi-generational families have lived together, which is not always the practice of choice, but is very often the only alternative because of the housing shortage which has existed since the war. It has been shown that the type of care offered by a family to the older person is, in general terms, equivalent to what the older person offers the family in return for this care (use of housing, care of grandchildren, financial assistance) [14]. In recent years, it is even possible to observe an increase in the financial assistance offered to children by their elderly parents [18,34] in return for the expected care offered by the children during times of illness or disability. This testifies to the closeness of family ties and the mutual obligation of one generation to another.

Regular financial assistance on the part of children to help their elderly parents is usually completely voluntary and affects around 7-12% of the population of older people in the communities in which the research was carried out [19,34].

Polish legislation ensures that children are obliged to make maintenance payments in respect of their elderly parents, who find themselves in difficult economic circumstances. In practice however, this law is invoked only in exceptional circumstances, although the newly introduced questionnaire used by social workers for the assessment of social circumstances takes into account the financial situation of all family members and may, in the future, provide a basis for invoking this law to a wider extent.

A basic form of assistance offered by families with respect to the older generations is to provide care during times of illness or disability. Around 80% of people over the age of 65 report this kind of support from their families [19]. A fairly common form of help on the part of the family is help with the activities of daily living (around 40% frequently, and around 20% sporadically). Among the population of elderly disabled people, help from the family is estimated to be of the order of 80% of cases (unpublished data from the Polish part of the SCOPE project).

Material help (clothes, food) is a form of support rarely required by older people from their families. Only 7% of people receive such help on a regular basis, and around 20% do so sporadically [19,34].

One of the most frequent forms of help which older people receive from their families is psychological support. Over 80% of older people declared this to be a form of support they received [19]. There is no research, however, either with regard to the satisfaction experienced by families in caring for their elderly relatives, or to the burden such caring may cause. The expectation would be that the burden for family carers of older people can only increase at present, as a result of the observed disintegration of life in multi-generational families. This area, however, is in need of further research.

As a result of the lack of any reliable data concerning the demographic characteristics of family carers, it is necessary to rely on indirect evidence. The people on whom older people feel that they are most frequently able to rely are their children and grandchildren (66%) and their spouses (25%). This last figure results from the fact that a great proportion of people in this age group are widowed. When this factor is taken into account (i.e. by questioning those whose spouse is still alive), then the spouse is most frequently cited as the main carer. [34].

No data exist to allow an assessment to be made of the attitudes of family carers to practitioners from either health or social services. On the other hand, there has been some research on the quality of family care for older people as assessed by doctors and nurses in the area of primary care. Only 21% of nurses and 14% of doctors regarded it as being of good quality, whilst 23% of nurses and 25% of doctors presented a negative opinion [23].

Assessment

The process of determining what kind of situation the older person finds him/herself in and assessing his/her needs (rarely that of family carers) is most frequently initiated by the doctor as one aspect of the routine medical assessment. It is undertaken only for those older people who have presented themselves with a health problem, or where someone else has asked for medical intervention. The method of assessment varies from case to case. No systematic or structured assessment instruments such as questionnaires are used in practice. Scales to measure functional performance are used only sporadically, mainly in rehabilitation centres. An exception exists in the assessment of aspects of performance on the activities of daily living, which are included in part of the medical application for placement in a care institution. The majority of the social needs of people living in the community are directed to the appropriate centre for social services, depending on the client's place of residence, and here the social workers are in direct contact with the doctor from the community health centre (it is often the case that the health and social services centres occupy the same building). The social workers are then able to carry out an in-depth interview concerning the client's home and family situation, based on an extensive questionnaire. This instrument assesses in particular the financial circumstances of the client and his/her whole family, with the aim of determining the extent to which the client will be required to pay for any services recommended by the doctor or negotiated with the client during the course of the interview. In addition, an assessment is made of the health status of the whole family (taking into consideration any disabilities, alcoholism, drug addiction) and the employment status of family members. Since one of the parties to the negotiations is the older person and/or his/her family, the questionnaire offers the possibility of helping to identify the main family carer. In cases where the aim of the assessment is to determine whether the older person should be placed in a residential home, the questionnaire is extended to include other assessment instruments. It is worth mentioning that the instrument is used to determine the home situation of all potential clients of social services (irrespective of age). It was introduced one year ago and its use is obligatory in all cases of applying for help from public sources.

Case Studies

Case 1

Female, aged 76, with osteoarthritis of the hips and knees, poor vision due to macular degeneration, and hypertension. Mobile with a frame within her home except for the stairs. Needs help with mobility outside, shopping, cooking and housework.

Social circumstances (A): Older person living alone in an isolated farmhouse. Widowed. Little money. Daughter and son-in-law unemployed with four children, aged 9 months to 7 years, and live 5 kilometres away. Two other children of the older person live over 100 kilometres away.

The role of the family carers In this case, the main burden of care for the older person would fall upon the daughter living close by. It is most likely that she, together with her unemployed husband, will try to help her mother by taking over all the tasks she is unable to take care of herself (cooking, shopping, housework). The level of care that can be delivered "at a distance" however, is unlikely to meet all of the older person's needs and will inevitably lead to a reduction in her quality of life.

If the daughter is not able to provide all of the essential care that her mother needs (bearing in mind that she has her own home and four children to look after), she will be forced to look for someone to care for her mother. This person is most likely to be employed on a purely private basis and not to have any training in the care of older people (a young unemployed person or a middle aged woman who has brought up her own family and is looking for ways of increasing her income, most likely in an informal way (i.e. avoiding tax and national insurance contributions)). The daughter and son-in-law are thus taking on an additional expense which, depending on relationships within the family, may be met in part or in full by the other children, living further away. In view of the tradition of being able to rely, above all, on family help in difficult circumstances and, to a lesser extent, awareness of the legal obligation that children have to take care of their parents, it is most likely that the children will come forward spontaneously to offer financial help to their mother.

If the family are indeed willing and able to offer financial support, making it possible to employ a paid carer, once the housing arrangements have been adapted as necessary, it may be possible for the older person to continue living in her own home and have her basic needs met. There is also the option of older people mother going to live with one of the children living further away, if only for the winter period.

If, in the vicinity of the older person's home, there are other households, it is possible that the neighbours might offer to help since, in rural areas, communities live very close-knit lives and it is common-place for people to help each other as a matter of course. Should it be the case that the members of the family have real financial difficulties, or show no interest in their mother, it is likely that neighbours would see to the older person's instrumental needs (on an entirely voluntary basis, or with social services meeting some of the costs). It is likely that a neighbour of an older disabled person would help her to prepare a meal, do her shopping and spend time with her.

Professional care In the situation described above, it is unlikely that the older person would be eligible for support from social services. Although most local authorities have social services centres, they are unable to serve all the villages in their catchment area. Very often, these centres employ only one person. In cases where an older person is referred to the Community Centre for social services by a health centre doctor, by the family or by neighbours, because of finding themselves in very difficult circumstances, there exists the possibility of applying for financial support (in the form of permanent or temporary benefits, or those designed to meet a particular need), which is means tested. In this situation it is likely that the older person would be granted financial support, which would make it possible to pay for the services of a carer. There is also the possibility that social services would pay in part for the services provided by neighbours, to the extent of two hours per day.

Assessment and support of family carers There is no formal system for assessing the needs of carers. No form of organised help is available (e.g. specialist advisory services regarding care provision, psychological advice, information services) to carers living in rural areas.

The social services interview for assessing the social circumstances of the older disabled person, which has recently been introduced, is designed to be the same, irrespective of the reasons for referral or the age of the client. As far as the family is concerned, its main interest is with regard to the financial circumstances, in order to determine their liability to pay for the services negotiated.

Social circumstances (B): Older person lives alone in a ground floor flat in town. Widowed. Daughter and son-in-law are both teachers in full-time employment, with 2 children aged 7 and 11, and live within 1 kilometre in the same town.

The role of family carers The family carers of the older woman living closeby in the same town have an easier task than that described in the previous case. They are able to visit their older mother more frequently. This means that they can supply hot meals which they cook in their own home, and help with the heavier household tasks, as well as assisting the older person with walking outside, and they are likely to find it easier to take her to their own home, so that she can spend at least part of the day with them. Maintaining contact with their elderly mother is also likely to be easier, as both households are more likely to have a telephone, enabling the older person to call for help in emergencies. In this case, it is possible to help by re-organising the immediate environment of the older person, to assist her in maintaining her independence to a maximum and thus in carrying out essential household tasks.

The family carers also have greater possibilities at their disposal for organising more institutionalised help for their mother (either from social services or by employing a paid carer). It is also possible that certain services (such as shopping, preparing meals) might be provided by neighbours living in the same block of flats. In many areas neighbourly help still plays an important role, especially in older areas of towns and cities, where residents know each other very well.

Professional care In this case, it would be possible to seek assistance from social services, from charitable organisations, or from the self-help groups which are gradually beginning to be formed in larger towns and cities throughout Poland. Centres for social services receive referrals from community health centre doctors or general practitioners, requesting care services from a Polish Red Cross nurse or a carer from the Polish Committee for social services. They would provide some of the following services, as necessary: delivery of hot meals to the person's home, help with household tasks such as cleaning, shopping and washing. These services are provided on a means tested basis. The costs may be covered in part by the client, and in part by social services. There is also the possibility of taking advantage of the services provided by a Day Care Centre or a Community Centre if one exists in the town.

Should the client or his/her carer make an application to the state Fund for the Rehabilitation of Disabled People, they can count on getting professional help in the form of assistance with carrying out the necessary changes to the person's home to make coping with their disability less cumbersome (e.g. handles around the bath, appropriate lighting, removing hazards and dangerous equipment around the home). The client is required to make a contribution to the cost of these services.

Assessment and support of family carers In towns, as in rural areas, no formal assessment is made of the needs of family carers. Family carers needing help in different situations are left to seek assistance on their own. They can turn to charitable organisations which are concerned with older people and to health service facilities for specific advice on dealing with the organisation of care for their older relative.

Social circumstances (C): Older person lives with spouse in 2-storey house. Retired with savings. Spouse is fit and well. No children. Bedroom, bathroom and toilet are upstairs.

The role of family carers It is most likely that the main carer of the older person in these circumstances will be her husband, who is in good health and physically fit. He will help her with managing the stairs and outside and will have to deal with all the household tasks which his disabled wife is unable to cope with e.g. preparing meals, shopping, cleaning. The good financial situation in which this couple find themselves will enable them to pay for services, as the need arises (hiring someone to help with the heavier household tasks, general cleaning etc.).

Professional care In this case, where the husband of the disabled older person is physically fit and the couple are financially secure, it is unlikely that social services would provide any kind of input in the form of services or benefits since, in practice, their interventions are restricted to circumstances in which the referred person has no family carer (or where the family carer is him/herself disabled), or in cases of difficult financial circumstances. The significant lack of personnel employed in social services means that they are unable to concern themselves with all those who are in need of help, and must restrict their services to situations in which the client has no other sources of help available to him. The husband of the older person has every right to apply for help with adapting their home to meet his wife's needs (e.g. ensuring there is a downstairs bathroom).

Assessment and support of family carers Once again, there is no system for the formal assessment of family carers and their needs. Should the husband of the older person be in need of assistance in the present situation, he will be left to rely on his own resources in looking for it. He may apply to have modifications made to their home to meet the needs of his wife in terms of mobility and using a walking frame. If he applies to the state Fund for the Rehabilitation of Disabled People, it is likely that he will get assistance with moving the bathroom and toilet downstairs, thus adapting the home to meets the needs of his disabled wife. Any help the carer may get in adapting his home in this way is not the result of a pro-active outreach policy the aim of which is to assess and then try to meet the needs of the client and his/her carer, but of the carer's own enterprise in seeking out information and help.

Case 2

Male aged 80, facing discharge from hospital following a stroke. Expected to be confined to bed or chair for several weeks with gradual recovery of mobility. Needs the help of one person for transfers, toileting, bathing and dressing.

Social circumstances (A): Older person living alone in an isolated farmhouse. Widowed. Little money. Daughter and son-in-law with four children, aged 9 months to 7 years, live 5 kilometres away. Two other children of the older person live over 100 kilometres away.

The role of the family carers In the case of a person awaiting discharge from hospital following a stroke, the social worker involved would carry out an assessment of the social circumstances of the client to determine whether the client will have the necessary care provided in his own home. This would be the case in the circumstances outlined above. If the immediate family is unable to organise help for their elderly father and, if the older person's condition promises to improve, then it is most likely that, at the family's request, he will remain in hospital for a longer period on either a Neurological or Rehabilitation ward. Nevertheless, this is unlikely to be for very long. Thus, if the disabled client, who may be disabled even in the most basic areas of the Activities of Daily Living (transferring, toileting, bathing, dressing) ,is discharged from hospital, then the most likely outcome for him will be that he will go to live with his children for a period of time. The client has three children, and they may take it in turns to care for their elderly father for a period of time sufficient for him to improve enough to return to his own home. The immediate family may receive 14 days paid leave from their place of work in order to take care of a sick member of the family.

Professional care Despite the fact that in the majority of local authority areas there are community centres for social services, the likelihood of being able to arrange help in the form of services from them (visits from a Polish Red Cross nurse, assistance with maintaining everyday hygiene, cleaning etc.) is virtually non-existent. These are not services which are provided on a wide scale and, in practice, in situations where the client lives at some distance away from the community centre for social services, he may not be provided with practical services of any kind and thus be forced to go into a social services residential home. The waiting list for residential homes may, in turn, be very long, as the demand for places is well in excess of the those actually available. Depending on the region of the country, the waiting time may be of the order of several weeks, months or even years.

In recent years, private residential homes have been set up which cater for clients who are able to pay for residency in these homes. The waiting period for a place is shorter, because the fees are much higher than in homes run by social services. Nonetheless, the likelihood that in this case the older person would have access to a private home in a rural area is very small, since they have arisen in large centres of population, which are relatively wealthy. For example, although a number of such homes exist in the vicinity of Warsaw, medium and smaller size cities are unlikely to have access to services of this kind. Bialystok, a medium sized city in the north-east of Poland does not have any private residential homes. It is possible to apply for help in the form of services, benefits to pay for nursing care and financial support for specific purposes in respect of any of the options discussed above.

Assessment and support of family carers In rural areas, even people whose needs are most acute have difficulty in gaining access to support from social services. There is no system in place for assessing and trying to meet the needs of family carers. It is likely to be the case that the client's family, finding themselves in difficult financial circumstances, are themselves in receipt of benefits from social services, and are therefore clients in their own right, and not just carers. It is therefore unlikely that their needs as carers will be met by social services.

Social circumstances (B): Older person lives alone in a ground floor flat in town. Widowed. Daughter and son-in-law are both teachers in full-time employment, with 2 children aged 7 and 11, and live within 1 kilometre in the same town.

The role of family carers In this case, should difficulties arise (e.g. because of the working arrangements of the family carers) in ensuring that the older person has adequate care in his own home (determined on the basis of an assessment carried out by a hospital social worker, who keeps in touch with the client's family), the most likely course of action would be to extend the period of hospitalisation to cover this period, in the light of the expectation that the older person is likely to improve over the next few weeks. This is relatively commonplace following stroke. If, however, the disabled older person is in fact discharged from hospital, then in urban conditions, it will be easier for the family to arrange care for him. In this case the older person lives close to his daughter, which means that she would be able to visit him frequently and to provide him with the necessary care. Another possibility would be for the older person to go to live with his family for the period required for him to regain sufficient independence to be able to return to his own home.

Should the family be unable to ensure that their father receives adequate care using their own resources, it is likely that they would employ the services of a paid carer, or of any support that social services may be able to offer.

Professional care In cases where an older, disabled person is ready for discharge from hospital, the hospital social worker will routinely carry out an assessment of the person's social circumstances to determine who is to provide further care for the patient. If the family is unable to take over this role, the older person will be referred to social services by the doctor in charge of the case, with a request for specific services. This may be the services of a Polish Red Cross nurse (to provide nursing care and maintain personal hygiene) or a carer from the Polish Committee for social services (to help with domestic tasks such as cleaning and preparing meals). The time available to provide these services may not exceed two hours per day. In the case of someone living alone, there exists the possibility of providing help in the form of the services of a community nurse from the community health centre. The range of help offered in this way and the frequency of delivery vary from one health centre to another. There is also a severe shortage of community nurses and social workers, which means that they have ever increasing caseloads with more and more demands made on their time. Typically, nurses will visit on an occasional basis to help with nursing care. If it is likely to be the case that the disability is only temporary, it is possible for them to intensify their input over this period.

Assessment and support of family carers There is no form of routine assessment for family carers. In this case it is most likely that the family themselves would initiate the request for professional help in organising care for their disabled father and adapting his home environment to meet his needs. The need to provide him with help in the personal activities of daily living might lead them to seek professional advice regarding the safest and simplest way of carrying out these tasks. The family carers will, however, have to seek this information out for themselves.

Social circumstances (C): Older person lives with spouse in 2-storey house. Retired with savings. Spouse is fit and well. No children. Bedroom, bathroom and toilet are upstairs.

The role of family carers In cases where the older person, awaiting discharge from hospital, has a spouse who is fit and healthy, it is most likely that the main burden of care will rest on his/her shoulders, as the closest family member. This is a very typical situation, in which one spouse fulfils the role of carer with respect to his/her partner (who is more sick or disabled). The wife's role will be to help her husband in carrying out all the tasks associated with the personal activities of daily living (transferring, toileting, bathing, dressing), with which he continues to have difficulty. It is likely that she will try to continue his process of rehabilitation as far as she is able, on the basis of practical advice she receives from the hospital doctor, the rehabilitation specialist and nursing staff.

Professional care If the family carer (wife) is able to help the older person with transferring, personal hygiene, dressing etc., as well as carrying out essential household tasks, it is unlikely that social services will become involved in this situation. Possible help might come in the form of adapting the home to meet the needs of the older person, or supplying necessary mobility aids (walking stick, crutches, walking frame).

Assesment and support of family carers In this case, as in all the situations discussed previously, there is no system in place for assessing the needs of the family carer. Should the family carer (wife) experience problems of an organisational nature, with which she would like to have help of a professional kind (e.g. rehabilitation) then she will have to take the initiative in looking for assistance. In most cases she is likely to turn to the health centre for help, and not to social services . If the couple's financial position allows, there exists the possibility of arranging for rehabilitation and physiotherapy sessions in their own home, on a private and therefore paid basis.

Case 3

Female, aged 86, suffering from dementia. Frequent wandering by day and night. Frequent falls. Incontinent of urine and faeces.

Social circumstances (A): Older person living alone in an isolated farmhouse. Widowed. Little money. Daughter and son-in-law are unemployed with four children, aged 9 moths to 7 years, and live 5 kilometres away. Two other children of the older person live over 100 kilometres away.

The role of family carers It is unlikely that the 86 year old person with advanced dementia will be able to live alone. Her family carers will have to ensure that she receives the required support and care necessary in her condition. The most likely scenario would be that one of the children would take their mother to live with them. Alternatively, she might live with each of the children in turn. They will have to care for their mother themselves, or ensure that she receives the 24-hour care that is essential in this situation. If they are unable to provide this, it is most likely that they will initiate the procedure for placing their mother in a residential home run by social services. Another possibility is for their mother to be placed in a psychiatric hospital on a long-term basis; since the care provided would be under the domain of the Health Service, it would be provided free of charge.

Professional care In this case the family could expect to receive help from social services in the form of incontinence pads and other articles for maintaining personal hygiene, should their mother remain in their care. They would also be eligible to apply for social security benefits in respect of providing 24-hour care, which might be granted on either a temporary or a permanent basis. No specialist services are likely to be available in rural areas. The only other alternative is to place the older person in a social services home, for which the waiting lists, as already mentioned, are very variable.

Assessment and support of family carers No formal assessments are made. The most likely scenario is that the family carers will be left to their own resources. They cannot expect help from social services in their own right as this is not a routine consideration.

Social circumstances (B): Older person lives alone in a ground floor flat in town. Widowed. Daughter and son-in-law are both teachers in full-time employment, with 2 children aged 7 and 11, and live within 1 kilometre in the same town.

The role of family carers In these circumstances, the family may try to care for their mother, so far as they are able, until alternative arrangements can be made. The family carers are likely to engage other members of the family in the care process. As the daughter is working full-time, she will be forced to make significant changes to her own life, maybe even giving up her job, to care for her mother. Since the older person exhibits some of the most difficult symptoms to deal with, in particular wandering, she requires 24-hour care. This means that her daughter may have to take her into her own home, or go to live with her, thus disrupting her own family life significantly. The services of a paid carer are unlikely to prove helpful here, as it will be almost impossible to find an untrained person willing to take on this kind of responsibility, 24 hours a day.

Professional care There are no specialised services for older people, either in the area of general medicine or in psychiatry. This means that the older person would remain under the care of her community health centre. Although a community nurse from the health centre might become involved in her care, this may not necessarily be the case, as community nurses were, until recently, allowed to refuse visits to psychiatric patients in the community, as they have no specialist training in caring for those with psychiatric disturbances. Recent legislation, however, now obliges community nurses to visit all patients irrespective of diagnosis. It is highly unlikely, however, that either the services of a community nurse or a paid carer, even if provided under the auspices of social services, would provide this lady with the level of care that she needs to ensure her safety and optimise her level of functioning in the light of her condition. Social services would thus, in fact, be unable to maintain this lady in the community without very intensive care and support from her family.

The alternative of a social services residential home exists, but waiting times are very varied, from a few months to several years, and this may not be a realistic option in practice. This leaves long-term hospital care or care provided by private homes which, as already mentioned, are not only expensive (the monthly cost is of the order of twice the average monthly salary), but may simply not exist in some areas of the country. Social services day care facilities would not be available to this lady in view of her symptoms. Few community psychiatric services exist.

Assessment and support of family carers No routine assessments are made. In many towns self-help organisations which bring together the families of people suffering from various conditions (e.g. Alzheimer's disease) are beginning to be formed. Their aim is to provide mutual support, possibilities of help in caring for the older person, counselling and advice on how to cope with specific difficulties, as well as providing a forum in which carers may exchange experiences. It is not always the case, however, that information about the existence of these organisations is readily available to those who might benefit from their services.

Social circumstances (C): Older person lives with spouse in 2-storey house. retired with savings. Spouse fit and well. No children. Bedroom, bathroom and toilet are upstairs.

The role of family carers Once again, in this situation, the full burden of care will rest with the older person's husband, the family carer. He will have to help her with personal hygiene and toileting, and provide 24-hour care, especially at times when she is disorientated or wandering. Given the age of the couple concerned, it is unlikely that they will be able to count on help from other family members, especially as they have no children themselves. The burden of care in these circumstances will be enormous, and will be borne by older people spouse.

Professional care Help from social services might be available in the form of occasional visits from community nurses, who will help with general household tasks and others which the family carer may be unable to carry out himself. Financial help is unlikely to be offered in these circumstances, since the couple have their own savings, though incontinence pads would be supplied free of charge.

Assessment and support of family carers No assessments of family carers are routinely made. The community nurse who makes regular visits to the homes of all geriatric patients would try to offer help and advice to older people carer in coping with his disabled wife. This may include advice on nursing care, help in adapting the home environment (providing easier access to the toilet, securing equipment which might provide a risk to the older person etc.). It is also possible that neighbours might offer help, which would provide the older carer with a break to help him to carry out his duties with regard to his wife.

Future Developments

Despite the fact that already eight years have passed since the change in the political system, Poland is still in a state of flux and transformation, and is rebuilding and developing its economic potential as a condition *sinequa non* for improving the effectiveness of its social policy. Legislative processes affecting this sphere of social life have not yet been completed, and economic realities would not appear to be a guarantee for achieving security in the area of health care and social services, not just where older people are concerned. Unfortunately, information regarding the details of health service reforms is still too little and too general to permit them to be fully applied to the needs of older people.

New health policies are directed towards the family, emphasising the role of the family doctor (general practitioner) whose services are available on a 24-hour basis and who is responsible for the health of the family in general. This is an opportunity not only for families, but for older people themselves, to receive help. Family doctors should therefore be extensively trained in geriatrics and social gerontology, knowledge of which they did not gain during their basic medical training. Gerontology is not a compulsory subject in Medical Schools and is taught in only 5 of the eleven Medical Faculties in the country. The lack of a common teaching programme both during medical studies and at a postgraduate level makes it impossible to introduce standard ways of incorporating the problems of older people into routine medical practice. Thus, education in the area of clinical and social gerontology creates a basic challenge and sets out the likely direction for any changes.

A further challenge for modern-day gerontology in Poland is to bring about an improvement in team co-operation between practitioners in the field of primary care in the area of recognising and helping to solve the complex problems and needs of the older person in his/her life environment. An essential condition for this kind of co-operation is the mutual exchange of information, based on objective and standardised instruments for the assessment of functional, psychological and social status. This would enable a standard approach to be developed with regard to the diagnosis and meeting of individual needs. Taking the opinion of the older person and/or his/her family carer into account when arriving at decisions would not only be a better way of finding out about and meeting their needs, but would also be a way of asserting their value in this situation. The development of pluralism in care provision, as well as providing support for family carers, might be a way of reducing the need for services from public sources, and at the same time help to improve quality of life for older people.

A further important challenge for health and social policy in Poland is the complex range of activities required to maintain and improve the functional status of older people. Multifaceted educational schemes, the promotion of healthy lifestyles, food consumption and recreation are not enough to compensate for geriatric rehabilitation. Deficits in this area should be tackled with the assistance of newly established Departments of Geriatric Rehabilitation and Extended Convalescence and widely accessible resource centres based in primary care centres, which could be used by people who are housebound [35].

Many of these, and other, recommendations have already been put forward several times in the form of expert advice, projects and reports by the Polish Association of Gerontology to the Ministry of Health. They have not, to date, been taken into account in health and social policies, nor have they been introduced into practice. It only remains to hope that, together with improvements in the economic situation of the country and the strengthening of local communities in the wake of the administrative reforms which have taken place in Poland, all of these recommendations will at last be realised.

References

[1] B. Synak, Ludzie starzy w warunkach przelomu systemowego: od dualizmu do pluralizu opiekuńczego. *Zeszyty Problemowe PTG*, **2,1** (1994) 6-23.

[2] B. Synak, Poland: Ageing and Integration in a Post-communistist Society. In: Elderly People in Industrialised Societies. Social Integration. In: H Mollenkopf (ed.), Old Age by or despite Technology, 1996,53-62.

[3] I. Svetlik I, The future of welfare pluralism in the postcommunistic countries. Eurosocial Report, **40/1** (1991) 13-23.

[4] B. Bień, Health Status and Health Care for older people in Bialystok, Poland: A 15-year Cross-Sequential Cohort Survey, 1979 - 1994. In: Social Welfare and Health Care for older people in Post-Socialistic Poland. Ed.: J.R. Rollwagen USA (in press).

[5] B. Bień, Wplyw pozaontogenetycznych uwarunkowań starzenia na zdrowotna i psycho-socjalna sytuacje ludzi starych: 15-letnie przekrojowo-sekwencyjne badania kohortowe ludzi starych w Bialymstoku. Praca habilitacyjna. Wydawnictwo Uczelniane, Bialystok 1996.

[6] K. Misko-Iwanek, Praca socjalna w pomocy spolecznej. W: Ubóstwo jako problem polityki spolecznej. Materialy z Ogólnopolskiej Konferencji Naukowej. Ustroń Wielkopolski, 13-16. VI.1993. Akademia Ekonomiczna im. Karola Adamieckiego w Katowicach, 1993,107-112.

[7] Z. Kawczynska-Butrym, Problemy wspierania rodzin z osobami niepelnosprawnymi. W: Badania nad niepelnosprawnoœci1 w Polsce 1993. Red.: A.Ostrowska, Warszawa 1994, 31-35.

[8] J. Coenen-Huther and B. Synak, Post-Communistic Poland: From Totalitarism to Democracy. New York, Nova Science 1993.

[9] GUS: Rocznik statystyczny 1997. Warszawa 1997.

[10] W. Piatkowski, Problemy spoleczne starych niepelnosprawnych mieszkańców wsi. Gerontologia Polska , **5,1**, (1997) 37-41.

[11] W. Pedich and T. Smolski, Rola szpitali w leczeniu i rehabilitacji ludzi starych. *Zdrowie Publiczne*, **87,2** (1976) 107-113.

[12] A. Zajenkowska-Kozlowska, Zdrowie w rodzinie i wydatki na ochrone zdrowia w 1994 r. Raport z badania modulowego przeprowadzonego w IV kwartale 1994r. w ramach Badania Budzetów

Gospodarstw Domowych. Główny Urząd Statystyczny. Departament Srodowiska i i Uslug Spolecznych, Warszawa 1996.

[13] J. Kopczynski and J. Halik, Zdrowie ludnosci i jego ochrona. W: A.Rajkiewicz (red.) Społeceństwo polskie w latach 1995/96. Warszawa, Fundacja im. F.Eberta: 1989 119-130.

[14] B. Synak, The Polish Family: Stability, Change and Conflict *Journal of Ageing Studies*, **4,4** (1990) 333-344.

[15] J. Piotrowski, Miejsce czlowieka starego w rodzinie i społeczeństwie. PWN Warszawa 1973.

[16] Sytuacja bytowa ludzi starszych w 1985 roku. 1985. Warszawa. Główny Urzad Statystyczny.

[17] B. Synak, Czlowiek stary i jego rodzina w zmieniajacej sie rzeczywistosci ekonomicznej w Polsce. *Problemy rodziny*, **1** (1992) 3-8.

[18] A. Kotlarska-Michalska, Analiza porównawcza wybranych wskazników wiezi rodzinnej wielkomiejskich malzeństw w starszym wieku. W: Z.Tyszka (red.) Analiza przemian wybranych kategorii rodzin polskich. Poznań 1990.

[19] M. Halicka and W. Pedich, Dzialania samopomocowe ludzi starszych. Badania panelowe w Bialymstoku. Mutual aid activity of older people. Report on the Bialystok Study. Akademia Medyczna, Bialystok 1997.

[20] Ekspertyza Polskiego Towarzystwa Gerontologicznego: Prawa obywatelskie ludzi starych w Polsce a Europejskie Deklaracje Praw Czlowieka. Materialy sympozjum PTG w ramach VI Euroforum, Bialystok 19-20 IV.1996. Gerontologia Polska 1996, 4, 2.

[21] W.C. Wlodarczyk, Reforma opieki zdrowotnej w Polsce. Studium polityki zdrowotnej. Uniwersyteckie Wydawnictwo Medyczne "Vesalius", Kraków 1998.

[22] M. Matlega, Sytuacja zdrowotna starszych mieszkańców Rzeszowszczyzny. W: Malikowski M. (red.): Problemy spoleczne w okresie zmian systemowych w Polsce. Materialy konferencyjne, Rzeszów 1997: 392-398.

[23] E. Fojt and G. Franek, Stan podstawowej opieki zdrowotnej nad ludzmi starszymi w województwie katowickim. Gerontologia Polska, **4(4)** (1996) 15- 19.

[24] A Wilmowska-Pietruszyńska and G. Wawrzyńczyk-Kaplińska, Aspekty organizacyjne rehabilitacji leczniczej w Polsce. Zdrowie Publ, CVII (8) (1997) 190-192.

[25] GUS: Stan zdrowia ludnosci Polski w 1996 roku. Warszawa 1997.

[26] Rozporzadzenie MZiOS z 17 wrzeœnia o nowych zasadach odplatnosci za leki, 1991

[27] Ustawa o pomocy spolecznej z dnia 29.11.1990. W: Dziennik Ustaw 1990, Nr 87, poz. 506.

[28] J. Kuleszyńska-Dobrek, Ludzie starzy i kombatanci - stan prawny. W: Pedich W.(red): Ludzie starzy. Centrum Rozwoju Sluzb Spolecznych, Warszawa, 1996: 53-63.

[29] A. Wisniewska, Polityka spoleczna wobec ludzi starych. W: Materialy VI Euroforum pt. "Ludzie starzy jako współtwórcy zycia rodzinnego i spolecznego", Bialystok 1996: 11-20.

[30] M. Przewoznik, Pomoc spoleczna w okresie przemian W: Malikowski M. (red.): Problemy spoleczne w okresie zmian systemowych w Polsce. Materialy konferencyjne, Rzeszów. 1997:452-465.

[31] A. Gajewski, Problemy socjalne ludzi starych w województwie bialostockim. W: Materialy VI Euroforum pt. "Ludzie starzy jako współtwórcy zycia rodzinnego i spolecznego", Bialystok 1996: 33-41.

[32] I. Klimowicz and L. Barylski, Od opieki do pomocy spolecznej. W: Malikowski M. (red.): Problemy spoleczne w okresie zmian systemowych w Polsce. Materialy konferencyjne, Rzeszów 1997 490-495.

[33] H. Kochaniuk, Opieka geriatryczna - zadania i przygotowanie zawodowe w opinii pielęgniarek srodowiskowych. *Gerontologia Polska*, **5(4)** (1997) 50-52.

[34] P. Czekanowski, Pomoc rodzinna i pozarodzinna w zyciu osoby starszej. Gerontologia Polska, **3(1/2)** (1995) 20-25.

[35] W. Pedich W., Wojszel B.: Health Policy and Practice for older people in Post-Socialist Poland: An Overview. In: Social Welfare and Health Care for Older People in Post-Socialistic Poland. Ed.: J.R. Rollwagen USA (in press).

Chapter 8

Portugal
(January 2000)

Daniela Figueiro
Universidade de Aveiro
Depart. De Ciencias da Educacao
Campus Universitario de Santiago
P-3810 Aveiro
Portugal

Liliana Sousa
Universidade de Aveiro
Depart. De Ciencias da Educacao
Campus Universitario de Santiago
P-3810 Aveiro
Portugal

Introduction

In Portugal, it is only since the 70s that the problems of the elderly and old age policies began to move into the foreground.

At present the Portuguese Constitution states that the elderly have the same rights and duties as all other Portuguese citizens since their judicial capacity is not in any way limited due to their age. Thus, article 72 states that:

1. The elderly have the right to economic security, to living conditions and family and community social intercourse which respect their personal autonomy and avoid and overcome personal isolation or marginalisation.

2. Third age policy includes economic, social and cultural measures which offer the elderly opportunities for personal fulfilment by means of active participation in the life of the community.

From these two points, the conclusion is that third age policy should not be based solely on the provision of material support (although such support is important for economic and social security) but also on adopting social and cultural measures which overcome isolation and social marginalisation (active participation in the life of the community, continuing links with the workplace and colleagues after retirement, creation of cultural clubs in third age centres, organisation of collective work in homes for the elderly, etc.)[1].

The recognition, socially legitimised and authorised in the Constitution of the Republic, of the need to introduce social policies specifically directed at old age constitutes a support for the creation of and further development of support structures for the elderly.

We can identify two missions for old age: the first is based on medical assistance; the second is based on social assistance. The organisation of these two types of support is different, although some signs of links are beginning to emerge between the social and health structures which provide support to people in this age group.

Regarding health services, the elderly Portuguese population does not have specific equipment and services, but rather resorts to the general care system which is designed for the general population, both in the sphere of primary health care as in specialised and differentiated care. In this context, the strategy which has been adopted is that of integrating specific responses to the needs of the elderly in the global health policy [1].

As for social responses, two types of support must be distinguished. In the first instance, institutions which provide collective accommodation for the elderly at greater risk of losing their independence and/ or autonomy, namely homes or residences.

More recently institutions were created which sought in principle to keep people in their own homes and to integrate them in the community. These are day centres, social centres and home help services, amongst other less generalised modalities. These modalities are preferred not only because it is considered that they give more respect to the dignity of the elderly, but also because it provides a less costly solution than accommodation. In all three of these responses the basic principle of respect is upheld by means of integration, provision of services to help the elderly meet their nutritional, health and entertainment needs by the organisation of walks and the widest variety of socio-cultural activities.

Country specific context

Like other countries in the European community, Portugal today shows a marked decline in fertility and birth rates, which, combined with the decrease in mortality rates, is the basis for the present process of demographic ageing (Table 1).

Table 1: Development of birth, fertility and mortality rates (1970 – 1987)

Year	Birth Rate	Fertility Rate	Death Rate
1970	19.2	79.9	10.4
1975	18.9	74.7	10.4
1980	15.9	65.7	9.6
1985	12.6	51.2	9.5
1986	12.2	49.2	9.3
1987	11.8	45.1	9.2

If the present tendency continues, the Portuguese population will go through a process of growing increasingly aged, as is the case already in many countries in Europe, with all the social repercussions on health, utilisation of services and cost of care. Thus, reading table 2, which draws a comparison between the elderly population and the total population of Portugal, allows us to conclude that in 1995, the number of people over 65 was already close to 14.7% of the total population, a figure, which, according to the prospective analyses of INE (National Statistics Institute) is tending to increase to 16%.

On the other hand, the table also shows us that the percentages of women relative to the total Portuguese population is in all elderly age bands higher than the percentages of men.

In effect, the problem of demographic ageing is linked to the economic, social and cultural transformations occurring in contemporary societies. They reflect the changes in demographic behaviour which are the result of the socio-economic development process, in which there are migratory movements, largely responsible for the spatial asymmetries evident in our country[1]. In fact, the socio-economic development of the coastal regions is a factor which attracts flows of migration which lead to the depopulation of the inland areas of the country, namely of their young working population. Thus, and although the regional asymmetry has been diminishing progressively, it is a fact that in our country there is a coastal zone which has a younger population, an intermediary zone which is average aged and an inner zone which is quite aged.

Table 2: Comparison of the elderly population with the total population (by sexes)

Age Groups	1995* MF	1995* M	1995* F	2000** MF	2000** M	2000** F	2005*** MF	2005*** M	2005*** F
65-69	5% (n=491 140)	4,6% (n=218 216)	5,3% (n=272 880)	5% (n=494 934)	4,6% (n=219 581)	5,3% (n=275 353)	4,8% (n=481 484)	4,4% (n=213 826)	5,1% (n=267 658)
70-74	4,1% (n=409 360)	3,7% (n=175 370)	4,5% (n=233 990)	4,3% (n=431 634)	3,8% (n=182 603)	4,8% (n=249 031)	4,3% (n=438 378)	3,8% (n=185 292)	4,8% (n=253 086)
75-79	2,8% (n=273 720)	2,3% (n=110 200)	3,2% (n=163 520)	3,3% (n=326 122)	2,7% (n=130 298)	3,8% (n=195 824)	3,4% (n=348 129)	2,8% (n=137 271)	4% (n=210 858)
80-84	1,8% (n=179 100)	1,4% (n=65 290)	2,2% (n=113 810)	1,8% (n=183 028)	1,4% (n=66 695)	2,2% (n=116 333)	2,2% (n=222 162)	1,6% (n=79 647)	2,7% (n=142 516)
85 e +	1% (n=103 230)	0,6% (n=31 010)	1,4% (n=72 220)	1,1% (n=111 579)	0,4% (n=35 031)	1,5% (n=76 548)	1,2% (n=118 202)	0,8% (n=37 400)	1,5% (n=80 802)

Age groups

H = Male
M = Female

Source: INE, Projections of the Resident Population

* The total population is 9,920,764; Men: 4,777,480; Women: 5,143,280
** The total population is 10,023,175; Men: 4,829,094; Women: 5,194,082
*** The total population is 10,111,864; Men: 4,873,232; Women: 5,238,632

In this way, Portugal today has a rate of ageing of about 15%, with some prospective analyses indicating values close to 20% in the year 2020 [2].

As for the main causes of death in this age group, in Portugal the main cause of death is cerebral vascular accidents (CVA), closely followed by cardiovascular illness. This situation indicates that probably in us there is a specific tendency to a high prevalence of arterial hypertension, which is the opposite of what is happening in other developed countries and namely in the European Union [2].

Regarding death from malignant tumours and chronic respiratory disease its position on the mortality table is identical to that of other countries [2].

Ermida [2] draws attention to other mortality rates in the aged Portuguese population which are quite significant and possibly less well-known. These are pneumonia and flu complications, accidents and suicides.

Legal situation concerning responsibilities for the care of older people

As well as article 72 of our Constitution, to which we have already referred, which explicitly states (no. 1) a specific right of the elderly, which is linked to certain state obligations and orders, we also find rules in Civil Law which are directed at protecting the elderly, particularly orders of Family Law relating to the Right to Food, a right which is very much protected in our judicial system.

This law (foreseen in articles 2003 and following of the Civil Code), encompasses everything that is necessary for maintenance, accommodation, clothing and food, obliging the descendants to provide food (article 2009, no. 1, line b), of the Civil Code).

On the other hand, as Guimaraes [3] refers to articles 138 (Prohibition) and 152 (Disqualification) of our Civil Code, although they are not specifically directed at the elderly unwell, nor do they even make any specific reference to the causes of prohibition or disqualification, none of the pathologies which, in terms of mental health, most affect the elderly, have come to be applied to situations of elderly unwell administrating their person or goods, including them in the concept of "psychic anomaly"[2]. According to Guimaraes [3], in this sense, Portuguese law solved one of the most delicate problems in the sphere of protecting the elderly, assuring the loan of its capacity, in cases of loss of mental faculties, guaranteeing the appointment of a suitable legal representative who is responsible for safeguarding the elderly person and for managing his estate strictly.

Health and Social Care for Older People: Structures and Functions

The Portuguese Social Security system comprises two areas: one of Social Action and one of Administration. At present, within the sphere of Social Action we can distinguish a series of social responses of support to the elderly, ranging from the most traditional to the most innovative. Thus we have:

Old People's Homes - these are units of collective accommodation, to be used on a temporary or permanent basis by old people most at risk of losing their independence and/ or autonomy. Their objectives are:
- Development of necessary support for the families of the elderly.
- Contribution to the stabilisation and delaying of the ageing process.
- Supply of suitable and permanent services for the problems of the elderly.
- Reinforcing interfamily relationships.

The services supplied by these units are:
- Accommodation.
- Food.
- Health care, hygiene and comfort.
- Companionship, recreation, animation and occupation.

Residences – these consist of apartment complexes for elderly people who are self-sufficient and can look after their own room, whilst also being able to avail of support services for their respective maintenance. The objectives of the residence are to:
- Encourage autonomy in the elderly, allowing them to have their own room
- Allow social integration and participation of the elderly in the community.

These living quarters are supported by some common services, for optional use, such as meals, domestic help, entertainment activities, library, television, etc. This type of unit is still very rare with us. However, in the city of Lisbon, Recolhimentos da Capital is considered as a Residence and it comprises five buildings [1].

Day Centres – these offer a range of services, provided in the unit, which contribute to the care of the elderly in their socio-familiar environment. Their objectives are:
- Meals.
- Care of hygiene and well-being.
- Recreation, social intercourse, occupation and animation.
- Holidays.
- Laundry services.

Recreation Centres – these take place in a local context and try to support the development of a series of activities of a cultural and socio-recreational nature and are designed for the elderly in a specific community area. They are more appropriate for an elderly population which, from an economic and family point of view, is neither very dependent nor needy, and they provide neither home help nor laundry services nor do they serve lunches. Their objectives are:
- To create a centre for meeting and social intercourse.
- To delay the dependency of the elderly.
- To promote leisure and occupation in free time.

The services they offer are:
- Encouraging recreational activities.
- Providing specific information on health prevention and autonomy in the elderly.
- Supplying light meals.

Home Support – this consists of providing individualised and personalised care in the home to people and families when, for reasons of illness, incapacity or other impediment, they cannot on a temporary or on a permanent basis take care of their everyday needs and/or activities. Their objectives are:
- To contribute to improving the quality of life of the elderly.
- To contribute to delaying or even to avoiding institutionalisation.
- To provide physical, psychological and social care to the elderly person to contribute to his well-being.
- To assure the elderly that their basic needs will be taken care of.

- To co-operate in the provision of health care.

The services offered can be:
- preparation, transportation and/or distribution of meals
- cleaning and tidying the home
- comfort and hygiene care
- company and recreation
- small repairs in the home
- obtaining necessary items for the home
- administering some medication
- laundry service
- various types of other help (attendance, outings, etc.)

Holiday Centres – these are social services, within a framework or not, which provide a programme of activities which aim to provide leisure and break the routine, thus giving the elderly physical, psychic, emotional, social and educational balance. Their objectives are:
- To provide a stay away from routine
- To promote a spirit of mutual help
- To provide contact with different communities and places
- To facilitate social integration through living together in a group
- To promote a creative capacity and spirit of initiative

In these places, priority is given to the elderly who have a disfunctional family environment, social and/or geographical isolation, who come from a degraded residential area, who have no opportunity to spend holidays with family and who are not very well (proven with a medical certificate).

Family Residence – this involves the temporary or permanent residence of elderly people in families considered to be suitable. Anyone can avail of this modality who has no family of their own or when their family does not have the means to take care of their needs.

Programme of Integrated Support to the Elderly (PAII) – this is a programme which developed out of the Dispatch Collection no. 259/97 of 21st of august. The Programme has the following objectives:
- To ensure the provision of care of an urgent and permanent nature aimed precisely at maintaining the autonomy of the elderly person in his own home and in his familiar environment.
- To establish means to ensure the mobility of the elderly and accessibility to benefits and services.
- To implement support to families who have to provide care and attendance to dependent family members, namely the elderly.
- To promote and support initiatives for the initial and continuing training of professionals, volunteers, family members and other people in the community.
- To promote attitudes and measures to prevent isolation, exclusion and dependency and to contribute to intergenerational solidarity as well as creating jobs.

With the support of PAII the following projects were created:

Support Centre for Dependants (CAD) – these are places with multidisciplinary services which provide integrated care on a temporary basis, directing support to different groups of aged to prevent, rehabilitate and reinsert them with people with dependence. They must develop primarily from already existing structures and preferably as resource centres.

Home Support Service (SAD) - this is aimed at keeping the elderly person in his own environment, along with his family, neighbours and friends and can also include people who are dependent. In this area, projects must develop bearing in mind the extent of the existing cover, namely the extension of support to cover the full 24 hours, the improvement in quality of services offered and the suitability of the home environment to the needs of the elderly people.

Training of Human Resources (FORHUM) – this is designed for family members, neighbours, volunteers, as well as for professionals, namely in the areas of Health and Social Services, and other members of the community, enabling them to provide formal and informal care.

Telealarm Service – this is a new initiative, on a national level, which as its objective aims to ensure the safety and support of the elderly, namely those who live in an isolated situation, trying to help them to maintain their autonomy. It is a complementary initiative, working via a national telecommunications network, which, on activating an alarm button, allows the social support network of each person to be contacted rapidly so they can respond more efficiently to the request for help. On the advice of the social support services, the Telealarm Service has an advantage over the telephone.

A permanent central service unit operates in the headquarters of the Portuguese Red Cross in Lisbon and the terminals are placed in the homes of the subscribers.

Health and Heat – this is designed to allow the elderly with more limited financial resources access to thermal treatments in the form of an allowance.

Technical Aids – technical aids for the elderly can range from wheelchairs to nappies, for example, since they compensate for the limitations of the elderly person and allow his social integration. As their objective they seek to achieve a greater degree of autonomy for the elderly person and allow his social integration. These aids include assistants for treatment and for training, ortotheses and prostheses, aids for mobility, for personal care and for hygiene, for communication, information and signalling, leisure aids, aids for domestic care, for furniture and alterations to the residence and other places, for handling products and merchandise and even aids to improve the environment.

There is also some financial assistance available for the elderly. Besides the programmes of social action provided in the aforementioned units and services, the Portuguese Social Security also ensures the social protection of individuals through social security schemes.

In this way the elderly can benefit from pensions in the Contributive or Non-contributive systems, according to whether or not they have paid contributions to the Social Security. In truth, whilst the Contributive Scheme presupposes contributions (deductions) and a certain period of professional activity which gives the right to a retirement pension, the Non-contributive scheme only gives access, for example, to the social pension, since the beneficiary has been unable to work in a professional capacity.

Thus, if they form part of the Contributive Scheme, the elderly will be able to have the right to:

- Old Age Pension – a monthly payment, for life, varying in amount, with the right to the 13th and 14th month, for people who have reached retirement age (65 years) and who have completed 15 years of continuous or interpolated contributions.
- Invalidity Pension – a monthly payment given during the life of the beneficiaries who, having completed a guaranteed period of 60 months of registered remuneration[3] and before reaching the age of retirement, find they are definitively unable to work due to illness or accident.
- Survival Pension – a monthly payment made on the death of a beneficiary of the General Social Security Scheme[4], by way of compensating the family of the beneficiary for the loss of income. Spouses, ex-spouses, descendants or the equivalent and ascendants, who, at the date of death have completed 36 months of contributions, qualify for this benefit.
- Dependency Complement – this is awarded in cases where the degree of dependency of the pensioner is such that he needs the assistance of a third party to attend to his basic needs. People on an invalidity, old age and survival pension who are dependent on the support of a third party can receive this benefit.

If they belong to the Non Contributive Scheme, the elderly will be able to benefit from:

- Social Pension – this is a monthly payment, for life, with the right to the 13th and 14th month for nationals resident in the country who are not covered by any other scheme of social protection, who have no gross income of any kind or which do not exceed 30% of the minimum remuneration guaranteed to workers in general in the case of a single person or 50% in the case of a married couple.
- Widow's Pension – this is a monthly payment to the value of 60% of the social pension, awarded to the spouse of the deceased pensioner from the social pension, if that spouse has no right to any other survival pension, provided their married status remains the same. To be eligible for this, the person must not be covered by any other contibutive scheme, nor receive any gross income in excess of 30% of the minimum remuneration guaranteed to workers in general in the case of a single person, or 50% in the case of a married couple.

The elderly can also benefit from some assistance with health care expenditure, such as in urgent cases, medication, disposable material and with travel to consultations. They also receive discount on telephones (60% reduction on subscription fee and 25 free units per month), on the price of tickets on public urban transport, buses and trains. Besides this, Inatel and Senior Tourism also give reductions or benefits to the elderly on holiday, thus making social intercourse and leisure easier for them.

Regarding health care, it is in this area that in terms of geriatric assistance, Portugal is practically "zero". In a general way, we can say that geriatric care in Portugal is supplied by technicians without any specialised training in geriatrics. The link between social and health structures to help the elderly is practically nil.

Given the (almost) non-existence of geriatricians and with the first nurses specialised in this field only just beginning to appear, we recognise that there are neither structures nor institutions offering geriatric care [4]. Thus the panorama of our country is as follows:

Table 3: Situation of geriatric support

Geriatricians (doctors)	0
Nurses for geriatrics	?
Hospital Geriatric Services	0
Geriatric assessment consultations	1
Geriatric Units	0
Acute Geriatric Units	0
Long Stay Hospitals	?

Source: [4]

Consequently, and except in cases of specialised pathology, the elderly person is treated, in most situations and at the level of both hospital and primary care, in a fragmented way [4]. Nevertheless, regarding psychiatric pathology, there is some organisation and care in this area, namely in the Gerontopsychiatric consultations available in some hospitals.

At present, the creation of geriatric units in general hospitals is a hypothesis defended by many professionals with experience in the area of care for the elderly. It is understood that these units will allow not only a better quality of health care attention to the elderly but will also facilitate the development of scientific and technical knowledge in this area.

Recently a legal diploma (Dispatch Collection no. 407/98 of 18th of June) was created which supports the creation of a working group comprising representatives from the General Health Management (Ministry of Health) and from Social Action (Ministry of Labour and Solidarity), with the task of diagnosing and analysing situations whose solutions must come from the combined intervention of these areas. This joint intervention of social support and continuing health care is directed at people who are dependent, among whom are some of the elderly.

Within the range of this diploma there is foreseen the creation of a type of innovative responses, named integrated responses. This type of responses is of a preventative and rehabilitative nature and supportive of people in a dependent situation, and they aim essentially at the following objectives:

- To improve the quality of life and to encourage their social and community insertion, as well as developing processes of social evaluation.
- To encourage and promote keeping them in their own home and in the social and family environment.
- To collaborate with families, reinforcing their capacities and abilities, giving them the necessary help and access to appropriate technical aids.
- To create and promote conditions which favour autonomy and well-being, stimulating participation of the people involved in the solution to their problems.

Integrated responses include:
- Integrated Home Support – this is a service providing home assistance which comprises a range of multidiscipline, flexible, inclusive, accessible and combined action from social support and health.

- Integrated Support Unit – a unit with a maximum capacity for 30 users, whose aim is to provide temporary, global and integrated care to people who, because of their dependency, are unable, in the assessment made by the integrated care team, to be supported in their home, but who do not need the clinical care of hospitalisation.

There are also other support structures for the elderly, such as:

Elderly Citizen Line – this is a free telephone line which provides information to the elderly on a wide range of rights and benefits, in such important areas, as, for example: health, social security, accommodation, equipment and services, free time. If the elderly person has any query he can ring this line and will find an interesting and attentive voice at the other end who will do everything to listen, advise and inform.

Elderly Card Foundation - as its general objective this aims to develop and promote initiatives designed to encourage well-being, personal fulfilment and full social participation of the over 65s, and as its specific goal, to launch and manage a card for the elderly as a means and access to goods and services in specially advantageous conditions for the respective users. For this purpose Card 65 was created, with which the bearer can take advantage of discount in services or in the purchase of goods in various sectors of activity.

Policies on family care

In the case of Portugal, the problem of care provided by families with the responsibility for elderly people is an important question for politicians, researchers and public opinion in general.

Undoubtedly, the lack of public debate about this question and the absence of political measures in this area rise, above all, from the fact that the family is considered "the centre of the tradition of collective responsibility to provide care …"[5]. Indeed, the image of family solidarity, including its oldest members, caring for them within the family circle, is deeply rooted in Portuguese society's cultural values, and so whilst the family continues to provide care for its old, it has not yet been the object of any specific political measures. A reading of table 4 below shows that there are people aged 65 and over living in 30.8 % of families in this country.

Table 4: Families with and without people aged 65 and over, in Portugal

Families without elderly	2,177,830
Families with elderly	967 904
Total number of families	3 145 734
% of families with elderly	30.8%

As we see from a survey carried out by Quaresma [1], in Portugal there are no specific support services for families providing care for the elderly. Units from the area of Social Security, namely the Day Centres and Health Centres with family doctors, provide forms of indirect support in so far as they try to create conditions conducive to maintaining the elderly person in his own familiar environment.

Meanwhile, some experiments have been developed, such as [1]:

- Temporary accommodation in Homes, to allow families holiday periods, or to replace them in cases of hospitalisation or other;
- Organisation of voluntary groups which, although they are mainly focused on supporting old people who are alone, in certain circumstances, they also play a complementary part in interfamily care (company, looking after the elderly for short periods of family absence, for example).

A global analysis of a study carried out by the Commission for Equality in Work and in Employment [6], at the expense of the Ministry of Employment and Social Security, entitled Inquiry into the Support Measures for Workers Responsible for Elderly Persons, in which almost 1000 contractors and personnel managers from all sectors of activity (except agriculture, arboriculture, hunting and fishing) were interviewed, allows us to draw the conclusion that the number of companies sensitive to the question of implementing support measures for workers responsible for elderly persons is very small indeed. The great majority (84.3%) replied that they did not have any specific measures which sought to provide this particular type of assistance, whilst they do not consider to be relevant the negative effects which come from assisting the elderly.

Nevertheless, on analysing the group of companies which claimed to have supportive policies for employees who have to give this type of assistance, the study indicates that the only measure of any significance, because implemented by 13.8% of companies, is the application of flexible timetables. On the other hand, there is a very small percentage of companies which refer to the technical support of social services, probably because it is a type of support with some tradition in the company [7].

In effect, regarding financial support, it states that families which care for their elderly members are not given any type of support in this sense. However, as Quaresma [1] confirms, "the development in progress, namely the attempt to create conditions to delay and avoid the institutionalisation of the elderly, have contributed to a progressive change in the forms of action of community support services regarding the needs of these families". The author goes on to inform us of the existence of experiments in progress, namely of economic support, which are aimed at improving the domestic unit or living conditions as well as acquiring technical aids essential to increasing the comfort of the elderly and their carers, often, the daily provision of care.

As for the psycho-social support for the providers of informal care, in the Portuguese context there is no organised form of this type of support, since, as we have already referred to, "until a very recent past, this care formed part of a natural process, culturally justified and socially accepted" [1]. In the meantime, some innovative actions are beginning to emerge. In this sense, Quaresma [1] reports that, in some Day Centres, types of psychological support for the families of the elderly are beginning to develop, their objective being to improve the attention/relationship between the relative/ elderly person.

As a conclusive synthesis to this point, Morais [8] states, "Social policy regarding old age should have as its prime objective the planning and development of a support system for relatives who are trying to combine their intentions, along with organised institutional aid and resorting to professional services available, in an attempt to make the demands of everyday life compatible with the responsibilities of caring for elderly relatives".

Roles of Family Carers of Older People Living at Home

In the case of Portugal there is a notable lack of studies published in the area of family carers of elderly relatives. In fact, after exhaustive research for a bibliography we could only find two studies on this subject, both published in 1996:

- Quaresma [1], whose main objective is a possible diagnosis of the Portuguese situation in terms of interfamily care of the very elderly, drawing its sources of information from professionals in Health and Social Action, and from 24 cases selected for interview in different regions of the country, the analysis of which allowed for a comparison to made between the aforementioned data and data of everyday life supplied by family carers of their elderly dependent relatives (> - 75).

- Rebelo [9], who made a descriptive cross analysis to establish a character profile of informal carers of the elderly aged 80 and over, in a small parish in our country. 56 carers of the elderly aged 80 and over were identified and they constitute the total population of the study.

The results obtained by both studies, although we consider them an important contribution to knowing more about informal carers, cannot be considered representative of these situations in general because of aspects of methodological order. Nevertheless, the information supplied by these studies allows us to create an image of the role played by these relatives in caring for their elderly.

Schematically, these papers refer to: total support of the elderly relative; partial support, complemented by support from community services (this situation more frequent in urban areas).

As for the sex and age of these carers, both studies are unanimous in establishing that, within the family, the main carer is a woman (wife, daughter or daughter-in-law), whose age is between 40 and 70 and above, depending on whether it is the wife or daughter/daughter-in-law. Quaresma [1] states that when the spouse is the main element for providing care and support, her advanced age and state of health make it difficult for her to do so.

The study carried out by Quaresma [1] informs us that the frequency and type of daily care given by family to their elderly relatives depends on the following factors:
- Degree of dependency of the elderly person
- Type of cohabitation
- Socio-economic situation
- Inter and extra family support

The analysis of the data based on these indicators allowed the author to state that the socio-economic situation and the inter and extra family support condition decisively the day-to day element of the family which assumes the responsibility of care in terms of the type of daily tasks.

Thus, in situations where there is effective cohabitation and a high degree of dependency in the elderly person, the completion of daily tasks can fall completely on the carer when she is unable to obtain services and does not receive them from within the family or from institutions [1]. Nevertheless, the author confirms that in the aforementioned situations – high degree of dependency and effective cohabitation – the demand on time available daily is, in all cases involved in this study, almost constantly permanent.

Schematically, this study allows us to verify that when there is no other form of help on a daily basis, the cohabiting family takes care of:
- Personal hygiene of the elderly person
- Preparation of meals
- Shopping
- Administering medication
- Household tasks
- Supporting the person's mobility

As for situations of cohabitation at a distance, the study indicates that the type and frequency of care given vary depending on whether or not there is inter or extra family support. In this way, in most cases of cohabitation at a distance interviewed in urban areas, it was found that the support given by relatives appears clearly to be complementary to services provided by local institutions, which take care of basic, daily needs. In cases of cohabitation at a distance interviewed in rural areas, it was found that the carers assumed all or most of the daily tasks, given their effective presence in most of these cases.

Another aspect which is worth highlighting is the repercussions that the task of caring for the elderly has on relatives. In fact, both at social, economic and health levels, both studies are unanimous in claiming that caring for the elderly has repercussions on the lives of those relatives who support them. So, in most cases, the situation is felt to reduce social life greatly, in other words, the studies completed allow us to see that most carers saw their social relationships greatly diminished. On the other hand, from the economic and professional point of view, the study by Rebelo [9] shows that many of the carers who were working had to give up their job, whilst Quaresma [1], in her investigation, confirmed that these carers expressed the need to improve their economic situation, not just to be better able to meet the needs of the elderly person but also to acquire medicines and technical aids to facilitate care. As for health issues, the repercussions of this type of task are felt to be detrimental in most cases.

Assessment

The evaluation of the situation of the elderly and their respective informal carers in an attempt to determine a social response is the responsibility of Social Security (more specifically of Social Action Services), a body subject to the Ministry of Work and Solidarity. In fact, the fundamental objectives of Social Action are the prevention of situations of need, disfunction and social marginalisation and community integration. On the other hand, Social Action also aims to ensure special protection for the most vulnerable groups, namely children, young people, handicapped and elderly, as well as other people who are in a situation of economic need or under the effect of disfunction or social marginalisation, in such cases which are not or cannot be met by social security schemes.

According to the Law of Bases of Social Security (Law no. 28/84 of 14th of August), social action follows the priorities and lines of direction established by the Government, keeping in view particularly:
a) meeting the basic needs of families and people most in need;
b) elimination of overlapping action, as well as geographical asymmetries in the implementation of services and units;

c) diversification of social action available, to allow for the appropriate development of forms of social support directly available to people and families;
d) guaranteed equality of treatment for all potential beneficiaries.

Specifically regarding the elderly population, the Social Action Services resort to methodologies, namely interviews, which enable a social diagnosis of the situation. The methodology used attempts to evaluate competencies and abilities as well as difficulties and obstacles to the elderly person, family and community, by means of contacts established for attending/ receiving, home visits and attention in the community.

Nevertheless, what transpired from some contacts which we established with certain social service operators, is the lack of a systematic methodology to evaluate the situation of the elderly person, thus making it difficult to make a diagnosis. In other words, in reality, other professionals when faced with the lack of evaluation methods for use with the elderly, which have been properly ratified for the Portuguese population, resort to various, different methods, based, in part, on evaluation scales drawn up by themselves, thus making it impossible to compare data and giving occasion to the loss of information in situations where the elderly person will have to "go through" various operators with different training.

Regarding informal family carers, they will be able to be supported punctually with technical and/or financial assistance. In fact, there is an attempt to carry out a combined and continuous assessment of families and situations, reformulating the life project of the elderly person whenever necessary.

In parallel, other services and responses will be given to them by institutions concerned with the elderly in the area, namely, Private Institutions of Social Solidarity (IPSS). These are institutions without any lucrative purpose, created on the initiative of individuals, whose purpose is to address the moral duty of solidarity and justice among individuals and since they are not administered by the State or by an autonomous body, by means of concession of wealth and offers of service, they aim to achieve, amongst other objectives, the following:

- support for children and young people;
- support to the family;
- support to social and community integration;
- protection of citizens in old age and illness and in all cases of lack of, or diminished means of, subsistence or capacity to work;
- promotion and protection of health, namely by providing preventive and curative medical care and rehabilitation;
- education and professional training of citizens;
- solution of people's housing problems.

To accomplish the objectives of social action, the State accepts, supports and values the contribution of these institutions in rendering social rights effective, through joint co-operation agreements.

In fact, the assessment of the elderly person's situation goes through an analysis focused on the social scale. However, in situations of specific health problems, the elderly person will be directed to the appropriate organisation – National Health Service (an organisation protected by the Ministry of Health) – where he will receive appropriate treatment, in a concerted action with solutions offered by Social Action Services.

In any case, the solutions depend on the willingness of the elderly person, offering him a normal and integrated life and enabling him, wherever possible, to remain in his normal environment.

Case Studies

In obtaining data regarding solutions to be offered in each of the following case studies, we opted to collect information from professionals working in the area of social action, namely social service workers responsible for units or support services to the elderly population in the community. It is important, however, to highlight that the solutions suggested for each case presuppose the existence of all the responses and units contemplated in our legislation, which does not mean to say that, at the moment, they are all fully operational and/or established all over the country.[5]

Case 1

Female, aged 76, with osteoarthritis of the hips and knees, poor vision due to macular degeneration, and hypertension. Mobile with a frame within her home except for the stairs. Needs help with mobility outside, shopping, cooking and housework.

Social Circumstances (A)
- Establish if the elderly lady feels motivated to remain in her home or not.
- Find out about the availability of the daughter, taking into account how close she lives, to take care of her mother in her mother's home or in her own.
- Direct to Social Pension, if the income from the Survival Pension is lower than the amount indicated by Social Pension.
- Direct to Dependency Supplement.
- Combine care with the other two children, gaining their economic and financial collaboration.
- Install a Tele-alarm system in her home, to be used in cases of danger, essentially during the night.
- Technical Assistance Concession for equipment to be prescribed by the doctor in attendance.
- If the lady expresses a preference to stay in her own home and if the daughter is unable to look after her, seek a solution from Integrated Home Support Service.

Social Circumstances (B)
- Depending on the motivation of the elderly lady to remain in her home or not during the day, the course of action could be via the social solution of the Day Centre or Home Support Service.
- If she gets help from the Home Support System, the situation will have to be clearly indicated for the volunteer service working in the environment, so as to promote the development of recreational activities and/ or assistance with small domestic tasks and transport.
- Direct to Dependency Supplement.

Social Circumstances (C)
- If the lady intends to remain in her socio-familiar context, accommodation would be subject to possible alterations (bedroom and WC on the ground floor), expenses to be met from her own income.
- They will be able to avail of the services offered by the Home Support Service or attend the Day Centre.

- If they agree to leave their home, the couple will go to live in a T1 type apartment, integrated in the Private Institution of Social Solidarity.

Case 2

Male, aged 80, facing discharge from hospital following a stroke. Expected to be confined to bed or chair for several weeks with gradual recovery of mobility. Needs the help of one person for transfers, toileting, bathing and dressing.

Social Circumstances (A)
- Request the collaboration of daughter and son-in-law to receive the elderly man in their home. Likewise, he could avail of the integrated health and social action care, through the social response of the Integrated Home Support Service.
- Award technical aids to facilitate movement in accordance with medical prescription.
- Request Dependency Supplement.
- Request the involvement of other children, namely through affective and economic support.
- Grant contingent subsidies to meet the expense of medico-social action (nappies, medication).

Social Circumstances (B)
- Temporary placement in an Integrated Support Unit, until he regains some capacity.
- Later, the elderly man will be able to avail of Integrated Home Support.
- Technical aids clinically prescribed to be paid for.
- Application for Dependency Supplement.

Social Circumstances (C)
- Direct to the Integrated Home Support Service.
- If the elderly person wishes to remain in his own home, alterations will have to be made to have the WC and a bedroom on the ground floor. As he is receiving an Integrated Response, as is the case with Integrated Home Support, the couple will be granted the technical equipment and finances to carry out the alterations to ensure their autarchy.

Case 3

Female, aged 86, suffering from dementia. Frequent wandering by day and night. Frequent falls. Incontinent of urine and faeces.

Social Circumstances (A)
- Assess the motivation and circumstances of the family to receive the elderly lady into their family unit.
- If she is taken into her daughter's home, support financially expenses of medication and incontinence nappies, through contingent subsidies and supplement this measure with services from the Home Support Service.
- Request a Dependency Supplement.
- Involve the rest of the family in care, seeking their affective and economic collaboration.

- If the daughter is unable/unwilling to attend her, she will be taken into the Old People's Home in the Private Institution for Social Solidarity.

Social Circumstances (B)

- Given the characteristics of the elderly lady and the unavailability of her daughter and son-in-law, the most suitable course of action would be to place her in an Old People's Home.

Social Circumstances (C)

- Direct to the Home Support Service.
- Make the family aware of the need to make the home safe, avoiding situations where she would be at risk of falling.
- Support/ attendance of informal carers (neighbours, friends, volunteers, etc.) who, following a Concerted Plan of Action, would help both elements of the family unit (social intercourse, recreation, obtaining goods and services, accompaniment to medical consultations, support in emergency situations).

Future Developments

In fact, until very recently, we can say that in our country there were almost no links between the social and health structures which assist our elderly.

Nevertheless, we cannot continue to ignore the demographic, social and family transformations occurring in Portuguese society which are giving rise to new needs for certain groups of the population, namely the elderly. The growing need to provide continuing services to these people, either because of an ageing population or because of changes in the social structures, is slipping away in particular from the family structure.

The provision of home and ambulatory services seems to be one of the most humane responses, but it requires the establishment of integrated support social networks which can guarantee the effective continuity of necessary care and which aspire to be global. It was with a view to achieving this objective that, as we have mentioned earlier, a legal diploma (Dispatch Collective no. 407/98 of 18th of June), was drawn up, with the precise purpose of creating responses to allow joint intervention of health and social action in the cases of dependent people in an attempt to respond to their needs, according to the type and extent of their dependency and to the socio-familiar contexts in which they live – articulated responses. This model of articulated intervention has as its fundamental objective the promotion of the autonomy of people who are dependent and the reinforcement of the capacity and ability of their families to deal with those situations, and as logic of intervention, to offer home care assistance.

However, it is only now that the first steps are being taken to implement this, as it is still not very much in evidence all over the country and it is hoped to extend it to all regions. For example, very recently, various social solidarity institutions from the district of Braga, in a concerted action with the Braga Sub-Regional Service and the Regional Health Administration, adopted the Integrated Home Support scheme which, in its first phase, will consider almost 50 elderly people in the municipalities of Famalicao and Vieira do Minho and will look to the creation of Integrated Support Units.

In general terms, we can say that from the point of view of quality, the initiatives and models in force in the area of Social Action are, in general, modern and adequate. However, in terms of quantity, we realise that we still fall relatively short of meeting the real needs. In fact, what is becoming urgent is the extension of the present solutions for assistance, namely of all those services which enable the elderly person to remain in his home environment, such as:

- The extension of the Home Support system as widely as possible and with the greatest number possible of users, for this service, if in existence, in many cases prevents confinement in a Home, thus allowing the elderly person to remain in his own environment, along with everything that is familiar to him, and to maintain his relationships with his neighbours.
- The extension of Day Centres and Social Centres all over the country, for these are extremely important for the help they give and for the prophylaxis of ageing which they practise, allowing the most autonomous people to remain in the heart of their community, increasing their ability and independence.

The multiplication of some recent experiments, namely the Programme of Integrated Support to the Elderly (PAII) which have very innovative projects and, according to Ermida [4], also have some very encouraging results, as seen in the evaluation of those already in operation.

Nonetheless, the emergence of specific questions regarding the problem of the provision of interfamily care to elderly people is extremely recent, probably due to the deeply rooted cultural model of family values which qualify the family and make it responsible for the provision of care to its elderly members.

In fact, social policy on old age should contemplate the planning and development of a support programme for family members who wish to combine their efforts with organised institutional aid, and with resort to professional services, to make the demands of actual life compatible with the responsibilities towards their elderly relatives [8].

Considering that these responses are not exempt from monetary contributions, it would be interesting and necessary to implement certain political measures which should take account of the following aspects:

- To ensure financial support to those providing informal care;
- To promote the training of those providing informal care, through short courses, to improve the quality of the care given; note that PAII, through its programme FORHUM (Training of human Resources) is already contemplating this type of training, nevertheless, it is necessary to extend it to all parts of the country, as well as increasing this type of measures;
- To guarantee forms of support which allow carers periods of rest
- To encourage forms of psycho-emotional support.

In this context, the implementation of this type of measure, clearly demands a research strategy which will provide a deep understanding of the problems faced by those who care for elderly relatives in the Portuguese situation.

Regarding health care for the elderly, it is in precisely this area that, as we have already mentioned, Portugal still falls relatively short of those countries where health care of the elderly is a reality. In fact, there are practically no specialists in geriatric care in Portugal, and it is only now that the first nurses specialised in this area are beginning to emerge, there are still no geriatrician doctors, nor institutions which provide geriatric care.

Considering specifically the hospitalisation of the elderly person whose situation needs a diagnosis and specialised therapy, it presupposes the existence of Geriatric Units with structures and their own environment, where the geriatric team will assess the elderly person and will give him suitable guidance [2]. In fact, this desirable situation does not occur in Portugal. In fact, most General hospitals are as yet unprepared to treat and assist the elderly who are ill [2].

This being the case, one of the greatest challenges facing the competent authorities, is, at least for the moment, the institutionalisation of geriatric training to make it more feasible to improve the health care given to the elderly.

Acknowledgements

Despacho Conjunto n.º 407/98 de 18 de Junho: Cria as respostas integradas.
Despacho Conjunto n.º 259/97 de 21 de Agosto: Cria o Programa de Apoio Integrado a Idosos
Lei n.º 28/84 de 14 de Agosto: Lei de Bases da Segurança Social.

Notes

1. Commentaries taken from Canotilho [12]. Constitution of the Portuguese Republic Annotated. Coimbra: Coimbra Editora.
2. According to Ana Prata [11], in Dicionario Juridico, "psychic anomaly" is understood to be "a permanent change in the mental faculties of an individual, which renders him incapable of governing his person and goods or, at least of managing his estate properly. According to the greater or lesser degree of psychic anomaly, the person can be prohibited or disqualified".
3. For all schemes, excluding the voluntary social security scheme in which the period is 72 months from the start of contributions.
4. And also Special Social Security Scheme of Agricultural Activities and Voluntary Social Security Scheme [12].
5. We are grateful to the very valuable collaboration of Dr Julia Rato (Regional Centre of Social Security – Aveiro) in the preparation of these case studies.

References

[1]   M. Quaresma, Cuidados Familiares às Pessoas muito Idosas. Lisboa: Direcção-Geral da Acção Social, 1996.
[2]   G. Ermida, Envelhecimento Demográfico, Doença e Cuidados de Sa~ude. In: Sociedade Portuguesa de Geriatria e Gerontologia (ed.), Temas Geriátricos – I. Lisboa: Parismédica, Reciclagem e Informação Médica, Lda, (1995) 53-67.
[3]   P. Guimarães, O estatuto dos idosos no direito português ou o fim do idoso crepuscular. *Geriatria*, **11** (1998) 11-20.
[4]   G. Ermida, Assistência ao idoso em Portugal. *Geriatria*, 12 (1999) 5-9.
[5]   R. Anderson, Prestação de Cuidados Informais. O Papel da Família. In: Comissão Nacional para a Política da Terceira Idade Actas da Conferêmcia Europeia «As Pessoas Idosas e a Família – Solidareiedade enre gerações». Lisboa: Ministério da Solidariedade e Segurança Social (1992) 52-74.
[6]   Comissão para a Igualdade no Trabalho e no Emprego, *Inquérito às Medidas de Apoio aos trabalhadores com Idosos a cargo*. Lisboa: Ministério da Solidariedade e Segurança Social, 1995.
[7]   Comissão Nacional para a Política da Terceira Idade, *65 e mais anos – Os números em Portugal*. Lisboa: Ministério da Solidariedade e Segurança Social, 1995.
[8]   L. Morais, Apoio familiar ao idoso. *Geriatria*, **12** (1999) 28-30.
[9]   A. Rebelo, Prestadores de cuidados informais – A idosos com 80 e mais anos, na freguesia de Moreira da Maia. *Geriatria*, **9** (1996) 22-28.
[10] G. Canotilho and V. Moreira, Constituição da República Portuguesa Anotada.Coimbra: Coimbra Editora, 1993.
[11] A. Prata, Dicionário Jurídico. Coimbra: Livraria Almedina, 1994.
[12] INE – Instituto Nacional de Estatística (s/d). Projecções da população residente 1995-2005. (documento policopiado).

Chapter 9

Spain
(December 1999)

Arantza Larizgoitia Jauregi
C/Sabino Arana 7, 3D
48100 Mungia, Bizkaia
Spain

Introduction

Elderly care in Spain is the responsibility of the family. Usually, a woman, the spouse or a daughter, tends to be the principal carer of the dependent elderly. Except for health care services that are available to all citizens by the public health system, formal support acts in a subsidiary role to family support. The regional welfare administration, under Autonomous Communities Governments, is responsible for providing social services to the elderly and their families. However, although formal support is significantly higher than some decades ago, is still insufficient to meet most of the needs. Access to basic services and to a minimum financial pension has being extended to almost all citizens. However, because of financial constraints and a little interest on expanding social expenditures, in practice, access to social services is limited to the poor, or to persons with adverse social circumstances and very low income. Conversely, the wealthiest may access some private services that in the late years are flourishing.

The current level of services is considerably higher than what it was conceivable a few decades ago. Although it is still far below the standard of most developed nations. The new emergent model of social services intends to provide to all Spanish elderly the services needed to maintain an acceptable quality of life. But access to those services is not considered a right of Spanish citizens, thus it can not be claimed. Decisions on the quality and content of the social services to be provided is left to municipal and provincial governments, that usually govern under tight economical constraints. Thus, there is room for large inequalities in the accessibility to services by Spanish elderly and their families. A further reason for concern is the lack of mechanisms to facilitate the co-ordination with the health care system in order to provide an integrated approach to elderly care.

The final result is that of a scarce, insufficient and fragmented service provision for the dependent elderly, with high levels of inequality across regions and localities. Care for carers of dependent elderly is an issue only marginally addressed.

This report is an attempt to provide an overview of the formal and informal care services for dependent elderly and their carers in Spain. The current level of services is considerably higher than what was available a few decades ago, but it is still far below the standard of most developed nations. But changes did not occur in isolation. They were the result of deeper social, political and economic changes that affected many aspects of society, and that had significant impact in lifestyles and even in the type of urban and living arrangements. A comprehensive overview of the social provision today needs to include at least a minimum understanding of the recent past and its evolution.

Social protection evolved from being associated to charity during the first three quarters of this century (the Spanish dictatorship) towards a more democratic concept of welfare system during the eighties. However, the "crisis of the welfare system", of which the constraints imposed by the European economic convergence and the economic crisis of the early nineties are significant contributors, reached Spain before the welfare system itself had consolidated. Policy makers, planners and professionals need to produce a great effort of research, imagination, prediction and risk taking in order to adopt sound initiatives within a sometimes difficult environment. Sometimes it is all at all avoided by adopting easy solutions that prove not be efficacious in the medium or long term.

Today, there is an ongoing debate aiming at improving the current welfare system, adapting its principles, financing, and structure to a more individualist, privatised model. However, the discussion on social policies and efficacious and efficient social programmes is confronted by the weight of traditional values, the scarcity of disposable resources, and the lack of social consciousness and of long term commitment of some policy makers (this is exemplified by the sometimes compulsive need to provide certain "care" in a mimetic reaction with foreign policies as seen with the "Viagra" phenomenon).

The following report is organised according to a scheme that begins by a general review of Spanish demography, and that summarises the main policies and care practices for elderly people. The second section provides a more detailed description of specific programs and policies. It is followed by an analysis of family support in the third section and by an evaluation of care programs in the fourth section. The fifth section describes some case studies, and finally, the report ends with an assessment of the main challenges for the future.

The report is based on an analysis of the main recent Spanish publications on elderly care. The Spanish journals specialised in elderly care have been reviewed as well as some grey literature (government and institutional reports and statistics). The report tries to provide an accurate summary of its sources, any inaccuracy is the responsibility of the author. I wish to transmit my gratitude to all Spanish researchers who have contributed to produce the information used in this report.

General overview of policy and practice

Policies for social protection have evolved significantly during the past century, as the country has experienced profound political, social and economic changes. The evolution of social policies could not have been separated from the general political climate. As such, in the period going from the end of the civil war (1939) and during the dictatorship, protective policies were understood as charities directed towards providing the most basic needs for the destitute. Slowly, by the second half of the dictatorship the higher economic and social development led to the institution of a social security scheme (1963) directed firstly to workers and their beneficiaries, but that later encompassed the basic needs of most of the elderly. The subsequent evolution of the social security system in the seventies (1974), resulted in the separation of the healthcare activities from the other protective areas leading eventually to two different administrations, the Ministry of Health and the Ministry of Social Welfare. Both administrations evolved separately and differently, with little points of encounter. The Ministry of Health enacted in 1986 a national regulatory framework, the General Health Act, by which access to healthcare became a right of all Spanish citizens and entitled residents.

The Social Welfare administration became responsible for all types of protective services other than medical (and other than financial pensions associated to the Social Security), but there is not a regulatory framework that defines the content and extent of the basic services to be provided. The political decentralisation initiated during the eighties led to the establishment of 17 Autonomous Communities, or regional governments. All of them are fully competent to regulate and manage the social welfare administration within their territory, and 8 of them are fully competent to regulate healthcare. In the absence of any national legal framework for social care, the development of social services is unequal across different regions and cities. Furthermore, social services have usually been ranked in the last position among social protection policies, after retirement pensions, health care and unemployment benefits, thus this sector tends to be the least pressing for policy makers, and the least financed.

Despite all these threats, social protection for the elderly has increased considerably in the past twenty years. Although it is still insufficient. In this evolution, the scarcity of resources has been a constant hindering a sufficient deployment of services, and threatening the sustainability of a future equitable "welfare system".

Cultural and demographic context

The demographic profile of the Spanish population changed dramatically in a short period of time. The proportion of people over 65 years increased rapidly during this century. In 1900, this group accounted for a mere 5% of the total population with an average life expectancy at birth of 34.8 years, while in 1981, this group reached to 11% and its life expectancy at birth was 75.7 years. In 1991, the over 65 years approached 13.7% of the total population and it is estimated that by the year 2026 they will reach to 21.2%, while those over 80 years of age will go from 2.9% in 1991 to an estimated 5.7% in the year 2026 [1].

The proportion of elderly people has more that doubled during this century, as well as its life expectancy. The ageing process is growing so that in thirty years one out of five Spaniards will be over 65 years, and one out of twenty will be more than 80 years old. This trend will undoubtedly affect the needs and demand for social care[1].

According to some data from 1989, most of the Spanish elderly remain at home living with some relatives, and approximately 20% of the elderly are living alone. The latter figure seems to have increased significantly in the past decades (in 1970, only 10% of the elderly were living alone), perhaps reflecting a trend or a change in living arrangements. The principal carer of dependent elderly, tends to be the wife or any other female relative, who in most cases (70%) lives in the same house as the elderly (17% living in separate homes). In only 12% of the cases, the main carer is not a close relative of the elderly [2].

As a consequence of the ageing process and its associated increase in morbidity, the use of healthcare services, including hospital admissions, has increased considerably; having a significant impact in some efficiency parameters, such as increases in the overall length of stay (close to 67% of the elderly, and 87% in the group over 85 years of age, report suffering from at least one chronic condition, but only 21% of them report having physical disabilities). Another significant factor for healthcare services is derived from the increasing prevalence of Alzheimer disease and its related health needs and expenditures [3].

General overview of policy and practice

The traditional response adopted in Spain to poverty, disease, or social inequities up to the recent decades of democracy, has been Charity. Starting with the civil war (1936-1939) and subsequent dictatorship (1939-1975) the first institutions of social protection that emerged were based on charity to tackle the needs of the destitute. Initially, they were led by religious institutions that with time were followed by social and political groups, and later by the State. After the war, there were a few charitable institutions, most of them managed and led by the Church, the victorious and only political party ("*El Movimiento Nacional*") and the only trade union ("*Organización Sindical*"). These institutions provided some basic help to the destitute (food, lodging, and some basic healthcare). Very slowly, the main charitable organisation (the "*Auxilio Social*") led by the victorious party moved from very selective policies which focussed on those who clearly accepted the political regime, towards a system orchestrated by the State, the *National Institution for Social Assistance (Instituto Nacional de Asistencia Social, INAS*), where the political affinity was not as much stressed. Charities still were mixed with some educational activities to obtain the political and social acquiescence of the destitute. This scheme prevailed until the early sixties as the only social policy.

During the second half of the dictatorship, new political trends and an impulse for economic development ("*el desarrollismo*") led to the institution of the Social Security system (1963) for workers and their beneficiaries to protect them against disease, work injury, disability, unemployment and death. A system of health care and maternity care, worker's compensation, pensions and retirement benefits was then instituted. The system included some discretionary social services. Retired workers and beneficiaries over 65 years of age were protected financially as well as in terms of health and social care.

A parallel movement in 1970, complemented the social services provided by the Social Security, by creating the "*Social Service for the Social Security of the Elderly*" (*Servicio Social de la Seguridad Social al Anciano*). This service enabled the creation of a national network of social institutions from a mix of public and private financing. A series of facilities, directed mostly to healthy elderly, were then created, such as social clubs in most large cities, at least one residence by province, and one geriatric centre in every region. With the exception of the social clubs, these facilities instituted co-payment schemes. These services were very popular but with the economic crisis of the mid-seventies and the political changes with the democratic transition, most of them were dismantled [4,5].

In 1978, a reform of the organisation of the Social Security marked a point of inflexion of significance for social policies. The reform tried to gain in administrative efficiency by separating the management of the Social Security economic benefits from all other non-economic services. It implied the separation of Social Security services into different associated administrations. Four separate institutes were created: the National Institute for Social Security (*INSS*) dedicated to aspects dealing with affiliation and economic benefits of the social security (worker's compensation, maternity leave, retirement pensions, and so on); the National Institute for Health (*INSALUD*) responsible for providing healthcare to beneficiaries, the National Institute for Employment (*INEM*), that deals with unemployment, and the National Institute for Social Services (*INSERSO*) dealing with social protective services, especially for the pensioners. In addition, there was a Treasury Department (*Tesorería de la Seguridad Social*) supervising the financing of all four institutes [4,5].

A short time later, the new political system represented by a democratic government assumed the principle that the State was responsible for ensuring social protection to all citizens. The Spanish Constitution (1978) in its 50th article affirms that "the State will ensure through an adequate pension system, the economic sufficiency of all elderly citizens. Likewise, with independence of familiar duties, the State will promote the elderly welfare through a Social Services System directed to meet their needs in terms of healthcare, accommodation, as well as cultural and social needs" [6].

To implement the new scenario, the existing institution that was dealing with social services for the elderly, the *INSERSO*, became the referent institution in the field, by assuming all Social Security responsibilities as well as the State charity institutions that still remained to protect the destitute (the *National Institution for Social Assistance,* and other religious or civic charities). The new *INSERSO* goals declared that the "*Spanish Welfare State*" was the sum of all public activities addressed to ensure access to basic protective services in order to procure an acceptable quality of life for all citizens [4-6].

Social expenditures raised subsequently, so that between 1975 and 1982 the number of new entitled pensioners (or elderly covered by the *INSERSO*) increased thirty times the number of contributors to the social security system. However, in 1982 there were approximately 14,5% of the population outside the social security system, and almost eight million of Spaniards were living in poverty, four million of them in extreme poverty. The Social Security system faced imminent bankruptcy and it was in need of a profound reform.

The change came with a major political reform. The organisation of the Spanish State was transformed with the democracy towards a decentralised State formed by 17 Autonomous Communities. The decentralisation was conceived as a gradual process, and it included as one of its first transfers, the devolution to Autonomous Communities of legal competencies dealing with "social services provision". The responsibilities assumed by the *INSERSO* were thus transferred to the Autonomous Communities. The *INSERSO* dissolved into the Ministry of Welfare and remained as an advisory body for social services for the elderly.

The late eighties and nineties have seen the development of Regional Acts for Social Services established by Autonomous Communities. Despite some regional differences, these Acts have in common certain significant features. Although they reject the concept of "charity" as an axis for social protection, they do not yet recognise the right of citizens to a basic social protection, nor they do specify the type of services citizens are entitled to receive. The application of those Acts is left to the judgement of consecutive regional governments. Furthermore, the management of social services is usually being passed to provincial or local governments. The latter tend to be who decide the level of protection for the elderly in their community. Thus, in practice, the implementation of social protection policies collide with other, many times more pressing, needs at provincial or municipal level. The combination of these factors leads to a limited system of public social services accessible only by the poor, and to another network of mixed private and public services (especially in hospice care) where the elderly need to contribute financially. Because of the high costs of hospice care, only a few of the elderly can access private care, thus, most of the low and medium class elderly are left with little or none formal care.

The evolution of the welfare administration was independent of and separated from the evolution of the healthcare administration. The latter evolved from another institution, the *INSALUD* (or *Spanish Institute for Health*), that was created from the Social Security administration such as the *INSERSO*. The *INSALUD* was conceived as the healthcare provider institution for social security beneficiaries but with time, and after subsequent reforms, it provides health care to almost all Spaniards. In 1986, the General Health Act sets a common national framework for the organisation and provision of healthcare and states the right to access to healthcare for all Spanish citizens. Following the political decentralisation process, competencies for healthcare regulation have been gradually devolved to some regions. So far, 8 Autonomous Communities have full competencies for the management and regulation of health care provision, covering to approximately 60% of the Spanish population. The remaining regions are still under the INSALUD administration, but they will receive full competencies in a short future. The historical separation of functions between the INSERSO and the INSALUD is maintained in most Autonomous Communities, with isolated but significant exceptions. The healthcare administration is characterised by its strong medical focus, the lack of a comprehensive integrated approach to elderly care, and the scarcity of mechanisms to co-ordinate with other providers and administrations, such as the Welfare administration. In practice, elderly care is fragmented between the two administrations, with medical and nursing needs being provided by the healthcare system, and social needs, with the limitations already mentioned, being addressed by the social services system. The intersection bears the risk of not being properly addressed by none of them.

One early and institutional attempts to reduce the isolation of both, the healthcare and social services administration, was the establishment of the so called "*Geriatric Assessment Teams*" proposed in the early nineties by the Ministry of Health. Those teams were conceived as multidisciplinary groups, staffed with at least one geriatrician, one social worker, and a nurse trained in multidisciplinary geriatric care, that would support the primary health care teams in a comprehensive assessment of geriatric needs. It was expected that those teams would facilitate the co-ordination of different providers, programs and services dealing with elderly needs, and that would promote the development of specific non-medical activities directed to promote the well being of the elderly. Despite the interest of this initiative, its implementation has been very scarce. In 1996, there were 15 Geriatric Assessment Teams in the whole territory, all of them located in hospitals Another 25 hospitals had some geriatric unit, and there were 15 Geriatric Day Hospitals. In a few occasions, some mixed social-&-health committees are emerging around hospital based geriatric units, but again their scope is very limited. Only the Autonomous Community of Cataluña developed a comprehensive program to provide integrated social and health care, the "*Life to Years*" program ("*Vida als Anys*")[7], that because its significance will be described later.

A significant initiative of the Ministry of Social Welfare (1992) was the creation of a National Gerontologic Plan in co-ordination with all the Autonomies to serve as an strategic planning for comprehensive elderly protective policies [6]. It was an attempt to set a framework to overcome the insufficiency of social provision as well as the fragmentation and limitations of elderly care. The Gerontologic Plan addresses long term policies covering four main issues: health, the elderly carers and relatives, community and institutionalisation services, and users' financial contribution. One of its basic principles consists in the design of policies to maintain the elderly autonomy and to keep the elderly in the community. The Plan assumes that the elderly relatives are those who hold the highest responsibility for elderly care, while the State plays a subsidiary and complementary role. This is specified in two ways: by establishing services in support of carers and by ensuring accommodation in hospice institutions for the elderly with special needs. The Plan expects that users will contribute financially to the services according to their payment ability [8].

A recent development of the Gerontologic Plan (1995) establishes the services that need to be provided to ensure a comprehensive strategy:

- Home Care (including home help and home assistance, medical and nursing healthcare, tele-alarm and other tele-services, and assistance to improve the home living conditions.
- Intermediate Social Services (including day care activities and day care centres, as well as temporary stays in residence accommodations).
- Informal support program.
- Programs for social and health co-ordination (to establish common grounds for an efficient co-ordination).
- Institutional Care (it aims at ensuring the availability of rest homes to all elderly people in need) [6].

Despite the interest of the Gerontologic Plan as a strategic and consensuated framework, it has not been successfully implemented. As an example, aids services to families, although increased substantially are insufficient to cover the major needs, and waiting lists for rest homes are excessive. The Plan did not solve the problem of increasing unmet demand among the elderly, the insufficiency of social services provision, the collapse of acute beds by dependent elderly in hospitals, as well as the scarcity of trained qualified personnel to respond to elderly needs.

In summary, the evolution of public policies in Spain, since the democracy, are directed towards the universalisation of social protection, although this tendency is only more complete in terms of the pensions system and health care. The progressive improvement of the public system of social services goes in the same direction but it remains very incomplete. The main axes that have followed recent public policies are the following:

- The universalisation of two key public systems: healthcare and pensions. Both systems, although with limitations, can be considered universal in coverage. Currently, almost the totality of elderly over 65 years of age receive a pension, that on average is 20% above the minimum income wage [9]. It is expected to evolve in the future towards a moderate income level [10].

- A series of services and equipment in the area of gerontology care (social and health care), that try to keep and support the level of autonomy and functional independence of the elderly. They are structured according to the following scheme: home care, increasingly diversified, and institutional care [11]. However, these services are only accessible by the poor (the public system), or by those who can afford the private ones.
- The "integration, prevention, and personal autonomy of the elderly" through the provision of information, tourist activities, training or education. A series of activities, services and equipment directed to the youngest segments of the elderly population.

The main contribution of the recent Gerontologic policies is at the level of establishing a framework for social provision. But this framework is not yet fully implemented due to the scarcity of financing and the lack of a definitive concerted government action to place comprehensive elderly care as a priority of the political agenda. The GDP share of social protection policies for the elderly in 1997 reached a 7,8%, and close to 31% of all social expenditure. But, close to 50% of the dependent elderly over 65 years of age are below the minimum income wage, and another 35% receive an income that is between 1 and 2 times the minimum income wage. Only 15% of the elderly earn more than twice the minimum income wage [11]. This data points out to the fact that many elderly are in need of extra economic support as well as of public assistance. The late adoption by the Spanish State of welfare policies has contributed to a late awareness and public debate over its future. A recent debate is starting over the future of the pension system, and it is likely that some time soon, the provision of social and health services for an increasingly aged population will be in the political arena. In line with this prevision, the private sector is emerging as an important provider of services [11].

Social and economic context, regional variations, and responsibilities for elderly care

The political decentralisation of Spain has contributed to the increase of inequalities in the organisation and content of social services provision. An important reason for this is the existence of significant differences in economic, geographical and demographic terms across regions and the lack of sufficient compensatory mechanisms across Autonomous Communities [10].

This phenomenon is of great importance since the organisation of service provision is decentralised. Autonomous Governments are responsible for regulating, managing and providing health and social services to their inhabitants, although the level of competence is again unequal across Autonomous Communities. The Regional Health Departments are the responsible institution to regulate, manage and oversee the provision of health care. The Regional Welfare Departments are responsible for the regulation and provision of social services within the Autonomous Communities, however, the management, and implementation of social policies is in fact transferred to Provincial or Local governments. Thus, as a result social services are managed by local and provincial governments, whereas healthcare is managed by Autonomous Governments [3].

Social expenditures for social services provision differ as well by Autonomous Community, resulting in differences in the services received by the elderly across regions. As an example, the percentage of the dependent elderly receiving formal care in the Basque Autonomous Community is around 18,4% [12], while the State average is close to 3,8% [1]. The knowledge about social services among the elderly varies as well. It seems higher among the youngest old and with the highest educational background,[2] in those living in urban settings, and among men.[3] But furthermore, there are many elderly in need for social services (especially of financial help) who are unfamiliar with the services available and with the procedures required to benefit from them [13]. However, most of the care received by the elderly is provided by their families, and family behaviour patterns with regard to elderly care seem to be similar across all the territory.

Another issue that explain regional differences in the use for services is the unequal demand generated by the migratory movements of this century that increased the inequalities in the demographic composition of regions. While the inner and rural regions of Spain (with the exception of Madrid) lost population, the coastal and wealthier regions accepted inhabitants. Thus, distorting the population pyramids in almost all Autonomous Communities, either because of an excess of persons in the labour force or because of scarcity of population in the active age periods.

Health and Social Care for the Elderly: Structures and Functions

Organisational structure and responsibilities for care

Formal care for dependent elderly is fragmented into two different administrations; the National Health Service that provides health care services and the Social Welfare administration responsible for the provision of social services. There is not a clear delimitation of the two fields especially where functional, cognitive and rehabilitative aspects collide. Nevertheless, because of the strong medical focus of the healthcare system, and its rigidity in personnel policies (it is basically staffed by medical doctors and nurses), most aspects dealing with the elderly wellbeing but that do not require of physicians or nursing care are not considered part of the healthcare system, and thus, may be assumed by the social services sector. The social services administration assumes by default all aspects not tackled by the medical sector, but because of the lack of a explicit regulation defining the basic services to be provided, the formal care available tend to respond to a mix of local tradition within the disposable budget. The economical constraints of the past years, imposed by a financial recession in the early nineties and the measures taken to adapt to the European economic convergence have translated into significant reductions in the welfare administration.

The Healthcare provision is regulated through a national law (the General Health Act of 1986) that sets the right to healthcare for all Spanish citizens and entitled residents as well as the principle of equity in access to care as the basis of the National Health Service. The Act sets the basic organisational principles of the National Health Service, and as such it establishes a structured network of health care institutions, organised into different layers of complexity. Individuals have access to the primary level and access to more complex services is mediated by the primary care practitioner. This model is consistent throughout the country and regional variations in management or organisation do not affect the level of care a citizen is entitled to receive.

The organisation of care provision differs significantly among the two systems of care. The health care system offers a primary care level that deals with most of the common problems, including elderly needs. In fact, almost 95% of the Spanish elderly are regular users of the healthcare system [1], especially of the primary care services, where care to elderly people accounts for almost 40% of its activity [14]. Thus, the impact of the healthcare system on the elderly welfare can be easily understood. In the social sector however, there is not such organisation of service provision. Although, there had been attempts to establish a system of primary care for social services that have led to the creation of some municipal offices for social services. However, these services are not the entry to the welfare administration, nor do they refer patients to other settings such as residences or day care centres. Thus, there is not a hierarchical organisation of social services provision even within the same municipal or provincial administration.

The financing models for the two administrations are also different. The healthcare system is financed through general taxation, whereas the social services are subsidised according to provincial or municipal policies, but users must co-finance the services. Elderly under certain level of income are exempt from payment or may benefit from tax deductions, according to local policies as well. In fact, because of the scarcity of social services, most public services are only available to the poor. The low, middle and upper classes of elderly people must use private or mixed services which they have to pay out of their pocket, or in some occasions they may receive some subsidy. Due to these financial constraints is not uncommon that the social services are not only faced with the elderly care, but also with the direct consequences of the financial demands imposed on carers and the elderly by the incompleteness of the welfare policies [3,15].

Furthermore, there are not mechanisms (law or regulations) on a nation basis to ensure an adequate co-ordination between the health and welfare administrations. The result is the co-existence of two different cultures of service provision, but also of confrontation and duplication among the two systems of care [15].

Role of professionals: who does what in elderly care and carers support. Policies on familiar support.

The system of social services provision tries to alleviate the elderly needs as well as family carers' burden. Social services are considered as subsidiaries to family care, thus, in fact they are considered as support services for carers. However, despite the apparent importance of carers for the social service administration, little attention is paid to measure the actual burden of care or the effect of caring on carers' health status and wellbeing [16,17].

There are two big categories of social services and family support programmes in Spain: respite services and psycho-social aid programmes. All of them try to reduce the negative consequences of caring [18].

As formal respite services there are the following:

Home Assistance Service (HAS). Home Assistance Service is the range of home services to address the domestic needs of elderly with problems to perform the activities of daily living. The coverage of home help services in Spain in 1991 was around 1% of all the elderly in need of such services. The Gerontological Plan aims at reaching to 8% of all dependent elderly by the year 2000.

The Autonomous Community of the Basque Government was the first region in developing such service, and it is actively promoting its expansion. Since its inception, this programme was developed as an attempt to create job opportunities for low educated, unskilled, women. The programme opened opportunities for unskilled women to enter in the workforce by taking care of the dependent elderly. However, one of its main problems lied in that it was not accompanied by any specific training, nor it did require special qualifications by potential candidates, thus the quality of the service was low in many instances. This issue together with problems of financial solvency, as well as with legal difficulties in integrating the new workforce into the rigid labour regulations of the public service, led to several conflicts that threatened the continuity of the programme. The situation was settled in 1990 with the creation of intermediate provider companies that established service contracts with the administration, and with the introduction of training programs for women. As a result, however, the service became more expensive and less accessible to many people. Today, the programme is facing a new crisis due to the to the long waiting lists for hospice care that keep highly dependent elderly in the community and increase the demand for home services. Thus, the HAS, that was designed to assist semi-dependent elderly, is not attending their target clientele since it is collapsed by elderly with high levels of dependency to whom is not prepared to provide the care they require [12,19].

The Central Government is proposing the expansion of those services with the following measures:
- By developing national regulations for HAS, including the financial contribution of the elderly and conditions for exemption.
- By specific and permanent training for HAS professionals.
- By developing criteria to assess the level of need, as well as a scoring system to measure and rank needs.
- By establishing mechanisms for co-ordination between social and health services in the local area.
- By promoting private initiatives as well as the associative movement
- By increasing the co-ordination between institutions with competencies in social services [9].

Day Care Centres. These centres started to be implemented in some communities during the late 80's. Day care centres have the mission of maintaining the levels of functional capacity of the dependent elderly so they could remain in the community, providing an intermediate service between home care and institutional care. They are staffed primarily by social workers, nurse assistants or aid workers.

Users of Day Care centres are elderly people who want to remain in their homes, but that have severe physical or cognitive impairment that limit its autonomy. Again, the level of coverage by those centres is very low [12] although it is increasing. It is expected to reach a rate of 0,5% of people over 65 years for the year 2000. It is considered as a very important resource to relieve the burden of caregivers [20].

Support to Family Caregivers. The Central Government recommended in 1991 the establishment of a specific program to support family caregivers. Its main lines were the following:
- Tax deductions for families caring a dependent elderly.
- Support for carers through continuous training and access to technical aids and to new technologies.
- New rest-home opportunities for temporal stays for dependent elderly [9].

These recommendations are commonly present in most regulations established by regional governments [12].

Temporary Stays in Rest Homes or Hospices. This program was designed with the purpose of ameliorating the quality of life of the dependent elderly as well as of supporting family carers by offering respite opportunities through temporary stays of the elderly in residential settings.

Rest Homes, Hospices, Residential services. Rest Homes try to provide accommodation for those elderly who can not live within their families. Traditionally, two types of Rest Homes have been distinguished, those for autonomous elderly, providing common facilities and hotel services, and those for dependent elderly, which in addition to hotel services provide different types of care. The experience has shown that with time, residences for autonomous elderly become residences for dependent elderly.

In the last years, there has been deployed a great effort by public and private initiatives to increase the availability of residential facilities in Spain. In 1994, the proportion of residential beds was of 2,38 beds per 100 people over 65 years, although there are large geographical differences. The highest concentration of residential beds is in the Communities of Navarra, La Rioja and the Basque Country, where the rate in 1994 was around 3,4% [12,21].

Recent developments or new designs to provide support to family carers. Is there any evidence of impact?

The Role of the Associative Movement. There is an increasing number of associations of family caregivers or of other civic groups (usually subsidised by the public administration) that act in practice as the single source of support for family carers. As seen previously, formal social services are scarce and healthcare services do not understand enough the complex needs of the dependent elderly and their families [17,22,23]. Most of those initiatives focus on senile dementia and Alzheimer caregivers, and most of them include the following components:

- Group interventions.
- Psychological interventions.
    1. Support (training, group dynamics, socialising, mutual support, sharing experiences, understanding perceptions, learning coping).
    2. Counselling, insight therapy, cognitive therapy, relaxation therapy, stress management.
    3. Understanding and overcoming emotional impact, stress, aggressiveness, grieving, blaming.
    4. Self-help.
    5. Interpersonal relations and communication.

- Introduction to pedagogical and educational programmes.
    6. Information.
    7. Skill improvement for home care.
    8. Development of therapeutic skills, problem solving, behavioural techniques.
    9. Emergency planning: legal, financial.
- Promotion and development of support networks.
    10. Family-Personal level.
    11. Community level.
    12. Professional level [16].

Some significant institutional initiatives

Despite the insufficiency of wellbeing policies in Spain, there are a few examples of comprehensive approach to elderly care that are worth mentioning. The Catalan

Autonomous community is most likely the leading community in addressing elderly care from a comprehensive, integrated strategy. This is the first community in developing an integrated programme for elderly care, the programme called "*Life to Years*" (or "*Vida Als Anys*"), which is not only characterised by its innovative and comprehensive approach, but also by its financial contribution to elderly care. This community has been followed by others, such as the Basque Region, the Canary Island, Valencia and Galicia.

The "Vida als Anys" program. In 1988, the "*Vida als Anys*" program was created in the Catalan Autonomous Community as the regional strategy to address the elderly care. It is a program managed jointly by the Regional Health Department together with the Regional Welfare Administration. It started with a definition of the functional and structural criteria that residential institutions should provide in order to be accredited as appropriate residences for elderly care. It thus, reunited the existing centres (private health centres, chronic hospitals, and welfare institutions) and adapted them to meet those requirements, in order to enable them to contract services with the Health Department. Potential users were assessed and categorised according to their level of need (elderly, chronically dependent, terminal patients, psychiatric patients, drug abusers). Finally the types of services offered were also defined and categorised (convalescence, palliative services, long stay). Referral mechanisms between the healthcare and residential institutions were established. A comprehensive community service was developed as well, with the creation of Home Support programs, managed by the *PADES*, a designated structure at the primary care level that manages and co-ordinates all care for the elderly. The *PADES* support the primary health care services by providing home healthcare to needy elderly, and co-ordinates with a network of social services: the *UFISS* or Interdisciplinary Units for Social Services, that liase with acute hospital care, and with day care centres.

The purpose of the programme is to maintain the quality of life of the dependent elderly, through a comprehensive understanding of care, being sensitive with the physical, emotional and spiritual needs of the elderly. Family support is understood as a key element to enhance the benefit of therapies. The programme offers respite and training services to families.

The programme is financed by both, the health care administration as well as the welfare administration, through a complicated allocation formula that tries to recover the cost to the pertinent authority [24].

Sendian (Care for families of elderly people in Gipuzkoa) Another program of interest is Sendian. This is a program created by the Provincial Administration of Gipuzkoa in the Basque Autonomous Region in 1996 with the aim of providing support to family carers. Despite its youth, it can be taken as a model since it is one of the few programs that address comprehensively the needs of carers. Its goal is to serve as a source of support for family caregivers so as to alleviate the burden of care-giving. The programme provides the following services:
- Family training in caring and coping skills.
- Psychological support to the elderly, the family or both.
- Voluntary aid, in co-ordination with the associative movement of elderly caregivers.
- Residential care, and Week-end day care centres.
- Technical help.
- Financial support.
- Self-Help groups.
- Tax deductions.

After finalising a successful pilot experience, the program will be expanded to cover the whole Province of Gipuzkoa in the Basque Autonomous Community [25].

Alternatives for health and social services co-ordination

The experiences previously described are exceptional arrangements in the Spanish service provision for the elderly. Its generalisation to other settings and regions although desirable faces many difficulties. It will undoubtedly need of a profound reorganisation of the current welfare and health administrations including profound changes in the prevalent culture of the two organisations as well as of providers in order to enable the establishment of common strategies and policies. But furthermore, any attempt for reform will face the restrictions imposed by a continuous limitation of resources, by the rigidity of some of the prevailing regulations and the centralisation of decision making, but also by the lack of a defined political responsibility at any of the administrations related to elderly care. Despite all of these constraints, the few experiences described seem to have accomplished success in terms of providing quality and comprehensive services to elderly people; partly due to a high level of commitment by the staff involved [26].

The Role of Family Carers of Older People Living at Home

Financial, social, personal, age and gender issues

According to some data of 1995, up to 72% of the elderly people who need regular assistance are helped by their relatives and acquaintances; another 5.4% are cared by private home care professionals, and only 3.8% are cared by the social services.

Up to 83% of informal caregivers are women who in general (61.5%) do not receive any assistance. Those women tend to be between 45 and 69 years old. They tend to be married (76.6%), and to live in the same lodging as the old people they care for (58,7%). Another group of women seems to have moved temporarily to the elderly home (12,9%), and a final group (14%) are taken care of elderly who live in their own. The educational status of these caregivers tends to be low (65,6%), and the majority of them do not do any other regular work (75%).

It is likely that this profile may change in the following years as demographic patterns, and the increasing participation of women in the labour force, together with a reduction in family size are changing [1]. However, there are studies that suggest that women caregivers are motivated by a strong morale imperative to take care of their old relatives and that this attitude will be transmitted from this to the next generation, despite social changes. While this theory may or not prove true, it seems plausible that the caring attitude of women will be confronted by the economic and societal dynamics [22].

Attitudes towards professionals

According to some theorists, the tendency towards caring seen among Spanish women is due to the traditional gender role division in society, coupled by an intense perception of self-blame, sense of duty and stress-reaction in the face of disease and disability. According to this theory, it seems justified that social services would play a subsidiary role, and needed only when the natural informal network failed, thus there is no the need for an early intervention [16].

Institutionalisation of the elderly is perceived as the last resort to cope with disability. This belief is fostered by the late development of a long-term care policy that would have contributed to keep the elderly in the community. But especially, it is reinforced by a prevalent cost-containment policy that results in an insufficient social service network to meet the needs of the population. The unequal supply of community services tends toward a medical, rather, than social or comprehensive, care for the elderly [27].

Studies on informal carers show that only 7% of them are receiving any type of help, half of whom receive support from private sources, and only the other half receive assistance from the public service. It has been reported that up to 61,5% of informal carers would like to receive some form of financial support, another 30,7 would prefer some home assistance, and another 11% some respite aid, in the form of a day care centre, or a temporary stay in a rest home [1].

Stress

The experience of caring is increasingly becoming an usual step in the life of most adult Spaniards. Most Spaniards accept caring for their elderly relatives as part of their family obligations, rooted in beliefs and feelings of reciprocal duty, emotional debts, and based in the strong belief that familiar care is always preferable to formal care. It is also suggested that informal care is more satisfactory in general for the elderly, due to the higher affection and emotional wellbeing involved [12]. The fact that caring may act as a "taboo", may hinder a more fluid communication between the carer and the cared person. Thus, the carer tends to act in isolation. The carer tries to achieve imprecise objectives, such as: avoiding the institutionalisation, caring for the elderly needs, and avoiding the elderly falling into depression and self-blaming [16].

Studies on family burden derived from caring show a series of disadvantages on carers such as: economical difficulties, housing problems, distress of carers and their families' lifestyle, new and sometimes overwhelming requirements and duties, and psychological distress characterised by feelings of insecurity, impotence and lack of control or self-blaming, and limitations on the social role of carers.

The carers' family life may result deeply disturbed by the change of roles and duties among their members. It is common to find alterations in the level of communications, reduction or lost of sexual activity, and changes in their usual emotional feelings of family members due to all of these factors. Close to 75% of carers is suffering from some degree of stress derived from caring, and almost 45% describe some associated physical problem due to caring [16].

Evaluation: How the Social Service Network Works for the Elderly and Their Carers

The rapid ageing process experienced in Spain, together with an also rapid and intense change in social and cultural values in Spanish families has caused difficulties for the articulation of an adequate and prompt response from the welfare administration to meet the new needs of the elderly. The response given was slow, insufficient, unequal and fragmented. Support services for carers have not been articulated either, thus increasing the demand for formal social services for the elderly. The private initiative has not been able yet to provide an affordable package of services for the majority of the population [10].

Social policy

For the past 20 years, there has been a significant increase in the provision of services, with the construction of new centres and residencies, availability of equipment, new professionals and programs. However, their level of achievement seems far away from that of other European countries. It is significant, that care for the elderly ranks fourth among social expenditures, after retirement pensions, healthcare, and unemployment coverage.

The insufficient policy on elderly care seems unsustainable. Furthermore, it is causing a negative effect financially, since adequate social policies alleviate the financial burden in other spheres of society. Another source of concern is produced by the lack of a common regulatory framework for social policies across all Autonomous Communities, that is the cause of high inequity in social protection for the elderly. There have been unsuccessful attempts to define a minimum package of basic social services across regions, as well as of accessibility criteria for entitlement.

The very poor are in most instances the only segment of the elderly with access to the social service network. The majority of the population does not have access, except by paying, which increases the financial difficulties for the low and middle classes (too wealthy to access the formal public network of services, too poor to pay for private services).

Another weakness of the formal services is the lack of mechanisms to articulate with informal carers. Although recently there have been attempts to advance in this area. Similarly, important efforts have been made recently to improve the qualifications of professionals and of resources [1].

Due to the fragmentation between health and social services, and the high degree of discretion in the classification of needs (disability is considered under the domain of social services, while rehabilitation and medical care is under the healthcare area) there is room for more inequity since the healthcare system is universal and more developed, but that is not the case of the social service system [1]. As it has been mentioned previously, the Catalan Autonomous Community is the only region attempting to solve this problem through the integration of the two administrations [28].

Health and social services co-ordination

In the past years the concept of health and social services integration became prevalent among policy makers, professionals and social scientists. However, the reality is that this is an unachieved objective in Spain.

The proportion of hospital beds classified as geriatric or long-stay was less than 7% of the total number of hospital beds in 1997. Excluding the four autonomous communities with the largest share (the Catalan Region, Madrid, The Canary Islands, and the Basque Country) the proportion is less than 3% of all hospital beds. The increase seen in the last years, although significant, is less than 10% and it is concentrated in a few regions. At the same time, the provision of residential beds has grown in the past 4 years in more than 20% (there were 22,684 beds in 1998). Although it is difficult to measure, community services (day care, home care and others) grown approximately in 7.8%.

The evolution of social and health services can be categorised as follows:
- The social sector for elderly care is growing and getting consolidated.
- The growth is heterogeneous, and follows unequal patterns across regions. The amount of resources, the quality of services, and the degree of participation of the different administrations is also unequal.
- Given the administrative rigidity of the healthcare sector, it may face difficulties in trying to adapt its resources towards the field of elderly care, although again there are large differences across regions.
- The co-ordination of health and social services is a recurrent topic for debate among policy makers, scientists and professionals [29].

The Gerontologic Plan that aimed at creating a common health and social space for elderly care has not been implemented. However, the provision of social services is becoming increasingly important and there are expectations that it become an important economic sector in the future, with potential for employment.

Evaluation of carer support programmes

The main fact is that there are not efficacious measures in support of carers, despite the evident need. Private help initiatives, of recent irruption, tend to focus on institutional beds, while they provide scarce home care or day care centres, other respite services, or tele-alarm services. A characteristic of private services is the high level of comfort and service quality of some of them that are unaffordable for the majority of the population; while more affordable services tend to be low quality and provided by low qualified staff.

Tax breaks offered to carers are in fact of very low quantity to exert any significant impact on carers' disposable income. Furthermore, tax exemptions are small and flat, not adapted to carer's incomes thus their impact on people of middle and higher income is even of lower significance.

Training and support programs on coping and methods and skills for caring have started to develop very recently. Its impact and level of coverage is still very limited so that for many families, the only service available is the institutionalisation of the elderly people [10].

The Home Assistance Service (HAS) seems to have exerted very low impact on carers and on the elderly because of its high cost and low coverage, resulting in a insufficient service provision. However, it is perceived as a basic service, thus it needs to expand keeping its double character of social service for the recipients, the elderly or their carers, but also of employment alternative for the workers, the low skilled or unskilled women [19].

Similarly, support services for carers are criticised by being insufficient and of low coverage. Another reason for complaint both from their customers as well as from the staff, lies in that due to the general scarcity of social services and support programs for carers, the existing programs need to respond to needs other than the ones they are designed for, thus overwhelming the staff and resources and providing low quality service.

Specific evaluations of support programs for carers of Alzheimer's sufferers suggest that it is difficult to establish a link between those programs and improvements in the cared person's functional status or well being. It seems that interventions improve the specific knowledge and skills related to the disease among carers, decrease the perception of burden, and improve their problem solving abilities. It is not clear, however, that depression among carers is improved or that their social functioning is improved [16].

It has been suggested that carers' support programs should have a more comprehensive psycho-social approach, and that they should include a broader range of objectives, including stress reduction, skill development, family support and training, as well as being adapted to the specific disease level and progression, to exert a higher impact on carers [16].

It has been found that up to two thirds of the carers that use day care centre as respite services show high levels of stress. Up to half of all of these carers refer being overwhelmed and exhausted by their caring activity. Half of them refer being depressed and close to a third of all carers report showing social and family functioning problems. In many cases, day care centres are being used as an unsatisfactory surrogate for the residential accommodation, thus increasing the perception of lack of success of these centres [17].

In the Basque Autonomous Community in 1993, close to 3,3% of people over 65 years were using HAS (home assistance services), 0.2% were using residential accommodation, another 0.2% attended day care centres, and another 0.2% used tele-alarm services. At this time the waiting list for social services exceeded the current capacity in:
- 26.4% for home services.
- 49.6% for residential centres.
- 57.1% for day care centres.

The corresponding supply for residential beds was 3.4 beds per 100 elderly population (over 65). It was estimated that 14,800 elderly living in the community were home-bed and highly dependent but only a 16,8% of them demanded a residential bed [12].

The immediate conclusion after these data is that the overall coverage is scarce, insufficient to meet the needs of the elderly and their carers, and unable to cope with the current demand for services.

Case Studies

The basic features of the Spanish health system and social services system define the case studies that are presented below. These are: the health care system is homogenous across the State and it is accessible and free at the point of service for all Spanish citizens. A minimum of financial assistance is provided to all Spaniards, although the pension may be too low to cover the elderly needs. The provision of social services is unequal across the State, but in general, the level of coverage is very low. Usually, only the poor are entitled to receive public social services. The low, middle and upper classes need to purchase private or mixed services with different levels of co-payment. The main source of care is provided by family caregivers.

Case 1

Female, aged 76, with osteoarthritis of the hips and knees, poor vision due to macular degeneration and hypertension. Mobile with a frame within her home except for the stairs. Needs help with mobility outside, shopping cooking and housework.

This is the case of an elderly woman with chronic health conditions and associate disability. It is likely, that the health care needs of this woman (medical and nursing care) will be covered by the healthcare system. Both the nurse and the doctor will visit the elderly for periodic check-ups of their health condition. If she needs to be seen at the health facility she could request a medical transport (an ambulance).

Social Circumstances (A): Older person living alone in an isolated farmhouse. Widowed. Little money. Daughter and son-in-law unemployed with four children, aged 9 months to 7 years, and live 5 kilometres away. Two other children of the older person live over 100 kilometres away.

Because of the little income of this woman and of her close family, she is a likely candidate for the local social services office. Most likely, the local budget for social services will be scarce, and there will not be many services available (day care centre, social workers…). However, she may get financial aid to purchase a frame, glasses, or a wheelchair if needed, as well as to do some works at their home in order to adapt it to her disability. Most likely, if this woman has lived for a long time in the same town, she may be known and get some help with shopping and the house from her neighbours and acquaintances, as well as from the town's church. Her unemployed daughter, who lives nearby, may become her main caregiver. According to the local availability of social services and waiting lists, the elderly woman may get some home assistance, and a tele-alarm device. If she gets more dependent she can enter into a hospice waiting list. According to local availability as well, her daughter may become a candidate for financial help from the social services, because of her many family burdens and scarce resources.

Social Circumstances (B): Older person lives alone in a ground floor flat in town. Widowed. Daughter and son-in-law are both teachers in full-time employment, with 2 children aged 7 and 11, and live within 1 kilometre in same town.

As in the previous case, this woman may have neighbours and acquaintances in the neighbourhood that may help her with the house and other domestic issues. Since she seems to have some money, the church and other religious groups will not help her specifically. Her daughter will most probably take care of her mother by visiting and calling her often, and will become her main caregiver. Nor this woman, nor her daughter as caregiver, will be clear candidates for the local social services. They will need to buy the prosthesis needed by themselves (glasses, frame, works at home). They may purchase private aid, such as some home care, or may join a day care centre if it is available in town and they can afford it.

Social Circumstances (C): Older person lives with spouse in 2-storey house. Retired with savings. Spouse is fit and well. No children. Bedroom, bathroom and toilet are upstairs.

This woman will not be entitled to receive any assistance from the public service. Most probably, they will receive some emotional support from some relatives, but the spouse will become the main caregiver. They may hire a person to assist with the home, and with other domestic duties. They may also hire if needed a nurse assistant. Probably, because of their age, they may not know of the existence of any other social services available in town, and may not join a day care centre or other facility. With time, they may enter a private rest home.

Case 2

Male, aged 80, facing discharge from hospital following a stroke. Expected to be confined to bed or chair for several weeks with gradual recovery of mobility. Needs the help of one person for transfers, toileting, bathing and dressing.

This man, with a disabled chronic condition will be discharged to home from the hospital given the lack of rehabilitative services. Only, if he is wealthy, will be able to afford the very few facilities in the country. The primary care nurse and doctor will visit him at home periodically for check-ups of his condition. The medical doctor will write a prescription for a wheelchair.

Social Circumstances (A): Older person living alone in an isolated farmhouse. Widowed. Little money. Daughter and son-in-law unemployed with four children, aged 9 months to 7 years, and live 5 kilometres away. Two other children of the older person live over 100 kilometres away.

It is likely, that this man will be discharged directly to his daughter's home, so she will be able to take care of him. Similarly to the previous case, this man is a candidate for the local social services office. The same conditions of scarcity of resources at the local social services office apply in this case, thus, there will not be many services available (day care centre, social workers...). However, because of his higher level of dependence, financial difficulties of the family, and the extra burden of the daughter, this man will be given higher priority in getting home assistance and financial aid to do works in the house, or purchase some aids.

Social Circumstances (B): Older person lives alone in a ground floor flat in town. Widowed. Daughter and son-in-law are both teachers in full-time employment, with 2 children aged 7 and 11, and live within 1 kilometre in same town.

As in the previous circumstance, it is likely that this man will be discharged directly to his daughter's home. However, because they do not lack financial resources they will not get specific help from the social services. If the family can afford, they may get some private home assistance. The caregiver burden will not be assessed.

Social Circumstances (C): Older person lives with spouse in 2-storey house. Retired with savings. Spouse is fit and well. No children. Bedroom, bathroom and toilet are upstairs.

This couple will not be entitled to receive any public assistance. The spouse will need to hire a nurse assistant, or any other person, to live in the house and take care of the elderly. The caregiver burden will not be assessed. If the level of dependency increases, they may enter into a private hospice.

Case 3

Female, aged 86, suffering from dementia. Frequent wandering by day and night. Frequent falls. Incontinent of urine and faeces.

This woman will be living with another relative or else she will be taken to a hospice. If she is in the community, she will receive periodic visits of a nurse.

Social Circumstances (A): Older person living alone in an isolated farmhouse. Widowed. Little money. Daughter and son-in-law unemployed with four children, aged 9 months to 7 years, and live 5 kilometres away. Two other children of the older person live over 100 kilometres away.

This woman will have moved to her daughters' home. She will have entered the waiting lists for the closest day care centre. The family will receive some financial aid to purchase some equipment. Probably there will not be available any caregiver support program in the locality. It is likely, that the daughter is not familiar with the Alzheimer's sufferers association, and thus, she will not receive any support. The daughter will suffer a considerable level of stress.

Social Circumstances (B): Older person lives alone in a ground floor flat in town. Widowed. Daughter and son-in-law are both teachers in full-time employment, with 2 children aged 7 and 11, and live within 1 kilometre in same town.

In this case, the woman will move as well to her daughter's home, but most likely, the daughter will become familiar with the Alzheimer's self-help groups. She could get some emotional and psychological support from those associations, as well as training and skills to cope with the disease. They could also join specific day care centres for Alzheimer sufferers, as long as they could afford them. With time, they may join a private hospice for Alzheimer sufferers.

Social Circumstances (C): Older person lives with spouse in 2-storey house. Retired with savings. Spouse is fit and well. No children. Bedroom, bathroom and toilet are upstairs.

In this case, the spouse will suffer all the care burden with little assistance. It is likely that the spouse will not be familiar with the Alzheimer's association, nor of specific day are centres. If this is the case, the spouse will only get some relief by hiring a nurse assistant, or any other person to help in the home, and by joining a private hospice.

Future Development

Most likely scenario

Taking into account the characteristics of the new generations that are reaching the ageing period, one of the most likely scenario that may take place in the short future in Spain is the following:
- The percentage of elderly people over 65 years that will be in need for services will approach 30%.
- The share of people over 65 years in need for services receiving assistance from the informal sector will go down to 65%.
- The share of people over 65 years receiving assistance at their homes will go down to 80%.
- The percentage of elderly people with income less than the minimum wage will go down to 45%, while the percentage of elderly with income between one and twice the minimum wage will remain unchanged and will increase to 20% the percentage of elderly with more than twice the minimum wage.

As a result, the demand for services will increase significantly. If the current desired level of coverage by the formal service is close to 8% of the elderly, in a few decades this level will need to be increased at least up to 11%. In any case, the level of real coverage by social services is far below those levels [11].

In addition, there are some data that suggest changes in the attitudes of relatives towards caring pointing out to a new scenario with important implications for elderly care [1]. Families are showing increasing fear and reluctance to care for their elderly. It will be, thus, needed to develop a system of social protection for the elderly focusing direct service provision, coupled with financial and fiscal incentives for the elderly and their carers [30].

It seems imperative, that formal and informal care will increase their mechanisms for co-ordination and co-operation. Similarly, there are not clear divisions for the private and public initiatives. The public administration must find ways for increasing the efficiency of service provision, through increasing the efficiency of the informal networks, as well as of the private sector [19]. The analysis of scenarios for co-ordination between the public, private and informal sectors is basic to understand the mixed economy of welfare, and the plural venues for welfare services towards the Spanish welfare system seems to evolve.

Currently, one of the main problems, consists in the delimitation of appropriate roles, responsibilities, and activities for each of three agents. The increasingly limited capacity of the informal sector to respond to many situations, and with the scarcity of resources in the public sector, together with an apparently emergent private sector, are some of the variables for the new scenarios [11].

Another issue of relevance will be defined by a more clear delimitation of the responsibility of the two level of social service provision: institutionalisation and community services. As well as of the equipment and technology needed [11].

Issues that need to be addressed

An adequate response to elderly care requires of a significant expansion and improvement of current services, but also of their rationalisation, re-ordination and optimisation [10].

Support for carers

The importance of the role of carers needs to be recognised. This is a necessary step for developing the set of services carers as well as the elderly need. Subsequently, there is the need for carers' support through training, counselling, information and other mechanisms. Mechanisms for adequate communication between carers and social and health professionals are also needed in order to adapt the service provision to the evolving needs of carers and of the elderly. It is needed to develop strategies to solve the common problems that occur among family carers, including mechanisms to improve the social interaction between family members to reduce isolation and self-blaming; and to facilitate the exchange of emotional communication [30]. It is significant, the lack of a specific instrument to measure the extent of family burden caused by elderly care, to assist in the management of elderly care [1,10,17]. Another related issue is that of the employment situation of carers. There is the need to develop specific support mechanisms to keep carers in the labour force, or to return to the labour force after caring [1,10].

Consolidation of existing programmes for dependent elderly

Including the extension of coverage and quality improvement both in the community and residential institutions. It is important to facilitate the accessibility to care services, by reducing the sometimes considerable administrative processes. Furthermore, entitlement requirements to access those programs need to be revised and homogenised [10].

Financial assistance

Diverse programmes more adapted to the elderly socio-economic reality need to be put in place. Among these are specific subsidies to family carers, or tax deductions. In any case, they need to be of sufficient quantity as to alleviate families' economic burden and will contribute to keep the elderly in the community [1,10].

Development of integrated social and health services

One of the most urgent issues is the need for an effective co-ordination between the health and social services, so as to develop a specific common social and health field for elderly care [15]. The most important challenge derives from the current insufficiency of the Spanish welfare administration, which needs to evolve to an horizon of universality of coverage, according to the economic development and stability of the Spanish economy.

Any extension of the formal service sector will need to be articulated with the family support [1,3,10,31].

Main Challenges

The main challenges facing the construction of an integrated social and health system for elderly care are the following.

Planning, management and financing

With the current division of responsibilities among the health and social administration, it is extremely difficult to achieve an adequate level of planning for services. Both of them are organised around different principles: the health system universal and financed through general taxes, whereas social services are based on entitlement criteria, and incur in high levels of co-payment. Despite the difficulties, there are few successful experiences (Programme "*Vida als Anys*") where policy makers have been able to generate new administrative mechanisms for combining the planning and regulatory function, the provision of services and the financing.

Perhaps the three main options for an adequate financing mechanism are: a net increase in public resources for elderly care (this option does not seem highly viable given the financial constraints imposed by the European financial convergence), changes in the current resource allocation within the welfare administration, or an increase in financing through increasing in workers contribution to the social security. Combinations of the three options may conform potentially likely scenarios [10].

Co-ordination in the provision of care

One of the current major issues explaining the difficulties in providing adequate elderly care lies in the extreme rigidity of both administrations, in terms of tailoring services to needs, hiring personnel, and adapting the existing funds towards the needs of the elderly. The major challenge for an integrated social and health service provision lies in the ability to create models of care where both administrations could purchase integrated services in co-ordination.

Case management

Due to the lack of a common point of entry to care, the allocation of specific needs to the health or social sphere, is a source of inequality in the provision of services. A first step towards co-ordination can be done by establishing single points of entry at the community. Similarly, it will be important to develop mechanisms for case management at the clinical setting.

Information systems

One of the main challenges that we are facing today, is the difficulty of analysing, measuring, and identification the case-mix of elderly needs. Fortunately, there are initiatives to advance in this direction with the design of functional assessment instruments, evaluation systems, case mix instruments as well as resource analysis systems [29].

Notes

[1] According to the National Health Survey of 1995, approximately 26.6% of the elderly over 65 years need help to perform one or more activities of daily living. Out of these, 13% are living on their own, 43% with their spouse, and 44% with their children or other relatives.

[2] It is likely that the civil war may have exerted a significant impact in the educational status of different elderly cohorts.

[3] The differential on the knowledge of social services by gender is decreasing in the youngest cohorts of elderly, but it still remains in favour of men, perhaps due to the higher social activity of men.

References

[1] P. Rodríguez and M.T. Sancho, Nuevos retos de la política social de atención a los mayores. Las situaciones de fragilidad. Rev. Esp. Geriatri Gerontol; 30(3) (1995) 141-152.
[2] CIS Centro de Investigaciones Sociológicas. "Situación Social de los Viejos en España". Estudios y Encuestas 21, abril 1990.
[3] F.J. Leturia and J.J. Yanguas J.J, Dependencia y articulación sociosanitaria: un reto de futuro. Zerbitzuan 32 (1997) 76-82.
[4] D. Casado Ayudas económicas y servicios sociales en el Estado de las Autonomías. Política social y servicios sociales. Comité Español de Bienestar Social. Marsiega, Madrid 1985.
[5] J. Sánchez Jiménez, Realidades sociales y políticas de transformación (España, 1940-1980). Documentación Social n 109, Cáritas Española. octubre-diciembre 1997.
[6] M.A. Vidal M.A, El desarrollo legislativo de la geriatría en España. La protección de la salud de las personas mayores, Geriátrica 15(2) (1999) 71-77.
[7] F. Guillen and J.M. Rivera, Situación y perspectivas de la Asistencia Geriátrica Hospitalaria en España. Rev Esp Geriatr Gerontol 32(4) (1997)236-238.
[8] F. Beland et al, Perspectivas en la organización e cuidados de larga duración, Rev Esp Griatr Gerontol 31(5) (1996) 277-290.
[9] INSERSO "Plan Gerontógico". Ministerio de Asuntos Sociales, 1992.
[10] H. Maravall, La atención a la dependencia: el gran reto de la política social hacia las personas mayores de los próximos años. Intervención Psicosocial, Vol. 66n 1 (1997) 9-19.
[11] J. Vizcaino J, Aproximación cuantitativa a los usuarios potenciales de los programas de atención social al anciano. Rev Esp Geriatr Gerontol 32(4) (1997) 225-235.
[12] "Plan Gerontológico de Euskadi (1994). Gobierno Vasco. Departamento de Justicia, Economía, Trabajo y Seguridad Social. 1995.
[13] A. Saco, El conocimiento de los servicios sociales por parte del colectivo de la tercera edad: El efecto generación. Rev Esp Geriatr Gerontol 30(4) (1995) 263-266.
[14] M. Martin et al, El anciano frágil en la comunidad. Rev Esp Geriatr Gerontol 32(NMI) (1997) 39-44.
[15] J.A. Aguirre, La atención socio-sanitaria en la Comunidad Autónoma del País Vasco, Zerbitzuan 25 (1994) 14-24.
[16] J.A. Padierna J.A, Apoyos socio asistenciales a los familiares de enfermos de Alzheimer. La carga familiar, Zerbitzuan: 47-54.
[17] F. Gómez-Busto et al, Perfil del cuidador, carga familiar y severidad de la demencia en tres ámbitos diferentes: domicilio, centro de día y residencia de válidos, Rev. Esp. Geriatr. Gerontol, 34(3) (1999) 141-149.
[18] I. Montorio et al, Programas y servicios de apoyo a familiares cuidadores de ancianos dependientes, Rev Esp Geriatr Gerontol; 30(3) (1995)157-168.
[19] Ararteko "Informe extraordinario sobre la asistencia no residencial a la tercera edad en la Comunidad Autónoma del País Vasco 1994-1995". 1996.
[20] C. Sannino, Centros de día un recurso en franca progresión. Zerbitzuan 32 (1997) 46-49.
[21] J.L. Martinez and J.J. Artells, Objetivo 30: servicios comunitarios para atender necesidades especiales" Informe SESPAS 2000. La salud pública. Nuevos desafios ante un nuevo siglo. Documento de trabajo (1999) 207-208.
[22] M.T. Bazo, El cuidado familiar en las personas ancianas con enfermedades crónicas: el caso de los pacientes con enfermedad de Alzheimer, Rev esp Geriatr Gerontol, 33(1) (1998):49-56.
[23] J.C. Caballero, Importancia de las asociaciones familiares en el caso de los enfermos con demencia, Rev Gerontol 7 (1997) 110-112.
[24] M.D. Fontanals de Nadal et al, Evaluación de la atención sociosanitaria en Cataluña. La experiencia del

programa Vida als Anys. Rev Esp Geriatr Gerontol, 30(3) (1995) 1899-198.
[25] A. Manterola, Sendian. Zerbitzuan 32 (1997) 54-58.
[26] C. Lopez et al, Una experiencia de coordinación sociosanitaria: el Area 4 de Madrid. Rev Esp Geriatr Gerontol, 30(3) (1995) 199-204.
[27] L. Gil de ramales et al, Conocimiento, uso y previsión de servicios sanitarios y sociales de apoyo al cuidador de personas mayores con incapacidades. Rev Esp Geriatr Gerontol, 34(1) (1999) 34-43.
[28] H. Maravall H, La coordinación socio-sanitaria: una exigencia ineludible. Rev Esp Geriatri Gerontol, 30(3) (1995) 131-135.
[29] E. Carrillo and C. Illa, Objetivo 6: vejez saludable. Informe SESPAS 2000. La salud pública. Nuevos desafios ante un nuevo siglo. Documento de trabajo (1999) 46-51.
[30] D. López, familia Acogedora. 207-216.
[31] J.M. Bleda, Tendencias y líneas de desarrollo de las políticas de vejez en Castilla-La Mancha. Rev. Esp. Geriatr. Gerontol, 32(5) (1997) 291-296.

Chapter 10

Sweden
(August 1999)

Rolf Hässler
Motala Hospital
LAH-Kliniken
59185 Motala
Sweden

Introduction

A lot of discussions regarding the future development of social and health care services for the elderly in Sweden are currently being held. At the heart of the discussion lies the controversy between obvious economic limits and traditional Swedish politics.

After the Second World War, care of the elderly was prioritised and the public sector assumed responsibility for social services and health care. This development was facilitated by a favourable economic situation, which consequently allowed for the provision of care by specially trained and qualified staff. Today it is evident that resources are limited and that it is important to find ways of prioritising.

Important areas for the elderly in Sweden are regarded to be financial security, good housing, social services and need-driven health care provision. Irrespective of financial limitations, it is intended that the elderly have a degree of choice and influence over the public help they receive, and that standards are maintained at a high level. It is also endeavoured that elderly people, even if they are unhealthy and disabled, have the right to be provided with proper services and the help they need to allow them to remain in their homes. Government and Parliament legislation and guidelines on care provision for the elderly address potential care providers and care. The general principles of the Swedish welfare state regarding the care of the elderly are the same nationwide.

In December 1997 Sweden had a population of 8.8 million; 17.5 % of these were over 65 years of age, a very high figure in comparison to other countries. Most people in Sweden are healthy at the age of 65 and do not need assistance in their daily life. However, the 80+ and 90+ age-groups have substantially increased over the last decade - prognoses suggesting further increase. As a result problems are anticipated, since age is the single factor demonstrating the strongest link with the use of social and health care services. An increase in the elderly population will certainly be accompanied by a growing burden on the various services for the elderly.

Table 1: Pensioners aged 65 and above

year	% of total population	Number of individuals
1950	10	700 000
1980	16,4	1 360 000
1985	17,4	1 454 000
1990	17,8	1 526 000
1996	17,5	1 543 000
2000 prognosis	17,0	1 529 000
2020 prognosis	20,7	1 958 000

Table 2: Pensioners aged 80 and above

year	% of total population	Number of individuals
1950	1,5	107 000
1980	3,2	263 000
1985	3,7	313 000
1990	4,3	369 000
1996	4;7	420 000
2000 prognosis	5,0	455 000
2020 prognosis	5,1	487 000

The Swedish system of national pensions and housing allowances is designed to give elderly people financial security. The national pension scheme includes a basic pension (folkpension) based on time of residence in Sweden and a supplementary pension (ATP) based on income.

The normal retirement age in Sweden is 65. The pension is index-linked. In addition a special partial pension makes it possible for people aged 61- 64 to combine part-time work with a pension. It is also possible to choose to draw the old-age pension from the 60th birthday or to postpone receipt until the age of 70. The amount received every month is lower if payments started early and higher if they are delayed. A recipient of a basic pension may be entitled to a state housing allowance. This is a means-tested benefit and the rules are determined by the state. In 1994 30% of old age pensioners received this type of benefit. The combined basic and ATP pension for a person with an average industrial worker's salary amounts to just over 70% of the earlier net income. Parliament has approved a change in the pension system from the year 2000. The amount of ATP will be determined by an individual's contribution to the pension system during his or her working life. In addition there will also be a guaranteed minimum pension.

Sweden's smallest units of local government, the 288 municipalities, are responsible for the social services. Health care is run by the regional units of local government, the 23 county councils and the municipality of Gotland, which is not part of any county council area. The work of both the municipalities and the county councils is regulated by legislation.

In 1982, the new Social Services Act (Socialtjänstelagen) came into effect. This is a framework law (enabling act) which emphasises the right of the individual to receive social services, "if the needs cannot be met in any other way". A case manager employed in the municipality judges the individual's housing and care needs. The public services provided are based on this judgement. If the individual is not satisfied, an appeal can be raised in an administrative court. From the first of January 1998 this law has been extended and now stresses clearly that only people with appropriate education and experience are to carry out the work. It is also emphasised that the municipalities have to make arrangements to support informal caregivers and make relief and respite care available.

In 1983 the Health and Medical Services Act came into effect. According to this act, health care shall be available to everyone on equal terms.

The Swedish Government agency responsible for the supervision, evaluation and monitoring of social services, health care and medical services is called the National Board of Health and Welfare. The board's overall aim is to promote good health, social welfare and high quality care on equal terms for the entire population.

Sweden's municipalities and county councils have an unusually autonomous position within the state. The local politicians are directly elected at general elections. Both municipalities and county councils levy taxes. The laws on social services and on health care allow the municipalities and the county councils great freedom to plan and organise their own services and impose taxes in order to finance them. The autonomy of local government means that services for the elderly are prioritised and organised in different ways in different parts of the country.

In 1992 the "Ädel reform" gave the municipalities the overall responsibility to handle social care and health care for the elderly and disabled. The purpose of this reform was to create a better structure and make it possible to use the resources more efficiently thus making it easier to implement parliamentary decisions. The municipalities were also required to reimburse the county councils for the costs of providing continued short-term geriatric care to patients whose medical treatment had been completed, but for whom no municipal housing or institutional care had yet become available. This created a strong incentive for the municipalities to expand their own housing and care facilities for the elderly. The "Ädel reform" forced the municipalities to make health care available to residents of special housing and to visitors of adult day care units. The municipalities were also given responsibility for providing technical aids for the elderly. Each municipality was requested to appoint a nurse responsible for assuring the standards and quality of municipal health care. If a municipality and a county council agree, the municipality may take over all home nursing care within a municipality. Pilot programmes were also initiated to allow the municipality to operate the entire primary health care system. The experiences of these organisational changes varied significantly and some of the programmes have now been terminated.

Health and Social Care for Older People: Structures and Functions

In recent years it has become increasingly important to enable terminally ill or seriously disabled older people to remain at home. The development of both hospital-based home care for terminally ill patients and hospital-based home-rehabilitation for those who need help with rehabilitation at home has provided a way of vacating beds in institutions. The organisational changes with evident responsibility by the municipalities for patients whose medical treatment has been completed have been of even greater importance. The decline in the number of elderly people in institutions is an obvious result. Another is the increasing need for help for people living at home, especially during the evenings, nights and weekends. The benefits have been both human and financial but the strains on informal carers have become more and more evident. There is now the risk that financial interests are forcing this development to happen too quickly and too extensively.

Most elderly people in Sweden (92%) live in ordinary homes. The general standard of housing is high with centrally heated homes, well-equipped kitchens, hot and cold running water and in-door toilets. Nevertheless, the policy that as many elderly people as possible are to remain at home often requires ordinary dwellings to be adapted to special needs. The municipality therefore adapts homes to minimise obstacles to mobility such as stairs and thresholds. These services are heavily subsided or free. According to the Social Services Act, alternative forms of housing are to be made available to those who are not able to live at home. Since 1992 the municipalities have been responsible for all special types of housing. The most common of these are service houses, group dwellings for dementia patients, old people's homes and nursing homes. The assessment of group-dwellings for dementia patients has been favourable.

In December 1995 more than 135 000 people lived in special types of housing for the elderly. Only 3% of the 65-79 year-olds used this type of housing, whereas 25% of those over 80 and more than 50% of those older than 90 lived in special types of housing. In 1999 only 1% of the 65-74 year-olds but still more than 50% of those older than 90 lived in special types of housing..

The municipal social services are responsible for the home help services, which supply assistance with shopping, cleaning, cooking, washing and personal hygiene to those elderly who otherwise would not be able to manage. The fees charged for home help services vary from municipality to municipality. The charges are also dependent on the number of hours of help needed and income. There is a limit to the charge, which means that the individual is always able to keep approximately one third of his or her income. Help is also available during the evening, at night and during the weekend. Most municipalities provide night patrols including both nursing and home help staff. Over the last decade the total number of recipients of this type of care has dropped, but the total number of hours of home help has increased. This is a consequence of attempts to cut back and rationalise services and to offer the resources only to those who need it most. Twenty percent of those individuals over eighty living at home were in receipt of social services and/or home nursing services in 1995. Most of them were living alone (60%). Thirty percent had help every evening or night. This high figure results from a lot of people with high needs living at home. It is obvious that those with a considerable disability, living alone or without a family close by are given priority.

Other forms of service are often provided along with home help. Most municipalities offer alarm services, chiropody, hairdressing, food services, help with bathing, snow-clearing etc. A number of services are offered at day centres, which are either independent units in the community or incorporated in sheltered accommodation. Day centres function as meeting places where the elderly in the area can get together for meals or group activities. Initially all day centres were run by the municipalities. However, in some municipalities the elderly themselves or a voluntary organisation have taken over the running of the day centres.

Day care units have been established to take an active part in rehabilitation. These units are important also as a way of providing relief to informal caregivers.

Another form of day care has been established for cognitively impaired elderly people. Many senile people live at home and are looked after by their families, often constituting a heavy burden for the latter. The day care units for the senile can therefore play an important role in giving both supervision and care and at the same time allow the family some respite. In these units the number of patients at a single time is strictly limited and care is provided by carefully selected staff.

The special transport services (färdtjänst) have a vital function for the disabled who are unable to use ordinary public transport. Eligibility for this service is established according to a needs test, and charges vary from one municipality to another. In 1995 23% of all elderly received this kind of service. More than 50% of those older than 80 used the special transport service.

During the last twenty years the number of beds and the number of days of short-term care have fallen continuously. The table below shows the difference between the number of beds in long-term care between 1991 and 1992 (The 'Ädel reform'). At that time, responsibility for care was transferred to the municipalities and a large number of beds were transferred to nursing homes.

Table 3: The Number of Beds at Hospitals in Sweden (from the Federation of Swedish County Councils – 1998)

	Short term care	Long term care	Psychiatric care	Together
1985	38 689	51 521	20 906	113 411
1990	35 403	45 965	14 533	98 009
1991	33 943	45 091	12 960	93 679
1992	31 737	12 600	11 846	57 778
1994	28 171	6 284	9 797	45 837
1996	24 973	4 699	7 276	38 139
1997	23 801	3 740	6 267	34 885

The number of beds and the number of days of short-term care have fallen continuously. During the eighties the reasons were ideological, but in the nineties the efforts to cut down costs by minimising hospital care have become increasingly obvious. In the last five years almost four out of ten beds in hospitals have been cut. The result is that many patients remain at home thus relying on assistance from the family, other informal care-givers and volunteers. However, the proportion of days of care provided for the elderly in comparison with other age groups has increased. This is partially due to the increased number of elderly people, but also due to the advances in the field of geriatric medicine with larger numbers of older people benefitting from new forms of treatment.

A small proportion of special housing for the elderly is provided by private entrepreneurs (8% in 1995). Some of these are foundations or other non profit-making organisations. Recently more and more private alternatives have been used by the municipalities in order to encourage competition in the care of the elderly and to minimise the costs. The building of private sheltered accommodation to be run on a profit-making basis and sheltered housing owned and administered co-operatively are examples of the increased interest in alternatives to the public system. It is important to note, however, that even where services are supplied by private care organisations, their activities are still financed and supervised by the municipality.

Most elderly people living at home see the district doctor or nurse at a district health centre. Home visits to those who have mobility difficulties are carried out mainly by district nurses and assistant nurses. The home nursing services have expanded considerably since the mid-1970s. More than a threefold increase in the number of district nurses highlights this increase.

The National Board of Health and Welfare continuously evaluates the development of care for the elderly and disabled. Considerable efforts are made to identify those municipalities which have identified good ways of designing care for the elderly. These good examples are consequently made known to other municipalities.

In recent years some problems have been encountered. For example, there are some elderly people who do not visit a physician for financial reasons. There are also seriously disabled people living in special types of housing for the elderly who, although they are very frail, seldom meet a physician. There is concern that patients may not receive optimal treatment. Increasing fees for home services have also resulted in people not using this facility. This could be a problem for the future as it has been recognised that home service could have a preventative value especially for those who are isolated and would benefit from personal contact.

Another problem is medication for the elderly. Improved knowledge about factors such as dosage, frequency, duration of therapy and specific contraindications is extremely important. Moreover, there are risks if elderly people do not use their medications correctly. In addition there are difficulties in providing sufficient support to those who need it. In recent years fees paid directly by the patients have increased substantially. Some elderly people feel that they cannot afford the expense and instead prefer not to use any medication.

Due to shorter hospital stays, the needs of the frail elderly discharged from hospital are sometimes extensive. A lot of work has been done to improve the prerequisites of developing patient-centred processes and the exchange of information between the different caregivers. This is looked upon as important in every link of the care chain but an evident example is discharge from hospitals. When a patient with changed needs is about to be discharged from hospital a patient-focused meeting will take place, with representatives from primary care, the hospital and the municipality, the patient and his or her relatives. This meeting is endorsed by guidelines from the National Board of Health and Welfare, and enables everyone concerned to have an influence on the subsequent caring process at home. It is unfortunate that sometimes these meetings do not take place at all, or not all parties are invited to attend. Shortage of time and difficulties in prioritising these co-ordination meetings may lead to later problems. Any resulting consequences for the patients might have been prevented with better co-ordination and co-operation.

Roles of Family Carers of Older People living at Home

In Sweden the informal care provided by families and other volunteers is of great importance. Data suggest that if the home help services had to take over this informal, voluntary work they would have to more than double their staff. Lately it has been obvious that work carried out be the family has a tendency to increase, especially for those with family living close by. Many of them manage without any support from the help services. Home help resources are being channelled more and more to support those who live alone and who have greater needs. This implies that the work carried out by informal caregivers is the foundation of care-provision with the contribution from the public sector being merely complementary.

With increasing numbers of elderly people remaining at home it is obvious that in the future the informal caregivers will have to take on an even greater responsibility. In the late eighties the understanding of the important role played by informal caregivers grew rapidly. This process coincided with diminishing resources in hospital care. Now there is the fear that in future family members may have to take care of their relatives even if they do not want to or if they do not have the necessary prerequisites.

Several different voluntary organisations offer support and help to the elderly and their relatives. Examples are the Red Cross and the Association of the Demented. Studies show that the role of these organisations is comparable with that in other European countries, but in Sweden they do not provide hands-on personal care. Almost 50% of all pensioners in Sweden are members of pensioners' organisations. This is of great importance and has led to a direct influence on both national and local political decisions concerning the elderly.

It is perhaps partly because of the well-developed welfare system that the needs of family carers have only recently received attention. The physically demanding nature of caring is well recognised, while family caregivers often feel that professionals do not understand problems such as lack of private time and inability to maintain outside interests. The result is too little support. And only recently have the positive aspects of caring been given attention. An understanding of the dynamics of family caregiving is of course important if adequate services are to be developed.

Recently, the experiences of special patient groups have been used to improve both the caring process and the support of caregivers by allowing the patients to formulate their own and their carer's needs. Caregiver organisations have also co-operated to develop support for caregivers. For example, the Association for the Demented has played an important role both in the developmental process of caring for the demented and in the support given to caregivers.

Relatives who take care of their elderly family members can receive payment from the municipality on certain grounds. This, however, is a very small group. Moreover, it is a diminishing group, and it is obvious that the resources are limited, and there is a tendency for the municipalities to reduce their costs as much as possible. In 1982, 21 000 relatives received financial support, in 1995 the number was 7 000 and in 1997 there were 6 000. It is possible for the municipalities to employ relatives who have a considerable workload to do at home. Following this scheme 6 200 relatives were employed in 1994. However according to statistical information this number had fallen to 4000 one year later, and by 1997 the figure was 3 300. If a person has to take care of a seriously ill family member, there is also the possibility for the carer is to take time off work (care leave), with compensation from the social insurance system, for up to a total of 60 days per person.

As the importance of informal care grows, it is becoming increasingly evident that the support for caregivers must be improved. During 1997 the National Board of Health and Welfare distributed some money to projects to support informal caregivers. Publications have been produced to share information on the projects and the results. From 1998 it has been legislated that the municipalities have to provide support for informal caregivers and make relief and respite care available. The government has now suggested that over a three year period 100 million Swedish Krona a year are to be used to support the development of a better support system for informal care givers. Relief and respite care are looked upon as very essential but the possibility to benefit from such support differs a lot between various municipalities. An extension of the availability of relief and respite care within the care system will be extremely important for the functioning of informal family care in the future. Day care is also of great importance, but providing this kind of care from nine to four and from Mondays to Fridays is not appropriate in some situations.

In some municipalities informal caregivers are invited to participate in groups in order to get proper information, education and practical knowledge about caring. These groups enable discussions to take place with other people who sometimes perhaps have had similar experiences and this has been a great relief to many people. The groups can consist of carers of elderly with similar diagnosis, with relatives in a nursing home or other groups, with the task of caring as the common factor.

Caregivers have different ways of handling their caring. Some are adamant that society should not influence their caregiving process. Others want a lot of help. Many informal caregivers describe the positive aspects of caring. Although there may be periods of severe stress and trouble, they cannot even imagine giving up caring. But for those who do not have the ability, inclination or desire, this work could be very burdensome, leading to high dependence on support if they really were to manage. It is also difficult to assess what kind of support is best. Moreover, needs differ both from person to person and from one situation to another.

Providing the correct information to patients and caregivers makes an important contribution to the reduction of both the patients' and caregivers' stress. The hospital discharge "conference" provides the opportunity to share this information. Many informal caregivers feel that they make a significant contribution to enabling the cared-for person to remain at home. This is particularly satisfying to the caregiver especially when he/she is aware of the cared-for person's preference to remain at home. However, if the caring situation is too demanding for the caregiver and he/she would rather see the cared-for-person admitted to hospital there might be conflict of interests, which ultimately may lead to anxieties for the caregiver.

Assessment

At present there is insufficient knowledge about the support received by informal caregivers in Sweden. The research is primarily descriptive with hardly any research able to highlight the effects of any support given. Moreover, the aims of support to informal caregivers are not clearly specified.

Some studies have tried to describe what kind of caring the patients prefer. Only 20% prefer help from the family rather than help from society [1,2]. Another study shows that elderly people do not want to depend on help from their relatives under any circumstances [3]. It is difficult to explain these results, and is even more difficult to explain the contrast between the wishes of the elderly as shown in the studies and the growing demand for help from family caregivers.

A study focused on people living at home, using a questionnaire to a stratified selection of the population, shows that only 35% of people with needs have both informal and professional care-givers [4]. An interesting fact is that people who need personal help are given that primarily from a spouse. People who only need help in the home mostly have help from a child. According to this study, nurses are not very involved in the caregiving process. A follow up study is planned to better describe communication between the different caregivers. A study from 1996 evidently shows that home-help staff are not aware of which patients the nurses visit and vice versa [5].

There are obvious risks for the carers particularly if the perception prevails that the caregiving situation is becoming unmanageable, which may ultimately lead to feelings of guilt, shame, insufficiency, heavy burden, and a feeling of being bound and isolated [6-8].

The need for respite and relief care for the informal caregivers is obvious. Personal support in different ways is important. This support could also be combined with information and education in different ways [8].

The National Board of Health and Welfare supervises and evaluates the care of the elderly in Sweden. Recently the Board has tried to examine the situation of informal caregivers.

A report [9] suggests that new forms of support for informal caregivers must be developed and those already existing must be improved. The report also suggests that it is important to develop new ways within the public system for systematic ways of identifying those elderly people and their informal caregivers who have needs.

Judging from a national survey which set out to identify what support informal caregivers are given in the municipalities [10] there are only a few municipalities that have a systematic way of supporting the informal caregivers. Five per cent of the municipalities have decided on a plan for support. Fifteen per cent have written information about the support provided. In 40% of the municipalities work is being carried to develop support systems for informal caregivers. Forty per cent have selected a particular person responsible for this work with informal caregivers. Seventy-five per cent of the municipalities had processes to identify people with particular needs. The above study presents the findings of a survey on the support given, but no effort has been made to try to evaluate the quality of what has been done.

Informal caregivers of demented people have been identified as an important group with considerable needs [11]. This has led to numerous efforts and interesting results regarding the importance of day care, other forms of relief and respite care and group discussions and group activities with the caregivers.

Burden is described especially for carers of the demented [11]. Some studies have also shown the care giving process as a positive experience for the caregiver, giving meaning to their life [12]. In this study the caregivers are followed over a two year period. According to the author it was obvious that at the beginning of the study, caregivers were inclined to see caregiving more as a burden, but with repeated contacts it became more obvious that the positive aspects of care giving were being recognised.

In other studies submitted for publication, attention is focused on the gratification and meaningfulness of caring for the caregiver [13-16]. The author has used questionnaires validated in the UK and translated into Swedish (CamiCadiCasi), and describes sources of satisfaction for the caregiver. In another study, the same author has highlighted different behaviours associated with caring and suggested that professionals must be aware of, and seek to complement, carers' coping patterns. A subsequent study on support for family carers stresses that help with the physical aspects of caring is much better than support given to their social and emotional needs.

Case Studies

In Sweden there are a lot of different ways of helping the patient and supporting informal caregivers. But it is fundamental that the patient decides. Of course that means that the situation can totally change if the patient does not accept the suggested solution.

1. Older person living alone in an isolated farmhouse. Widowed. Little money. Daughter and son-in-law unemployed with four children, aged 9 months to 7 years, and live 5 kilometres away.
2. Older person lives alone on a ground floor flat in town. Widowed. Daughter and son-in-law are both teachers in full-time employment, with 2 children aged 7 and 11, and live within 1 kilometre in the same town.
3. Older person lives with spouse in 2-storey house. Retired with savings. Spouse is fit and well. No children. Bedroom, bathroom and toilet are upstairs.

Questions

For each of the nine combinations
1. What roles would the informal/family carer typically occupy in caring for the older person?
2. What services would typically be provided to support the older person?
3. How would the informal/family carer's needs typically be assessed (if at all), and What support if any could typically be provided for the carer?

Case 1

Female aged 76, with osteoarthritis of the hips and knees, poor vision due to macular degeneration and hypertension. Mobile with a frame within her home except for the stairs. Needs help with mobility outside, shopping, cooking and housework.

(*Social Circumstances A*) Older person living alone in an isolated farmhouse. Widowed. Little money. Daughter and son-in-law unemployed with four children, aged 9 months to 7 years, and live 5 kilometres away.

The female will be offered a consultation with a doctor. Perhaps there is a chance of improving her health by an operation, by medication or by rehabilitation. If this is not feasible she will be offered the opportunity of moving to another not so isolated flat without stairs.

If she decides to remain in her home, she will be offered appropriate alterations to her home. After a visit from a case manager from the municipality she will probably be offered transportation and home services. At the visit the case manager assesses mainly the needs of the old lady but probably the daughter also takes part in the meeting. The offers made may take into account what both parties have said. The woman herself decides how much help she wants.

Perhaps she will accept the help offered. In that case her relatives may assist with shopping and some other things in the home. But if the woman refuses the help offered, the situation will be quite different. The burden on the relatives will be much heavier and the family will have to take much greater responsibility. If the woman prefers not to have any help from the municipality, the family carer will probably not receive any support, unless she specifically asks for it.

(*Social Circumstances B*) Older person lives alone on a ground floor flat in town. Widowed. Daughter and son-in-law are both teachers in full-time employment, with 2 children aged 7 and 11, and live within 1 kilometre in the same town.

She probably will be offered an examination by a doctor. Perhaps there is a chance of improving her health by an operation, by medication or by rehabilitation. If not she will be offered appropriate adjustment of the home.

After a visit to her home from a case manager she probably also will be offered transportation and home services. At that visit the case manager assesses mainly the needs of the old lady but the daughter also takes part in the meeting. The proposals will be based on comments from both parties. The woman herself decides how much help she wants.

Perhaps she will accept the help offered. In that case her relatives may assist with shopping and some other things in the home. But if the female refuses any offers of help, the situation will be quite different. The burden on the relatives will be much heavier and the family will have to take much greater responsibility. In that case the family carer probably will not receive any support, unless they specifically ask for it.

(*Social Circumstances C*) Older person lives with spouse in 2-storey house. Retired with savings. Spouse is fit and well. No children. Bedroom, bathroom and toilet are upstairs.

Will be offered an examination by a doctor. Perhaps there is a chance of improving her health by an operation, by medication or by rehabilitation. If this is not possible discussions will be held regarding the wish to find and move to a one-storey house. If not she will be offered adjustments to the home.

A case manager will pay a visit to their home and talk to the old lady and her spouse. Perhaps they will come to a mutually beneficial agreement. In that case the old lady will be offered transportation services. The couple is offered further help in the future if needed. One month later the spouse phones the case manager. There are problems when he has to go shopping. His wife is very anxious when she is on her own. They discuss the possibility of the lady using the day care facilities one day a week between nine o'clock and four o'clock. This gives him the opportunity to do the shopping etc while his wife is not at home. He is offered more help if needed.

Case 2

Male, aged 80, facing discharge from hospital following a stroke. Expected to be confined to bed or chair for several weeks with gradual recovery of mobility. Needs the help of one person for transfers, toileting, bathing and dressing.

(*Social Circumstances A*) Older person living alone in an isolated farmhouse. Widowed. Little money. Daughter and son-in-law unemployed with four children, aged 9 months to 7 years, and live 5 kilometres away.

When it is decided that the patient should be discharged from hospital a conference will be held where a case-manager from the municipality, the hospital staff, the relatives and the patient discuss the options available. The man is offered the opportunity to move to a nursing home for a given period where he will receive help and rehabilitation. After a one month stay he will return home in a much better condition.

If he has not recovered enough he will perhaps be offered another period of rehabilitation or he will be offered the choice of different kinds of housing where suitable help can be provided. The daughter and her family are invited to take part in the discussions.

It is possible that the man will not accept the initial proposal but wants go home at once! In that case he will be offered some form of rehabilitation at home and a combination of social and care services night and day. He will also have an alarm installed. Even if he is offered a lot of help the stress on the relatives will be huge. Contact with the practitioners will be extremely important. Some form of assessment of the situation of the family caregivers will probably be carried out.

(*Social Circumstances B*) Older person lives alone in a ground floor flat in town. Widowed. Daughter and son-in-law are both teachers in full-time employment, with 2 children aged 7 and 11, and live within 1 kilometre in the same town.

When it is decided that the patient should be discharged from hospital it a conference will be held in which a case-manager from the municipality, the staff from hospital, the relatives and the patient discuss the future possibilities. The male is offered a place in a nursing home for a given period in order to receive help and rehabilitation. After having been in the nursing home for one month he needs as much help as a month ago.

After further discussions there are numerous possibilities. He can either stay for a few more months or choose between other kinds of housing where he can have the help he needs. Perhaps he chooses to move to an old people's home. The daughter and her family take part in the discussions about the future living arrangements and show him a number of different flats. The daughter's family helps with moving the belongings to the old people's home. The man is depressed and cannot cope with his dependency. The daughter visits daily but only stays for an hour and "there are twenty-three hours left" as her old father keeps saying. Like the old man, the daughter and her family are also quite unhappy.

After two months the daughter is invited to a meeting with the staff, other relatives and friends of the other persons living in the same housing to discuss their experiences. She feels comforted at being able to share her problems with somebody else and listen to other people's problems.

(*Social Circumstances C*) Older person lives with spouse in 2-storey house. Retired with savings. Spouse is fit and well. No children. Bedroom, bathroom and toilet are upstairs.

When it is decided that the patient should be discharged from hospital, there will be a consultation in which a case-manager from the municipality, the hospital staff, the spouse and the patient discuss the future possibilities. The man is offered the opportunity to move to a nursing home for a short period to receive help and rehabilitation. After having been there for one month he is better but still needs further help.

Before his discharge the house is adapted to take a lift to the first floor. He has received transportation services. Day care is arranged for three days a week for additional rehabilitation. At the same time the spouse has the opportunity to do something else and in that way feels a little relief.

A month later the spouse feels exhausted and cannot manage the situation at home any longer. She gets in touch with the case manager and asks for help. After discussion the situation they plan for a fortnight's institutional care within the nursing home. During this the case-manager has discussions with the spouse about the future need for support. They meet the patient afterwards and decide together how to continue.

Case 3

Female, aged 86, suffering from dementia. Frequent wandering by day and night. Frequent falls. Incontinent of urine and faeces.

(*Social Circumstances A*) Older person living alone in an isolated farmhouse. Widowed. Little money. Daughter and son-in-law unemployed with four children, aged 9 months to 7 years, and live 5 kilometres away.

The woman visits the general practitioner with her daughter. The daughter is very upset. She says: "we can't stand it any longer". The physician's judgement is unmistakable. This is a clear dementia. The municipal manager is contacted. If they are lucky, the following day the woman will be offered to live in a group dwelling for cognitively impaired persons. This housing will probably function well. But the family needs a lot of support of the staff. They particularly appreciate the meetings with relatives of other residents and the staff every second month. At these meetings they are given a lot of information about dementia and they have the opportunity to discuss with other relatives.

One day eight months later the daughter is very upset. She cannot recognise her mother any longer. She cannot sleep during the nights. One of the members of staff proposes that she contacts the Association of the Demented to get more information about the disease and to make contact with other relatives of demented persons. The woman makes contact and has in that way the opportunity to get a lot more information. After some weeks she is reassured. Later she will be very active herself to work for the association.

(*Social Circumstances B*) Older person lives alone on a ground floor flat in town. Widowed. Daughter and son-in-law are both teachers in full-time employment, with 2 children aged 7 and 11, and live within 1 kilometre in the same town.

The female will be offered housing in a group dwelling for cognitively impaired people. This arrangement will probably function well. Her daughter's family has the chance to visit her whenever they like and they can take a walk together with her to their own home whenever they like.

(*Social Circumstances C*) Older person lives with spouse in 2-storey house. Retired with savings. Spouse is fit and well. No children. Bedroom, bathroom and toilet are upstairs.

The municipality manager pays a visit. She has heard from the district nurse what a mess the home situation is. She wants to talk with to the husband. But it is impossible. The old lady follows them everywhere. The manager understands that it is impossible to talk at home. She instead tries to arrange a meeting in her office. But the spouse points out that it is impossible, since he can't leave the house. He never goes out without his wife. After some discussion they decide to accept help from the district nurse who is aware of the situation and is able to stay with the lady for an hour while he is talking to the manager.

Two days later they meet. The spouse is very tired but he can't even consider abandoning his wife. After some discussion everything is very clear. The spouse will go on taking care of his wife, but he needs some support. He needs information and someone to talk to (he is advised to get in touch with the Association of the Demented). He needs to have some time alone.

They decide to try day care for cognitively impaired people. A week later a man from the day care centre arrives and begins to talk to the couple. He wants to get to know as much as possible about the habits of the lady. He wants to get to know the husband too in order to be able to support him as much as possible.

A week later the lady is invited to the day care centre. She arrives with her husband who happily enough discovers that she seems to like being there. Some weeks later he is easy in his mind, the wife is in the day care unit twice a week from nine to four. He can visit her there but the most important thing is that he can do whatever he likes these two days. This makes it much easier for him to endure caring for her the rest of the time.

Future Developments

The tendency to decrease the number of beds in hospitals is expected to continue. This means that nursing outside hospitals, in the homes of the patients or in some casual living arrangements will increasingly become the norm. Further tests are needed in order to identify the best way of organising satisfactory care for the elderly efficiently and effectively. Different alternatives are already being tested. The main challenge is to find a way of optimising the co-ordination of care surrounding the patient. How can people in different organisations be encouraged to co-ordinate their efforts for maximum benefit to the patient? How can patient-focused care be best developed? A lot of research has still to be done.

Why should support to informal carers be prioritised in times of limited resources? There are both ethical and economical reasons. With increasing numbers of elderly people staying at home, it seems likely that families, other informal caregivers and volunteers will have to take greater responsibility in the future. If the support is not improved, a lot of problems are likely. Many informal caregivers describe the positive aspects of caring, but sometimes there will also be periods of stress and problems. In such periods it is especially important that the caregivers receive ample support to help them to continue providing care.

In the future, caregivers are likely to organise themselves into a stronger pressure group to have maximum influence on future developments in the caregiving process.

The National Board of Health and Welfare suggested in its report from 1997 that new forms of support to informal caregivers must be developed and those already existing must be improved. To succeed in that a lot of research has to be done, to highlight how important it is for public systems to develop new ways to of contacting representatives of the elderly and their informal caregivers .

With the January 1998 legislation requiring the municipalities to support informal caregivers, the future development of informal caregiving in Sweden will probably be influenced significantly. This law will be the basis for any future development. Moreover, the government has identified funds to stimulate projects on developing support for informal caregivers. The results of this research will be communicated to other municipalities to encourage their future participation.

Even if some clear caregiver needs have been identified, a lot of research still has to be done. The need to reduce the feeling of stress and burden is important. Different forms of support might help decrease levels of stress. So far three main forms of support have been identified, namely financial support, psychosocial support (networks, private discussions, discussion in groups) and practical support (relief and respite care), and ways must be found to improve the ways in which these supports can be made available.

There is insufficient knowledge regarding "best support". Moreover the aim of any support is not clearly specified. There are different ways of handling this problem but an interesting development is that some counties and municipalities have begun to organise special groups where caregivers and patients formulate their most important needs. This is a way of developing the health care provision but may also be used to identify the needs of the informal caregivers. The patients and the informal caregivers are given the opportunity to formulate their needs and suggest ways in which support can be given to caregivers. However, what needs to be borne in mind is the fact that the situation for each caregiver is unique and this makes it difficult both for the informal caregivers, the practitioners and "society" to find generally applicable solutions. The patients ask for more flexibility, they want to increase the influence of each individual and so do many informal caregivers. These ways of co-operation will probably be used more in the future in order to improve the situation for the elderly.

An extension of the availability of relief and respite care within the care system is an important prerequisite for the functioning of informal family care. The extension of day centres and adult day care units should also to some extent be seen as support for informal care. The experience of group dwellings for dementia patients has been favourable and the municipalities have expanded this kind of housing in recent years. Even more expansion is planned for the future. Day care units for those with cognitive impairment will also be expanded.

The care of the elderly in Sweden has to be improved. At present assessment of the care chain for the elderly is being carried out. But it is also necessary to identify what constitutes a care-team and a good and efficient working relationship. Developing co-operation between the different parties involved is a great challenge. Once this has been achieved, care of the elderly will improve, as will the situation of the informal caregivers.

A lot remains to be done to improve the situation for informal caregivers in Sweden, but a lot of prerequisites have been improved lately and this should make it possible to bring about important improvements within the next few years. The main challenge will be to co-ordinate all the good resources from public care and informal care and to individualise the care of each patient and support for each informal caregiver.

References

[1] E. Jeppson Grassman, Frivilligt socialt arbete. Kartläggning och kunskapsöversikt. SOU 1993:82.
[2] L. Andersson L and L. Johansson, Äldres behov av och inställning till hjälp och vård. *Socialstyrelsen, Ädelutvärderingen* **96** (1996) 6.
[3] T. Möller, Brukare och klienter i välfärdsstaten. Om missnöje och påverkansmöjligheter inom barn och äldreomsorg. Publica, 1996.
[4] Y. Hellström and I. Hallberg, Adults 75 years and Older living in their Own Homes and Depending on Help from Others. (not yet published).
[5] G. Olivius et al, Elderly Care Recipients in a Swedish Municipality living in their own Homes and being Cared for by their Families. Diseases, functional Health Status. *Health and Social Care in the Community*, (1996) 133-141.

[6] L. Johansson, Informal Care of dependent Elderly at Home – Some Swedish experiences. *Ageing and Society*, **11** (1991) 41-58.
[7] M. Grafström *et al*, Health and Social Consequences for Relatives of Demented and Non-demented Elderly: a Population-based Study. *Journal of Clinical Epidemiology*, **45** (1992) 861-870.
[8] L. Johansson *et al*, Familjen som vårdgivare till äldre och handikappade. Socialstyrelsen. *SoS-rapport* (1994) 22.
[9] National Board of Health and Welfare. Taking Care of the Elderly. Report, 1997.
[10] National Board of Health and Welfare. Taking Care of the Elderly. Report, 1998.
[11] M. Grafström, The experience of burden in the care of elderly persons with dementia. Stockholm: Karolinska Institutet, 1994.
[12] C. Sällström, Spouses Experiences of Living with a Partner with Alzheimers desease, 1994.
[13] U. Lund,. Perceptions of Difficulties and Support among Family Carers in Sweden, (submitted).
[14] U. Lund, Sources of Satisfaction among Family Carers in Sweden, (submitted).
[15] U. Lund, Coping Strategies among Family Carers in Sweden, (submitted).
[16] U. Lund, Supporting Family Carers in Sweden, (submitted).

Chapter 11

United Kingdom

(December 1999)

Kate Lothian
Research Assistant
University of Sheffield
Sheffield Institute for Studies on Ageing
Community Sciences Centre
Northern General Hospital
Herries Road
Sheffield S5 7AU
United Kingdom

Kevin McKee
Lecturer
University of Sheffield
Sheffield Institute for Studies on Ageing
Community Sciences Centre
Northern General Hospital
Herries Road
Sheffield S5 7AU
United Kingdom

Ian Philp
Professor of Health Care for Older People
University of Sheffield
Sheffield Institute for Studies on Ageing
Community Sciences Centre
Northern General Hospital
Herries Road
Sheffield S5 7AU
United Kingdom

Mike Nolan
Professor of Gerontological Nursing
University of Sheffield
Samuel Fox House
Northern General Hospital
Herries Road
Sheffield S5 7AU
United Kingdom

Introduction

Britain's ageing population

The United Kingdom, similar to many countries across Europe, is facing challenges posed by an ageing population. In 1994 there were over nine million people aged 65+ living in the UK. It is estimated that, with life expectancy increasing by around two years per decade [1], this figure will have increased to over fourteen million people by the year [2]

Although many individuals will feel healthy and fulfilled in their old age, it is acknowledged that at some point most older people will suffer health difficulties. The probability of suffering a physical impairment increases with age. Of those aged 85 and over, for example, 73% of men and 75% of women report at least one serious disability [1]. As a specific example, more than one-third of those over 65, and one-half of those over 80, are estimated to have a hearing impairment. Similarly, 75% of the 100,000 UK residents registered as blind are over 65 [3]. Other conditions common to the older population include mental frailty, incontinence, musculoskeletal failure, respiratory problems and cardiovascular weaknesses. Projecting current rates forward it is estimated that there will be between four and five million people aged 65 and over with chronic health problems such as these in the year 2025 [4].

The ability to cope with day-to-day activities such as personal hygiene and domestic chores is critical to the maintenance of an independent existence. Yet, the health difficulties common in an ageing population have obvious implications for the performance of these activities of daily living (ADLs). In a sample survey in 1996, for instance, 41% of those aged 65-74 and 52% of those aged 75 and over reported an illness that limited their lifestyle (compared with 22% of all age groups) [1]. As an example, Johnson [3] reports that an estimated 1.4 million people over 65 are unable to do their own shopping. Indeed, at least 15% of the elderly population are thought to be dependent on others for the performance of tasks that they would previously have performed independently. Although statutory authorities will provide support for some tasks, a great many tasks are supported by informal carers.

Britain's informal carers

The UK government reports that one adult in eight (13%) is providing care, indicating that there are about 5.7 million carers overall in Great Britain. Of these, 1.7 million (4%) devote at least 20 hours a week to caring and 0.9 million care for more than 50 hours a week [5].

Despite the realisation that "the great bulk of community care is provided by friends, family and neighbours" [6], informal carers have been largely undervalued. It is only in recent years, against a background of expansive academic research in the field of caring [7,8], that the government has announced "a shift in practice" towards greater recognition of carers and their opinions. Indeed, a recent Department of Health document reads, "The Government values carers and will support them in their caring role" [9]. Policy has been introduced with an aim to assessing and increasing the support available to users and carers, adopting an integrated family based approach and improving practice so that bureaucracy is minimised [10].

As evidence of their dedication to this shift in practice, the Prime Minister announced a *National Strategy for Carers* in June 1998. Policy builds on the earlier *Carers (Recognition and Services) Act 1995* and has three key approaches:

1) Information for carers	Providing wider and better sources of information about the help and services that are available to carers
2) Support for carers	Providing support via the communities in which carers live, in the planning and provision of services, and in the development of policies which will assist carers in combining employment with caring
3) Care for carers	Providing care that will help carers maintain their health, exercise, independence and will allow their role to be recognised by policymakers and the statutory services

The government does appear to be increasingly recognising the valuable role that informal carers play in the community. Altering the status of informal carers within society is, however, a major challenge. At present "the quality and type of support that carers receive remain a matter of chance" [11]. Governmental policy in this area is still young and will take time to be effectively implemented. Indeed, Banks [12] reports "a gap between policy to support carers and practice". In addition, limitations to recent Acts are already evident [13] and revisions may be necessary. Recent surveys of carers within the UK highlight that there is a great distance to go before carers feel that they are valued and supported in their roles [14,15].

Caring for carers

There are a variety of agencies within the UK that are responsible for the carer's, as well as the cared-for's, welfare. Primary among these is the National Health Service and the Department of Social Services. To a lesser extent, organisations within the voluntary and private sector also play a role.

Although policy is implemented at a national level through these statutory agencies, it should be noted that regional variations are evident. Particularly salient are the differences in services and support that carers in rural areas receive as compared to those living in urban regions. The Social Services Inspectorate, for example, acknowledges that those in rural areas suffer a paucity of service provision; higher costs in providing services, a lack of funding available to small rural voluntary organisations; and a lack of choice of services [16]. In response organisations such as the National Federation of Women's Institutes are calling upon the government and other relevant institutions to identify and provide for the needs of rural carers [17]. And indeed, efforts are being made to lessen the gap between rural and urban provision, such as introducing mobile day centres in North Herefordshire or establishing a home care co-operative for the rural communities of Nottinghamshire [18], but there is still much to do before consistency is achieved across the nation.

Legal responsibilities for care of older people

Legislation regarding the informal care of dependent older people is relatively scarce. Although various duties and responsibilities are imposed by statute upon professional or paid carers, informal carers are not legally obliged to either initiate or maintain their caring duties. For those who do 'volunteer', there are no rules in existence to dictate who can become an informal carer and what skills/resources they should possess. As a result, individuals are sometimes ill-equipped, at least initially, to cope with the demands of day-to-day caring. Subsequently, if not receiving an adequate level of care, the older person may suffer. In severe cases the law intervenes to protect vulnerable older people from maltreatment. Indeed, carers are liable for damages in respect of any assault upon the person cared for and, in serious cases, could be prosecuted if a criminal offence, such as neglect or mistreatment, has been committed [19].

For those who choose not to become an informal carer, decisions need to be made about whom will care for the dependent older person and where this care will be received. The social services authority, under the *NHS Community Care Act 1990*, will need to undertake an assessment of the needs of the older person. The assessment outcome will largely determine whether the older person remains in his/her own accommodation, supported by community services, or whether there is a need for residential or nursing care. If such care is deemed necessary, the authority, under the *National Assistance Act 1948*, has a duty to meet that need. The older person is able, in theory, to specify where they would like to live within the UK. In reality choice is restricted, with the authority deciding whether the 'preferred accommodation' is suitable and not too costly [20]. Those resident within accommodation provided by the authority will be charged a standard fee. Those unable to pay the standard rate will have a statutory test of resources applied and will be charged at a lower rate accordingly. Family members are not legally implicated in covering the costs of a dependant's accommodation fees. In some cases, however, spouses (who, according to the *National Assistance Act 1948*, are liable to maintain each other) may be requested to refund part or all of the local authority's expenditure on the residential accommodation [21].

Health care for older people

Health care services for older people living in the United Kingdom can be divided into those provided by the public, private and voluntary sectors.

The statutory sector

The United Kingdom's National Health Service (NHS) was established in 1948 to provide free comprehensive health care to all. Although the NHS is "constantly adapting to medical, social and political change" [22], its basic objective remains the same to this day.

The NHS is funded primarily through taxation and National Insurance contributions. Figure 1 depicts the basic structure of the NHS. Overall responsibility for the NHS lies with the Secretary of State for Health supported by the Department of Health. The Secretary of State sets the strategic direction for the NHS and answers to Parliament. Within the Department of Health is the NHS Executive, which implements the health policies laid down by the Secretary of State and manages the funding and the way the service operates. The NHS Executive aims to integrate health and social services policy to provide a fully comprehensive national service. NHS Executive Regional Offices were established to ensure that Primary Care Groups and Health Authorities work together to make proper arrangements for commissioning specialist health services at a regional level. Health Authorities are responsible for improving the health of their residents and overseeing the effectiveness of the NHS locally. Although local Health Authorities presently purchase health care for the local population, it is hoped that Primary Care Groups - comprising all GPs and community nurses in an area - will take over the responsibility for commissioning services for the local community. Once accomplished, Health Authorities will focus more on long-term Health Improvement Programmes - identifying the health needs of local people and specifying what needs to be done to meet them. Finally, almost all hospitals, community services and ambulance services run themselves as self-governing NHS Trusts. These too are planned to be party to the local Health Improvement Programmes allowing hospital clinicians to make a more significant contribution to service planning [23].

Figure 1: Current structure of the National Health Service

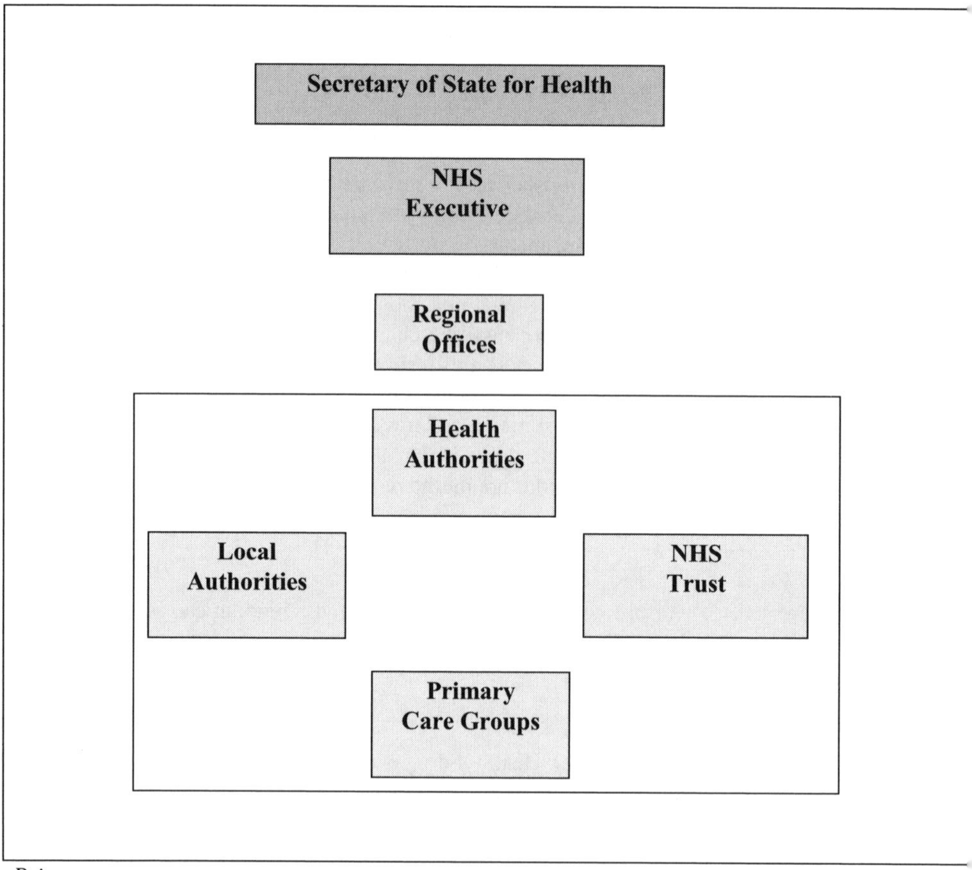

```
                    Secretary of State for Health
                              |
                         NHS Executive
                              |
                        Regional Offices
                              |
        ┌─────────────────────────────────────────────┐
        │              Health Authorities              │
        │                                              │
        │   Local Authorities          NHS Trust       │
        │                                              │
        │              Primary Care Groups             │
        └─────────────────────────────────────────────┘
```

Primary care

Access to the NHS system is predominantly through GPs who diagnose and treat many problems themselves or, where appropriate, make referrals to specialists and their services. In 1998 there were almost 30,000 GPs within the NHS, with the average patient list size being almost 1,900 patients [24].

Over 90% of older people are registered with a GP. As such, older patients absorb a great deal of GP time. Indeed, GPs are reported to have the highest professional contact rate with elderly people in the community [25]. Goddard and Savage [26] report that, in 1991, 57% of males and 55% of females aged 65 and over had utilised GP services in the three months prior to interview. Contact rates increase with age with percentages rising to 68% for males and 56% of females for those aged 85+. Annually it is estimated that approximately 75% of those aged 65 and over will visit their GP [4].

Such contact may take place in a variety of settings including the patient's own home. Indeed, it is reported that more than half of the contacts made with GPs take place in the patient's own home [27]. There is a clear trend for the number of older people receiving a home visit to increase with age. A 1996 survey found that 11% of people aged 65-74 and 27% of those aged 75 and over reported a home consultation in the previous two weeks [1].

The introduction of the GP contract [28], which came into force in April 1990, is likely to have increased the contact time between GPs and their older patients. The contract requires GPs to conduct an annual assessment of each patient on their list aged 75 and over. In return, the GP receives a monetary reward for every patient screened. (See *assessment* section). That said, the more recent introduction of *NHS Direct* and *NHS Direct On-line* is likely to have a reverse impact on GP consultation figures. *NHS Direct*, the health advice telephone service, took over 200,000 calls over the winter of 1999-2000. According to the Secretary of Sate for Health, "One third of callers were helped to care for themselves rather than having to go to the family doctor or the casualty department" [29]. Plans to provide pro-active care via such services are currently being revealed. For example, as well as taking calls, *NHS Direct* will soon be ringing out to remind at-risk groups, such as older people, to have an influenza vaccination or to check on the welfare of recently discharged patients.

Yet, many of today's older generation will not have the resources or confidence to access NHS phone, Internet and digital sites. Perhaps utilisation of these services by the older population will increase as today's younger, more technologically confident, generation grow old. Even then, it is unlikely that these remote health services will take over all of the duties performed by GPs. Indeed, it is probable that there will always be a role for GPs with regards to the health care of older people. GPs alone, however, are not equipped to deal with the multiplicity of medical and social problems that older people often present with. As such, the GP relies upon the support and expertise of a multidisciplinary NHS team. Service providers include geriatricians, psychiatrists, occupational therapists, physiotherapists and clinical psychologists. The majority of these specialists will be based within a hospital setting.

Hospital care

There are a variety of ways in which older people may access the acute hospital system: as an emergency, a GP referral, via an outpatient clinic or a waiting list. The majority enters as the result of an emergency or a medical referral [30]. Only 20% of admissions are via the waiting list [4].

Once admitted to acute hospital, the specialist seen will depend in part on the medical condition that the older person is presenting with and, in part, on regional variations in policy. Three principle models characterise the ways in which acute medical care can be shared between geriatricians and other medical professionals. In some regions/hospitals an integrated model is adopted whereby all physicians receive patients irrespective of age. An age-defined model, meanwhile, indicates that a patient's age determines whether they are admitted to a geriatric or a general medical ward. Finally, needs-based models refer to the allocation of patients on admission to either the specialist wards for older people or to general wards based on locally agreed criteria.

The average length of stay within hospital increases with age from approximately 9 days for a person aged 65-74 to around 16 days for someone aged 85+ [31]. According to the Department of Health [32], the average hospital stay for all patients, including older people, is decreasing. That said older people remain the main consumers of health care services, exerting greater demands as they age. As an illustration, of a sample surveyed in 1996, 24% of those aged 75 and over reported attending an outpatient or casualty department during the three months prior to interview, compared with 15% of all age groups [1]. Coni & Webster [33] state that "an elderly person costs the health service nine times as much as a young person". In 1995, for example, NHS expenditure per head was £703 for those aged 65-74, £1280 for those aged 75-84 and £2261 for those aged 85 and over.

Day hospitals

Day hospitals, usually located at district general hospital sites, allow provision of hospital-based services for patients living in the community who need further treatment and management. The operational policy of a particular day hospital will depend on local needs and arrangements. Flexibility is possible due to the availability of a multidisciplinary team including nursing staff, occupational therapists, physiotherapists and social workers, along with the input of other professionals including dieticians, speech therapists, chiropodists, dentists and continence advisors. The wide-ranging scope of care provided by day hospitals has been neatly summarised [34]:

- Provision of assessment & treatment for those who are not acutely ill and do not require in-patient supervision, especially for disabling conditions requiring rehabilitation.
- Provision of facilities for those requiring special procedures and investigations who may be too frail to attend a conventional out-patient clinic.
- Provision of supervision after discharge from hospital for those requiring further physical therapeutic or nursing care.
- To serve as a half-way house between hospital and home, providing reassurance to carers, relatives and patients in those cases when anxiety about the discharge exists (this is applicable to a minority of patients).
- Provision of a sufficient level of care to allow continued residence in the community for frail, old patients who might otherwise have to enter some form of residential care.

Traditionally the emphasis of day hospitals was, and to a large extent remains, on rehabilitative care. Yet contemporary day hospitals have developed to provide a wide variety of patient care ranging from specialist clinics, for example for Parkinson's disease, osteoporosis and memory difficulties, to endoscopy and blood transfusion [35]. Indeed, Reynolds & Allen [34] comment that "The value of day hospitals should not be underestimated". This is particularly true with regards to the health care of older people where day hospitals represent "a unique and important facet in health care" [36].

That said, recent research and reviews have critically scrutinised the cost-effectiveness of day hospitals. Indeed, a number of hospitals have been forced to close down as a result [35]. Yet, many believe that day hospitals fulfil an important role in the health care system and that they will survive so long as they address voiced concerns and demonstrate that they have a cost-effective niche in the delivery of health care.

Psychiatric hospitals

In addition to acute and day hospitals, older people represent a large proportion of the total number of patients resident in psychiatric hospitals and visiting psychiatric day hospitals. The likelihood of being admitted to a psychiatric institution is a third greater for females than males and tends to increase progressively with age [4]. Recognising this fact, there has been a rapid expansion of old age mental illness services in recent years. As an illustration, approximately 917 (12%) of the 7722 psychiatrists practising in the UK now specialise in Old Age Psychiatry [37]. With this in mind it is perhaps surprising that disorders common to older people, such as depression, often remain undetected and untreated [38,39].

Community care

Following discharge from acute hospital older people are often in need of follow up, continued care and rehabilitation programmes. "For the last thirty years or so it has been government policy that, wherever possible, sick and disabled people should be cared for in the community rather than in institutions" [5]. There is an increasing awareness of the value of community care in maintaining older patients within their own homes despite frailty or disability. Indeed, Bauer [40] writes, "Without a balance of effective and supportive community services many more people would become institutionalised". The value of community care was further emphasised with the publication of the White Paper *Caring for people* in 1989. The Paper, based on the Griffiths Review [41], adopts the assumption that community care is the best form of care available for most people. Victor [4] neatly summarises the proposed objectives:

1. To enable people to live as normal a life as possible in their own homes or in a homely environment in the community.
2. To provide the right amount of care and support to enable people to achieve maximum independence.
3. To provide people with greater say in how they live their lives and the services they need.

Informal carers such as husbands, wives, friends, relatives and neighbours undertake much care in the community. Professional care regimes, however, are often overseen by community health workers such as district nurses, health visitors, psychiatric nurses and community remedial therapists. Contact is made in a variety of settings including patient's own homes and community drop-in centres.

District nurses are funded by the District Health Authority (DHA) and are often based at a GP practice or District Health Authority health clinic. They provide a variety of services including hands-on-nursing; treatments such as injections, enemas and dressings; specialist care (e.g. stoma management and continence advice); and liaise with other services as appropriate. According to Coni & Webster [33] the elderly represent about 80% of the workload of district nurses. Once again, contact time increases with age. As an example, 2% of those aged 65-69 are in receipt of district nursing health care compared with about 15% of those aged 85 and over [26].

The community psychiatric nurse plays a similar role to that of the district nurse. Coni & Webster [33] comment that this is a small but expanding group in the field of community care. Community psychiatric nurses play an important role in supporting patients and their carers, monitoring progress or deterioration, and liaising with other services.

The work of both district and psychiatric nurses is complemented by that of the health visitor, who fulfils important duties in identifying needs, advising, counselling, educating and contacting other health and social service providers. It is estimated that 15% of health visitors' time is devoted to care of the elderly [33]. That said, health visitor contact with this age group appears to be declining. This is probably due to the training offered to health visitors which is largely focused around the health care of young children. Denham [42] comments that this issue should be tackled: "Given the proven effectiveness of health visitors working with older people, it might be appropriate to strengthen their training in this area".

Additional community health care support is provided by a number of professionals including physiotherapists, occupational therapists, chiropodists, podiatrists etc. In theory a comprehensive community health service is provided by the statutory sector. In reality there are flaws and limitations to the system. For example, there is general agreement in the literature that current levels of hospital and community chiropody/podiatry services for older people are inadequate [43-45].

It should also be noted that regional variations exist in the availability of community personnel and resources. Of significance is the contrast between services available to those living in urban areas and those living in more rural localities. According to Department of Health data [16] over 80% of rural parishes are without community health services such as a GP practice, a chiropodist, a dentist and an optician within their boundaries. Considering that only 51% of older households own a car, and that public transport is often scarce in rural areas or difficult for older people to use [46], these figures have obvious implications for older people's health and well-being. In response the government has recently proposed "to renew the NHS as a genuinely national service. Patients will get fair access to consistently high quality, prompt and accessible services right across the country" [23]. Improved service provision will either be obtained via increased availability of resources or improved access to facilities further afield. As an illustration, one English city, Durham, provides specialist day care in residential homes near to where service users live to avoid the need for longer journeys.

Residential care

Despite the increasing emphasis on maintaining older individuals in their own homes via community care, there is sometimes a need for the elderly to be placed in residential care. Residential homes provide regular, ongoing supervision and assistance for older people who are no longer physically or mentally competent.

The average age of residents within long-stay homes is around 82 to 83 years and appears to be rising [47]. Indeed, commenting on the age-related institutionalisation rate, Hall et al [48] report that half of all individuals over 95 years of age are in residential care at any one time. And, because longevity favours females, there are more women resident in long-stay homes than men.

Although residential care is increasingly being provided by the private sector, a large proportion remains the responsibility of the statutory sector. The Royal Commission on Long Term Care [49] estimates that 205,000 older people in the UK receive publicly financed residential care. With the average annual cost of residential homes being £12,844 (and £17, 524 for nursing homes), the expenses to be met by the local authority are not to be underestimated. Indeed, in 1995 statutory residential care is believed to have cost local social services close to £2,000 million. To assist in covering these costs, many of those accommodated in local authority residential care homes are obliged to pay means-tested charges towards their living expenses.

The private sector

The private sector of health care provision is by no means comprehensive or evenly distributed throughout the UK [47]. Private facilities do, however, allow those with sufficient resources to avoid the worst aspects - such as extensive waiting lists and busy wards - of the state system.

Although by no means as extensive as that in the statutory sector, private health care provision does appear to be on the increase. Laing [50], for example, reports that 11% of the UK population was covered by private health insurance in 1995 compared with just 4% in 1979. Similarly, the Laing Review [50] estimated that private hospital-based health care increased from 7.5% in 1984 to 20% in 1995. Between 1981 and 1993 independent hospitals noted a 58% increase in the number of in-patients treated and a 440% increase in the number of day cases [51-53]. Whether the private sector's dramatic increase will continue into the new millennium is uncertain. Baggott [54], considering the limitations of independent provision, writes, "It may well be that the private sector is nearing the limits of its expansion".

When older people utilise private health resources, it is generally in the form of continuing care. Indeed, Baggott [54] writes, "private sector provision is extensive in the long-term care of the elderly". Sinclair et al [47] report a 220% increase in the number of places in private residential homes in England and Wales between 1976 and 1986. Similarly, the Griffiths report on community care, presented to the government in 1988, draws attention to the fact the private sector contributes largely in the field of residential care [41]. Coni & Webster [33] report that 35% of residential home places were provided by the private sector in 1994; a threefold increase from figures in 1983. These increases can, in part be explained by recent changes in social security policy which widened the availability of board and lodging allowances [55]. That said, only half of the residents in the private sector are supported by social security payments. Sinclair et al [47] suggest that the social security alterations simply acted as a catalyst for further change in this area.

Salient among recent changes is the increasing number of older people possessing private health insurance. Traditionally, insurance contracts were designed only to cover short-term acute conditions and, as such, were not always appropriate for older individuals. An increasing number of companies, however, are now offering Long-Term Care Insurance (LTCI). Indeed, the Association of British Insurers estimates that there are now some 23,000 LTCI policies in force across the UK [49]. That said, with 10% of applicants being rejected on medical grounds, and the remainder being faced with high premiums, only a relatively small proportion of those aged 65 and over possess private health insurance [4]. As the Secretary of State for Health commented, "Elderly people are precisely those who need health care most but can afford private health insurance least" [29]. Thus, the majority of older people must rely on the public sector for health care provision.

The voluntary sector

The government reports that there are many thousands of voluntary organisations involved in health care that operate at a variety of levels [56]. A simple distinction can be made between formal and semi-formal voluntary organisations. The former are large, have a relatively substantial income, cover a large area, employ paid staff and have regular links with professionals in the statutory sector. This type of organisation is more likely to have projects running at a national level. Semi-formal voluntary organisations, meanwhile, are smaller, have little income and are more likely to focus on voluntary projects at a more local level.

Organisations that operate at a national level often play an important lobbying and policy development role. The Centre for Policy on Ageing, for example, is a charity established in 1947 to "formulate and promote... policies which will allow older people to achieve their full potential in later years" [57]. Other organisations involved in campaigning for health and social issues related to older people include Age Concern and Help the Aged. A similar lobbying role is undertaken on behalf of carers by voluntary organisations such as the Carers National Association. In addition, umbrella organisations such as the National Council for Voluntary Organisations (NCVO) provide a collective voice for lobbying issues key to its numerous member organisations.

The smaller, more locally based, voluntary organisations provide important health and social care services. Services provided by such organisations may substitute, complement or support those offered by the statutory sector. These may include hospice care, self-help groups, information services, advice centres and health research facilities. A number of health related initiatives have been nurtured by these sort of voluntary agencies. The Beth Johnson Foundation, for example, have established a Peer Health Counselling scheme whereby older volunteers offer health advice and support to older people. The Foundation report beneficial results in the field of health promotion amongst recipients of the service [58].

Much of the funding for such voluntary organisations is acquired through a variety of fundraising efforts. As well as encouraging individual donations, many organisations raise money through organising events and establishing fundraising services. Help the Aged, for example, have 378 high street shops selling donated goods [59]. In addition grants may be available from local authorities, health authorities/boards and charitable trusts. Indeed, Baggott [54] reports that "currently over £50 million is allocated to voluntary bodies in the field of health and personal social services, most funded by the Department of Health". As well as offering funding, the government also plays a role in regulating the activities of voluntary organisations. Following recent publication of the document *Regulating Private and Voluntary Healthcare* the government plans to introduce the Care Standards Bill. The bill is designed to regulate private and voluntary healthcare and social care services in much of the United Kingdom.

Health and Social Care for Older People: Structures and Functions

The statutory sector

Department of social services

In the UK the primary provider of social services to older people within the public sector is the Department of Social Services (or Department of Social Work in Scotland). Although there is variation across the four countries, the UK's Social Services tend to be run by the county/city/metropolitan borough council. Heading up the department is the Director of Social Services who oversees councillors and council officers.

When considering what help the Social Services Departments may offer, it should be highlighted that very little is enshrined in law. Under the 1990 NHS and Community Care Act, an individual has the right to ask for an assessment for community care services. Councils can, however, refuse assessment if they feel services are unnecessary [60] or that they are not obligated to provide for the individual [61]. If viewed as appropriate, an initial assessment is usually conducted by a social worker at the individual's home. A straightforward decision regarding an individual's needs is often made promptly. More complex needs, however, tend to be assessed by a care manager who will draw up a care plan.

Although charges are not made for an initial assessment, councils may ask for a contribution towards services offered. Regional variations exist: some councils ask for a flat rate contribution for services whilst others means-test individuals and ask them to pay according to their income. Others may not charge at all.

Once assessed there are a variety of services that the Social Services Department can provide. These may be provided directly by departments themselves or, as is increasingly becoming the case, by private and voluntary organisations that are contracted to provide on their behalf. Services offered may include environmental adaptations, home maintenance, housekeeping, food provision (Meals-on-Wheels and luncheon clubs), personal care, transport provision, day centres, recreational services, security checks and relief periods for carers of the older person. Needless to say, the assortment of services offered to older people is costly for the Department of Social Services. In 1996, for example, almost half of English local authority personal social services expenditure, 49% (£4070 million), was spent on services for older people. This compared with 8% for other adults and 24% for children [62].

Day care

Day care centres and hospitals were only introduced on any scale in the 1960s and 70s. Since then there has been a rapid growth in their availability and utilisation. At present approximately 5% of the elderly population attend day care centres around the country [33]. Although the private sector offers a proportion of the day care available, the majority is provided by the statutory sector. Regional variations exist but it is estimated that about 260,000 older people are currently in receipt of day care services, with current public spending on day care estimated at £360 million [49].

Social workers are the main bodies referring older people to local authority day centres. The centres themselves fulfil a number of roles such as offering meals, activities and social relationships, disseminating health education and advice, and providing a base for community and visiting professionals ranging from health care workers to hairdressers. In providing these facilities, day care centres allow carers a break from their caring duties.

Short-stay care

Alongside day care provision, local authorities organise a number of short-stay care services. Such services allow older people to stay for a limited period, either on a one-off or a rotational basis, in a local authority residential home. Generally homes catering for permanent residents are utilised. A number of short-stay breaks, however, are organised in specialist homes/units. Overall the provision of short-stay care is on the increase. Indeed, the government reports that there are now more short-stay than long-stay [63].

Short-stay care is seen as having a number of functions. As well as providing the older person with a holiday/rehabilitative break, it is often employed to aid in emergency situations or to prepare/assess an older person for entry into long-term care. Furthermore, the benefits are not limited to the older individual. One of the primary purposes of short-stay care is to provide relief for carers. Indeed, the government's *National Strategy for Carers* highlights relief for carers as one of the main issues to be dealt with and has allocated £140 million to be spent on carer breaks over the next three years.

The private sector

The private sector's contribution to the social care of older people is essentially encapsulated in domestic help and care. Sinclair et al [47] write that, in terms of its scale, the private sector of domestic help for older people is as important as the public home help service. This being the case, social service departments are gradually realising the benefits of adopting "a mixed economy of care" [64] whereby the statutory and independent sectors work together to provide the local community with the necessary services. To encourage social service departments to engage in such activity, a substantial proportion of the special transitional grant was restricted for provision of services in the independent sector. A report by the Audit Commission, which oversees the external audit of local authorities and the

NHS, comments that "the independent sector is a major player and it must be integrated effectively with the care system" [64].

The Voluntary Sector

Sinclair et al [47], report a lack of clear specification of the proper role and actual contribution of the voluntary sector in relation to the care of the elderly. That said, it is evident that voluntary services play a valuable role in the social care of older people and their carers. This is achieved via a number of services which may include providing practical help; offering reassurance, companionship and social relationships; giving advice/information; and campaigning on behalf of service users. Help the Aged, as an illustration, offer a variety of services which include a telephone advice line providing welfare rights advice to older people and their carers, a door to door transport facility for frail older people, a 'handyvan scheme' installing smoke alarms and locks, information distribution, and home help services. In addition, Help the Aged campaigns for improvements in social and health issues related to older people. Current campaigns include a call to prevent older people dying needlessly of cold related diseases in winter, and a programme enabling older people to advise technology manufacturers on how new developments can improve their quality of life [59]. Similar services, activities and campaigns are organised by voluntary agencies across the United Kingdom.

Such services may substitute, complement or support the social care services offered by the statutory sector. As an example, meals on wheels are generally provided by local authority social services but tend to be delivered by volunteers.

Roles of Family Carers of Older People Living at Home

According to the 1995 General Household Survey one adult in eight (13%) in the UK is providing informal care and one in six households (17%) contains a carer. Around 4% (1.7 million) of these adults care for someone in their own household whilst 8% (3.7 million) look after individuals living elsewhere [5].

Who is caring for whom?

There appears to be very little data relating solely to carers of older people in the UK. General data, however, allows insight into the generic characteristics of carers.

It would appear that females are more likely to adopt, or have imposed upon them, the caring role than males. The 1995 General Household survey found that 3.3 million women were informal carers compared with 2.4 million men. Among these carers, the peak age for caring has been found to be 45-64 [5,14]. The duration of care is often lengthy with 24% of carers having cared for their dependent for at least ten years and 23% having cared for between five and nine years [5].

As to who is being cared for, a survey of 1,346 carers who were caring for eight hours or more every day revealed that 50% were caring for partners, 24% for parents or parents-in-law, and 22% for children with special needs [14]. Focusing more on older adults, over half of all those being cared for are people aged 75 years and over [1]. Those between the ages of 45 and 74 are most likely to be cared for by a spouse/partner. Those aged 75 to 84 are equally likely to be cared for by an adult son or daughter as a spouse/partner. Meanwhile, those aged 85 and over are much more likely to be cared for by an adult child [14].

A substantial minority (18%) of carers report having to look after more than one individual. Coupled with this, over a third reported that no one else helped them look after their dependants [5].

The data available also provides insight into the type of duties that UK carers carry out. Of those carers with dependants living in the same household, just under 60% help with personal care; around 60% provide physical help; just under 70% provide practical help and nearly 80% provide general supervision. Carers of dependants in other households were much less likely to provide personal care [5].

Becoming a carer

The literature indicates that, more often than not, carers find themselves assuming the caring role without having made a conscious decision to do so: "...it is wrong to assume that informal carers have chosen this role....often they are *involuntary* carers" [19]. In the survey of 1,346 carers, 70% of those aged 16-64 reported not being asked if they could cope before an individual was discharged from hospital into their care at home. Similarly, only 9% of individuals within this sample mentioned receiving any form of training [14].

The literature suggests that carers generally feel ill-informed. Nolan et al [65] write, "Family carers...are lucky to receive even basic information or advice when they take on their role". This opinion is supported by surveys of carers who voice dissatisfaction at the lack of information they receive regarding, for example, the dependant's medication [15]. Similarly, Taraborrelli [66] writes of many carers' initial ignorance of the task at hand.

Recognising these issues the government's *Carer's National Strategy* gives carers a right to choose to care or not and, if they select the former, to be adequately prepared to adopt the caring role [9]. The intention is to provide carers with up-to-date information, training and adequate support throughout the period in which they adopt caring duties. Although commendable on paper, in practice such training and support has been introduced in a rather ad hoc manner with no definitive training/support protocols in existence.

Financial support for carers

It is estimated that informal carers save the Government £34 billion every year [14]. In return they are eligible, providing they are under retirement age and caring for more than 35 hours a week, for the Invalid Care Allowance of £38.70 per week. There are currently 373,000 recipients of Invalid Care Allowance [67], costing the government £800 million a year. Although this figure may appear large, for those caring for 20 hours a week this works out at under £2 an hour - considerably less than the minimum wage. This knowledge should be coupled with the fact that substantial expenditure may arise from regular caregiving. Items such as unprescribed medicines, incontinence aids, special diets and mobility/transport provision, as well as additional wear and tear on household appliances (such as washing machines/dryers), often prove costly. Furthermore, a great many carers must forsake a full-time career to allow time and energy for their caring roles. As such many suffer a major loss of earnings [68]. Thus, the Invalid Care Allowance clearly offers only a very limited contribution towards the costs of informal caring.

That said, the government is currently consulting on proposals which, according to the *National Strategy for Carers*, could mean that, by 2050, carers receive an extra £50 a week in today's terms. In addition a Carers Special Grant of £140 million is being made available over the next three years to allow carers to take breaks from their caring duties [9]. This is certainly a step in the right direction for carers, many of whom consider short-term breaks to be one of their key priorities, and yet local authorities have already reported that the

Carers Special Grant will only go a short way to meeting local demand for short-term break services [69]. Clearly more funding is necessary if the needs of all carers are to be met.

The impact of caring on carer's health and well-being

Data available suggests that caring takes its toll on carers' health and well-being. Figures collected by the Carers National Association, presented in Table 1, are alarming [15]. Much literature is available supporting the notion that caregiving is often detrimental to an individual's health. Haug et al [70] conducted a longitudinal study of 121 caregivers of the elderly. They write, "Both the physical and mental health of the caregivers declined significantly during the study". According to the General Household Survey, the average person consults their GP five times per year, yet one survey found that 16% of carers had visited their GP 6-10 times and 10% more than ten times in the last year [15].

Table 1: Impact of caring on carers' health, by age

Age of Carer	Carers physically injured as a result of caring	Carers treated for stress-related illness since being a carer
Up to 24	57%	88%
25-34	61%	57%
35-44	55%	66%
45-54	58%	60%
55-64	51%	53%
65-74	46%	47%
75-84	39%	40%
85+	46%	36%
Total	51%	52%

Assessment

Assessment of the caregiver

It is only in recent years that authorities have recognised the existence of informal caregivers and acknowledged their vital importance. Coupled with this awareness came the knowledge that caring can be a gruelling task, resulting in a multitude of needs which have to be met if carers are to remain sound in body and mind. In recognition of this fact, the government devised the *Carers (Recognition and Services) Act 1995*. The main feature of the Act is to commission social services departments with a statutory duty to assess carer's ability to care and their needs. The Department of Health suggests that a carer's assessment might cover the following:
- their perception of the situation
- the nature of their relationship with the user
- the tasks undertaken and consequent impact
- tasks carers would like help with
- their social contacts and support received from family, friends and neighbours
- their emotional, mental and physical health
- their willingness and/or ability to continue to provide care; options available to the carer, particularly carers who are in employment

- their understanding of the illness or disability of the patient, and its likely/possible development
- other responsibilities e.g. work, education, family/child care commitments
- carers' strengths and ways of coping
- any particular stress factors and/or aspects of the caring task which the carer finds particularly difficult

The Carers Act, which came into force in April 1996, is clearly an effort to enforce the government's assertion that "statutory service providers should do all they can to assist and support carers" [63]. Certainly, it "provides a sound platform on which to build" [13]. However, limitations of the legislation exist and should be recognised.

A key flaw of the Carers Act is that it is simply not being sufficiently enforced. Evidence suggests that many carers are not being offered an assessment nor do they know that they have a right to ask for one [11,15,71]. Secondly, assessment eligibility criteria are unclear [72]. The Act targets those who "provide a substantial amount of care on a regular basis". The terms "substantial" and "regular" are, however, undefined and, as such, are open to local interpretation. Indeed, Banks [12] reports evidence suggesting that, as financial resources are stretched, eligibility criteria become increasingly stringent. Thirdly, those assessments that are undertaken remain strongly focused on the cared-for with carer's needs being marginalised [12]. Indeed, Nolan et al [13] point out that carers are very rarely afforded an assessment independent of the cared-for person. Fourthly, assumptions are made about an individual's capacity and willingness to care. Carers from ethnic minorities in particular frequently experience a stereotypical expectation that their communities will support them [12]. Finally, no demand is made for the utilisation of a standardised assessment tool. As such, there is inconsistency in the methods adopted to measure carer needs [73]. In addition, assessments are likely to focus on the objective components of caring, such as physical demands, which may tell us relatively little about the degree of stress that a carer is experiencing [74]. Furthermore, Nolan et al [13] point out that all too often assessments focus on the negative aspects of informal caregiving to the detriment of "the neglected dimension": satisfactions of caring.

In recognition of these limitations the government launched the Carers National Project in 1998, which resulted in the, previously mentioned, *Carers National Strategy* being introduced in early 1999 [9]. The Prime Minister labels it "a decisive change from what has gone before", allowing carers to choose whether or not they wish to care; preparing them for the caring role; providing them with adequate support; and enabling them to care without detriment to their health or inclusion in society. With regards to carer assessments, the Paper recognises that the implementation of the Carers Act is somewhat "patchy" but that, when assessments are undertaken, "carers report satisfaction both with the process and with the results" [9]. It is stated that carers are entitled to expect at least an annual discussion of their needs, the resources available, the help they receive and the care provided. Nothing is said, however, about the manner in which this information is to be collected.

Assessment tools intended to measure carers' needs are in existence. Included among them are the Burden Interview [75], the Caregiver Strain Instrument [76], the Caregiver Appraisal Measure [77], the Carers of Older People in Europe (COPE) Index [78] and the Caregiver Hassles Scale [79]. Of course, concerns regarding tick boxes and one-off "hit and run" assessments [80] need to be considered. As to who should conduct the assessment, social services staff are legally obliged to do so. Governmental papers point out that, in addition, local health professionals should be aware of the carer's health needs [9]. It is not made clear which of the health professionals should be responsible for this task. Wright

[81] suggests that practice and district nurses are in a good position to assess the informal carer because of their familiarity with the role of individual family members. In addition, the *Carers National Strategy* notes that housing authorities may also need to assess the carer's circumstances [9]. Once again, when, where or how is not specified.

Clearly, headway is being made towards a statutory, comprehensive assessment of carers within the UK. Indeed, the *Carers (Recognition and Services) Act 1995* and *the Carers National Strategy* lay strong foundations. Yet, obvious limitations exist. Steps need to be taken to ensure that comprehensive, preferably standardised, assessments of informal carers are regularly undertaken by specified, skilled staff. Carers need to know that they have a right to such an assessment, independent of the individual for whom they care. Information gleaned from assessments needs to be processed and shared wisely so that appropriate resources may be supplied and care pathways adopted. It is hoped that, as the *Carers' National Strategy* is implemented and developed, these issues will be adequately tackled giving rise to an effective and comprehensive assessment of family carers.

Assessment of the older person

The government's 1990 contract for general practitioners [28] requires them to offer an annual assessment to patients aged 75 and over. The assessment, usually carried out by the GP or a practice nurse, should consider the older individual's functional needs, mental state and social circumstances together with reviews of medication, incontinence and sensory impairment [82].

Many studies have supported the concept of an annual health check for older people. They appear to be useful in detecting previously unreported problems [83]. Brown et al [84], for example, found that new problems were discovered in 43% of patients seen in Nottinghamshire. In addition, Chew et al [85] report that the majority of doctors and nurses regard routine assessments of the elderly as worthwhile. Similarly, older people themselves have been found to hold generally positive views of the assessment [86].

Despite these findings, the value of these annual assessments for all older people has been called into question [87,88]. An explanation is offered by Fletcher [89] who writes, "The UK health policy of regular assessment of people aged 75 and above to be carried out by general practice has been implemented haphazardly with little guidance on appropriate methods and levels of assessment". Indeed, considerable variations exist in the nature of checks undertaken due to a lack of standardisation.

Proposals have been made to initiate a standardised approach to enhance the efficacy of the annual health checks [90]. Indeed, the need for regular standardised and comprehensive assessments is among the guidelines set out in the Department of Health's National Service Framework for Older People, due for publication towards the end of 2000. Employing a standardised assessment instrument is just one method that is being considered in a bid to improve the overall efficacy of the assessments. Philp et al [91] for example, have designed a brief instrument "for rapid assessment of an older person's physical, mental and social well-being" which focuses on quality of life, and recognises the role of family carers. Although quick to administer, the instrument will highlight areas in need of further investigation in an individual's life. Other examples, although often more lengthy, include the Barthel Index [92], the Camberwell Assessment of Need for the Elderly [93] and the Duke OARS [94]. It is hoped that, in an effort to minimise inconsistencies, standardised and validated assessment instruments such as these will be introduced on a large scale across the UK.

Of course, it is important to consider who administers such assessment instruments and in which setting. Recognising that a tool's effectiveness may well alter according to the context of the assessment, instruments have been devised for sole use in specific settings. The Hospital Anxiety and Depression Scale [95], for example, was primarily designed to measure psychological distress within the context of a hospital setting. Meanwhile, assessment instruments, such as the Duke OARS [94], are probably better placed in a community setting. It is usually expected that assessments will be undertaken by individuals with at least a basic medical knowledge. Currently, the majority of assessments are conducted by practice nurses and, to a lesser extent, GPs. Fewer still are carried out by health visitors and district nurses [96]. Despite their medical background, however, concerns have been raised about the lack of training that assessors have received in administering regular health checks and in valuing general preventive care of the elderly [96,97]. Further concerns have been expressed with regards to a lack of smooth interaction and co-operation between bodies comprising a multidisciplinary health team across settings [2]. As such, older people may not be receiving the most comprehensive and individually-tailored health assessment and subsequent care pathway.

Case Studies

The following case studies aim to serve as an illustration of that discussed above.

Situation 1: Older person living alone in an isolated farmhouse. Widowed. Little money. Daughter and son-in-law unemployed with four children, aged 9 months to 7 years, and live 5 kilometres away. Two other children of the older person live over 100 kilometres away.

Case 1: Female, aged 76, with osteoarthritis of the hips and knees, poor vision due to macular degeneration, and hypertension. Mobile with a frame within her home except for the stairs. Needs help with mobility outside, shopping, cooking and housework.
- Likely to remain living in own home, downstairs.
- Help from family where possible although, because of the children, will probably need more assistance in the form of local authority home help (Shopping, housework, friendship). Home help may also cook or meals from Meals-on-Wheels. Depends if woman can afford to receive them.
- May visit a day centre for contact with others.
- NB. Rural area so limited resources
- Visited by GP and District Nurse

Case 2: Male, aged 80, facing discharge from hospital following a stroke. Expected to be confined to bed or chair for several weeks with gradual recovery of mobility. Needs the help of one person for transfers, toileting, bathing and dressing.
- Needs intensive care
- Either to family. Better in short-stay care. Will be in public sector since he doesn't have much money. Nursing, toileting, food etc. will be provided.
- Return home when mobile again

Case 3: Female, aged 86, suffering from dementia. Frequent wandering by day and night. Frequent falls. Incontinent of urine and faeces.
- Not safe on her own. Needs constant care and to be watched over.
- Long-term residential nursing home, statutory sector. (Means-tested charging).

Situation 2: Older person lives alone in a ground floor flat in town. Widowed. Daughter and son-in-law are both teachers in full-time employment, with 2 children aged 7 and 11, and live within 1 kilometre in the same town

Case 1: Female, aged 76, with osteoarthritis of the hips and knees, poor vision due to macular degeneration, and hypertension. Mobile with a frame within her home except for the stairs. Needs help with mobility outside, shopping, cooking and housework.
- Ground floor flat so no need to tackle stairs. Mobile in own flat so will remain there.
- Family close by will probably help in the provision of meals and taking her out.
- Lives in urban area so local authority resources more abundant and more easily accessible. May receive home help/transport services etc.

Case 2: Male, aged 80, facing discharge from hospital following a stroke. Expected to be confined to bed or chair for several weeks with gradual recovery of mobility. Needs the help of one person for transfers, toileting, bathing and dressing.
- Needs intensive help. Because daughter and son-in-law both work full-time will probably require outside help. Social services can help with home adaptations, home help etc. Alternatively he may be entered into short-stay residential care.

Case 3: Female, aged 86, suffering from dementia. Frequent wandering by day and night. Frequent falls. Incontinent of urine and faeces.
- To remain living at home alone would be unsafe. Likely to be admitted to a nursing home. May be private if she/family are capable/willing to pay. Otherwise will be a publicly funded home and woman will be asked to pay a means-tested charge.

Situation 3: Older person lives with spouse in two-storey house. Retired with savings. Spouse is fit and well. No children. Bedroom, bathroom and toilet upstairs.

Case 1: Female, aged 76, with osteoarthritis of the hips and knees, poor vision due to macular degeneration, and hypertension. Mobile with a frame within her home except for the stairs. Needs help with mobility outside, shopping, cooking and housework.
- Likely to be eager to remain in own home with spouse. Could live downstairs except for the fact that toilet and bathroom are upstairs. If spouse is able to help her upstairs then no problem. If not, consider moving.
- Main duties of caring will fall upon the husband. He is unable to receive Invalid Care Allowance however because he is over retirement age. Will be able to claim state pension for both of them. Disability allowance? Will have to make use of savings for living expenses and perhaps private home help for cleaning etc.
- Respite care will probably be needed but may be hard to get. May be easier if living in urban area.

Case 2: Male, aged 80, facing discharge from hospital following a stroke. Expected to be confined to bed or chair for several weeks with gradual recovery of mobility. Needs the help of one person for transfers, toileting, bathing and dressing.
- Will probably remain at home with wife adopting the caring role. May need extra help with lifting etc. Possible role for district nurse/health visitor here. GP will make home visits.
- May use savings to help with private nursing help at home until husband is more healthy and mobile.

Case 3: Female, aged 86, suffering from dementia. Frequent wandering by day and night. Frequent falls. Incontinent of urine and faeces.
- Husband may decide to take care of wife at home. Could employ private help with savings.
- Heavy duty task. He may decide that it is better for both of them that she is admitted into a nursing home for the elderly. Can use savings to pay for private care. Husband can visit her regularly and be with her for meal times etc.

Future Developments

The above discussion has raised a number of issues relating to carers and their dependants which now need to be consolidated. Trends in social and health care provision need to be summarised and likely future developments discussed.

Recognition of carers

Currently there appears to be a general trend, on paper at least, towards greater recognition and support of carers. The government's *Carers (Recognition and Services) Act 1995* and *National Strategy for Carers*, launched in 1998, are evidence of this. In short, carers are promised greater financial support, increased availability of information, effective health care and needs assessments, more opportunities to take breaks from caring, support in maintaining their independence, and valued involvement in the planning and provision of caring-related services. Indeed, governmental policy documents, accepted at face value, paint a rosy picture of the caring role.

Unfortunately, reality seems to be several steps behind this ideal. There is a general consensus among carers and carer support agencies that a gap exists between policy and practice [12,14,15]. Surveys reveal that a large proportion of carers feel unappreciated, misunderstood by health practitioners, not sufficiently supported by social services, and often are thrown into the role without consultation or training. Health problems are rife, as are financial difficulties [11,14,15].

Admittedly, policy in this area is young. Indeed, the government itself recognise that some issues will take years, even decades, to resolve. Yet, today's carers have unmet needs that need to be addressed here and now. Evidently positive steps need to be taken to bridge the gap between existing policy and current practice. Action needs to be taken to enforce policy so that carers feel valued, are sufficiently supported, have their health and social needs met and are able to maintain a sufficient level of independence.

Current problems and future development

In order to clarify the areas in which development is necessary, it is important to highlight key flaws in the current system. We begin by examining the main public agencies that support carers and their dependants: the National Health Service (NHS) and The Department of Social Services (DSS).

Although both the NHS and DSS have been designated a key role in supporting carers, there is a distinct lack of co-ordination and co-operation between the two. Indeed, each agency works as a separate body and only has limited interaction with the other. The carer and the cared-for, however, present with a rich conglomeration of health and social needs, that would be best met by a comprehensive interdisciplinary team. Recognising this fact, the government writes that members of differing teams all "need to see their own role as part of a wider network of support for carers and....all have a crucial role in referring carers to other appropriate sources of help" [32]. Cited as examples of good practice are GP practices, hospitals and social services departments that have issued carers with 'contact cards' listing telephone numbers of all the main carer support agencies, and assembled carer-designated notice boards to communicate relevant information to local carers. So, although the institutional boundaries are deep-rooted, effort is being made in some regions to encourage a more holistic approach to carer support. Albeit slow, developments need to continue in this manner if the diversity of carers' needs are to be effectively met.

Further problems arise when boundaries exist not only between organisations but also within them. Reporting solely on DSS practice, Fruin [11], reports that "variation occurred between individual social workers and care managers, between teams, between areas within authorities and between authorities". He concludes that carers are subject to "the lottery of location". Such inequalities are clearly not acceptable and standardised approaches to carer support, coupled with service monitoring, need to be established and maintained on a national level.

Related to the issue of inequality, this chapter has highlighted the existence of regional variations in service provision. Particularly salient are the variations between support available to those living in rural areas as compared to those living in urban regions. In England alone, more than ten million people live in what is formally classed as rural areas. Although this sample of the population has the same varied and wide ranging care needs as people living elsewhere, problems arise "associated with equity, access, isolation and geography" [16]. Fruin [11], following inspection of local authority support for carers, comments, "Support depends far more on where carers live and who they are in contact with in social services than on what they need". Future developments need to tackle these issues, adapting services in order to meet the needs of all carers and their dependants across the UK, thus eliminating the "lottery of location".

In addition to discussing the agencies in existence to support carers, one must consider the actual services that they offer. Assuming that future developments will build on current trends, it seems that carers and their dependants will be greatly involved in the planning and provision of relevant services. Henwood [15] suggests that carers should be "involved at all levels of primary and secondary care, in genuine partnership and co-operation". Similarly, Nolan et al [65] point out that, with their wealth of experience, carers should be regarded as "experts" in the field of caring and, as such, their input to carer services should be encouraged and valued. Such opinion is supported by governmental literature which states that "The government believes that all services used by carers should involve them in service planning" [32].

Presumably the expertise of carers and their dependants will be called upon to highlight areas of difficulty so as to best tailor services to fulfil unmet needs. At present assessments introduced under the *Carers (Recognition and Services) Act 1995* and the 1990 GP contract are the main means of detecting areas of need. Yet, as has been stressed earlier in this chapter, limitations exist in the assessment procedures for both carers and older people receiving care. Steps need to be taken to clearly define who is eligible, to ensure that assessments are conducted where individuals meet eligibility criteria, to determine exactly what should be incorporated into assessments for carers and their dependants, to introduce standardised assessment tools, to ensure that assessments account for cultural sensitivities, and to characterise clear care pathways overseen by professionals from a broad range of service agencies. Furthermore, those conducting assessments must recognise that, although individual carers and older people have personal issues to deal with, they also form a 'caring team' that needs consideration at another level. Indeed, the Department of Health points out that "Providers of the range of services and benefits which exist to meet the needs of the sick, disabled or frail elderly people must recognise that the patient or user of services and their carer are closely linked, and must not neglect the carer's existence and needs when they are looking at and meeting the needs of the patient or user" [32].

Clearly, there are a whole series of issues in need of consideration if future developments are going to favour carers and the older people they care for. Judging by current trends, the main carer support agencies do seem to be travelling in the right direction. Yet, much work remains before carers feel valued and fully supported in their role and dependent older people receive the health care and resources they feel necessary. Victor [4] warns that, aside from the detailed aspects of carer and older person care, there are more generic issues that may pose problems in the future. She questions whether the health service is equipping itself to meet the demands of an ever-increasing older population: "NHS changes are very concerned with improved management and 'efficiency' and do not seem to confront the need to increase resources simply in order to maintain the status quo". Furthermore she questions whether hospitals, which represent "technologically sophisticated institutions geared towards crisis intervention", are appropriate for dealing with the often chronic conditions of an increasingly old, and possibly frail, population.

Yet not all is negative. Although there are definite areas in which improvements need to be made, examples of good practice can be found. In Bradford, for example, the Department of Social Services have produced a comprehensive information pack for carers. In Islington specialist day centres have been made available to ethnic minority older people. In Merton the Social Services unit have departmental sessions focusing on carers issues and have provided training sessions for their own staff who are carers themselves [11]. Clearly then, trends are being established in the right direction for carers and the older people they care for. Yet, whilst examples of good practice remain isolated cases rather than the norm throughout the UK, the physical, mental and emotional needs of older people and their informal carers are not being adequately met. Steps need to be taken to develop and implement national and local policies so that the UK's 5.7 million carers no longer feel unappreciated and unsupported in their role.

References

[1]   Health Education Authority, Older People Fact Sheet 1: Older people in the population. London, HEA, 1998.
[2]   Health Advisory Service (The NHS Health Advisory Service), Services for people who are elderly, London: HMSO, 1997.
[3]   M.L. Johnson, Social Gerontology. In R.C. Tallis, H.M. Fillit, J.C. Brocklehurst,. Brocklehurst's textbook of geriatric medicine and gerontology, Fifth Edition, London: Churchill Livingston, 1998.
[4]   C.R. Victor, Health and health care in later life, Buckingham: Open University Press, 1991.
[5]   Office of Population Censuses and Surveys, Social Surveys Division, General Household Survey 1995, Informal Carers, London: HMSO, 1995.
[6]   Department of Health, Caring for people: Community care in the next decade and beyond, London: HMSO, 1989.
[7]   G. Parker, With due care and attention: A review of research on informal care, (Second edition), London: Family policy Studies Centre, 1990.
[8]   J. Twigg, Carers: Research and practice, (London: HMSO, 1992.
[9]   Department of Health, Caring about Carers, A National Strategy for Carers, DoH. 1999.
[10] Department of Health, A guide to the National Health Service, NHS Executive, 1995.
[11] D. Fruin, A matter of chance for carers? Inspection of local authority support for carers, Social Services Inspectorate/Department of Health, 1998.
[12] P. Banks, Carer support: Time for a change of direction? London: King's Fund, 1999.
[13] M. Nolan, G. Grant, J. Keady, The carers act: realising the potential, *British Journal of Community Health Nursing*, **1(6)** (1996) 317-322
[14] L. Warner, and S. Wexler, Eight hours a day and taken for granted? London: Princess Royal trust for

Carers, 1998.
[15] M. Henwood, Ignored and invisible? Carers experience of the NHS, Report of a UK research survey, London: Carers National Association. 1998.
[16] D. Brown, Care in the Country - Inspection of Community Care in Rural Communities, Social Services Inspectorate, 1999.
[17] National Federation of Women's Institutes, Caring for rural carers, London: NFWI, 1993.
[18] Help the Aged & Rural Development Commission, Growing old in the countryside, A case study practice manual, London: Help the Aged, 1996.
[19] G. Ashton, Elderly people and the law, London: Butterworths, 1995.
[20] Department of Health, National Assistance Act 1948 (Choice of Accommodation) Directions (1992) issued with DH Circular No. LAC (92)27, 1992.
[21] M. Mandelstam, An A-Z of community care law, London: Jessica Kingsley, 1998.
[22] R. Levitt, A. Wall, and J. Appleby, The Reorganised National Health Service (Fifth Edition), London: Chapman & Hall, 1995.
[23] Department of Health, The new NHS. Modern. Dependable, London: HMSO, 1997.
[24] Department of Health, Statistics for General Medical Practitioners in England: 1988-1998. Available at ttp://www.doh.gov.uk/pub/docs/doh/medprac.pdf.
[25] D.C. Kennie, Preventive care for elderly people, Cambridge: Cambridge University Press, 1993.
[26] E. Goddard and D Savage, People aged 65 and over, in *GHS*, No. 22, supplement A, OPCS, London: HMSO, 1994.
[27] Royal College of General Practitioners, Care of old people: A framework for progress. Occasional paper 45, 1990.
[28] Department of Health, Terms of service for doctors in general practice, London: HMSO, 1989.
[29] A. Milburn, The NHS: The case for modernisation, Presented at the King's Fund Seminar, 2 February 2000.
[30] Health Advisory Service 2000, "Not because they are old": An independent inquiry into the care of older people on acute wards in general hospitals, dLondon: HAS 2000, 1998.
[31] Department of Health, Shaping the future NHS: Long term planning for hospitals and related services, 2000. Available at http://www.doh.gov.uk/nationalbeds1.htm.
[32] Department of Health, Implications of shorter length of hospital stay, Priority areas: first round, 1999. Available at: http://www.doh.gov.uk/ntrd/rd/psi/priority/first/16.htm
[33] N. Coni and S. Webster, Lecture notes on geriatrics (Fifth ed.), Oxford: Blackwell Science, 1998.
[34] P.J. Reynolds and S.C. Allen, Rehabilitation of the elderly - an overview, in R.B. Shukla and D Brooks (eds), A guide to the care of the elderly, London: HMSO, 1996.
[35] R.B. Shukla (ed.), Care of the elderly. London: HMSO, 1999.
[36] G.C.J. Bennett and S. Ebrahim, The essentials of health care in old age (second ed.), London: Arnold, 1995.
[37] Royal College of Psychiatrists, Personal Correspondance, 2000.
[38] Audit Commission, Forget me not: Mental health services for older people, London: Audit Commission, 2000.
[39] R. Lasser et al., Diagnosis and treatment of geriatric depression, *CNS Drugs*; **9(1)** (1998) 17-30.
[40] D. Bauer, Care in the community. In M.W. Shaw, (ed.), The challenge of ageing (second edition), (London: Churchill Livingstone, 1991.
[41] R. Griffiths, Community Care: Agenda for Action, report to the Secretary of State for Social Services, London: HMSO, 1988.
[42] M.J. Denham, (ed.), Continuing care for older people, Cheltenham: Stanley Thornes, 1997.
[43] I. Harvey et al., Foot morbidity and exposure to chiropody: population based study, *British Medical Journal*, 315 (1997) 1054-1055.
[44] Q.D. Sandifer et al,. Foot morbidity and exposure to chiropody, *British Medical Journal*, 316 (1998) 1608.
[45] E.G. White and G.P. Mulley, Footcare for very elderly people: a community survey, *Age and Ageing*, **18(4)** (1989) 276-278.
[46] T. Harding, A life worth living: The independence and inclusion of older people, London: Help the Aged, 1997.
[47] I. Sinclair et al., The Kaleidoscope of Care: A review of research on welfare provision for elderly people, London: HMSO, 1990.
[48] M.R.P. Hall et al., Medical care of the elderly, (Third Ed.), Chichester: Wiley, 1993.
[49] Royal Commission on Long Term Care, With respect to old age, London: HMSO, 1999.
[50] W. Laing, Laing's Review of Private Health Care, London: Laing & Buisson, 1996.
[51] J.P. Nicholl et al., Comparison of the activity at short stay independent hospitals in England and

Wales, 1981 and 1986, *British Medical Journal,* **298** (1989) 239-242.
[52] J.P. Nicholl et al., Role of the private sector in elective surgery in England and Wales, *British Medical Journal,* **298** (1989) 243-247.
[53] B. Williams and J. Nicholl, Patient characteristics and clinical caseload of short stay independent hospitals in England and Wales 1992/3, *British Medical Journal,* **308** (1994) 1699-1701.
[54] R. Baggott, Health and health care in Britain, (Second Ed.), Basingstoke: MacMillan Press, 1998.
[55] A. Tinker, Elderly people in modern society (Third Ed.), London: Longman, 1992.
[56] Department of Health, Vouluntary organisations involved in health care, Department of Health, 2000.
[57] Centre for Policy on Ageing, Promoting informed debate about issues concerning older people, 2000. Available at www.cpa.org.uk.
[58] V. Ivers and K. Meade, Older volunteers and peer health counselling. A new approach to training and development, Stoke-on-Trent: Beth Johnson Foundation Publications, 1991.
[59] Help the Aged, Fast Facts. Information Leaflet, London: Help the Aged, 2000.
[60] L. Eaton, How social Services Work in S. Crompton, (ed.), The Carers Guide 1995, (Second Edition), London: MacMillan Magazines, 1994.
[61] A. Griffiths and G. Roberts, The law and elderly people, (Second ed.), London: Routledge, 1995.
[62] Department of Health, Health and personal social statistics for England, 1997, London: HMSO, 1998.
[63] Department of Health, Prime key indicators of local authority social services 1986/1987, SM16, DOH, 1989.
[64] Audit Commission, The coming of age. Improving care services for older people, London: Audit Commission, 1997.
[65] M. Nolan et al, *Understanding family care,* Buckingham: OU Press,1996.
[66] P. Taraborrelli, Exemplar A: Becoming a carer. In N. Gilbert (ed.), Researching social life, London: Sage, 1993.
[67] Department of Social Security, ICA Statistics, 30 September 1998.
[68] R. Hancock and C. Jarvis, The long term effects of being a carer, London: HMSO, 1994.
[69] Carers National Association, Give us a break. A study of the impact of the Carers Special Grant in the north of England. Summary and Recommendations, London: CAN, 2000.
[70] M.R. Haug et al, Effect of giving care on caregivers' health, *Research on Ageing,* **21(4)** (1999) 515-538.
[71] E. Holzhausen, Still battling? The Carers Act one year on, London: Carers National Association, 1997.
[72] L. Clements,. A real act of care, *Community Care,* 14-20 March: 26-27, 1996.
[73] H. Arksey et al, Carers' needs and the carers act: An evaluation of the process and outcomes of assessment, Executive Summary, University of York: Social Policy Research Unit, 1999.
[74] R.A. Kane and J.D. Penrod, Family caregiving in an ageing society: Policy perspectives, Thousand Oaks: Sage, 1995.
[75] S. Zarit et al, Relatives of the impaired elderly: Correlates of feelings of burden, *The Gerontologist,* **20** (1980) 649.
[76] B.C. Robinson, Validation of a caregiver strain index, *Journal of Gerontology,* **38** (1983) 344-348.
[77] M.P. Lawton, Measuring caregiving appraisal, *Journal of Gerontology,* **44** (1989) 61-71.
[78] M. Nolan and I Philp, COPE: Towards a comprehensive assessment of caregiver need, *British Journal of Nursing,* **8(20)** (1999) 1364-1372.
[79] M.J. Kinney and M Stephens, Caregiving hassles scales: Assessing the daily hassles of caring for a family member with dementia, *The Gerontologist,* **29(3)** (1989) 328-332.
[80] S. Hunter et al, The inter-disciplinary assessment of older people at entry into long-term institutional care: lessons for the new community care arrangements, *Research, Policy and Planning,* **11(1/2)** (1993) 2-9.
[81] M. Wright, Taking Care, *Community Care,* **17** (1990) 14-16.
[82] C.A. Wilkieson et al, Standardisation of health assessments for patients aged 75 years and over: 3 years' experience in the Forth Valley Health Board area, *British Journal of General Practice,* **46** (1996) 307-308.
[83] K Brown et al, Problems found in the over-75s by the annual health check, *British Journal of General Practice,* **47** (1997) 31-35.
[84] K Brown et al, Health checks on patients 75 years and over in Nottinghamshire after the new GP contract, *British Medical Journal,* **305** (1992) 619-621.
[85] C.A. Chew et al, Annual assessment of patients aged 75 and over: general practitioners' and practice nurses' views and experiences, *British Journal of General Practice,* **44** (1994) 263-267.
[86] D Wilkin et al, GP assessments of patients aged 75 and over: consumer survey, Manchester: Centre

for Primary Care Research, 1994.
[87] S. Iliffe *et al*, Assessment of elderly people in general practice. Part 1: Social circumstances and mental state, *British Journal of General Practice*, **41** (1991) 9-12.
[88] S Iliffe *et al*, Assessment of elderly people in general practice. Part 2: Functional abilities and medical problems, *British Journal of General Practice*, **41** (1991) 13-15.
[89] A. Fletcher, Multidimensional assessment of elderly people in the community, *British Medical Bulletin*, **54(4)** (1998) 945-960.
[90] P. Wallace, Linking up with the over 75s (editorial), *British Journal of General Practice,* **40** (1990) 267-268.
[91] I. Philp *et al, EASYcare,* Elderly Assessment System, UK version 1999-2002, Sheffield Institute for Studies on Ageing (SISA), The University of Sheffield, 1997.
[92] F I. Mahoney and D.W. Barthel, Functional Evaluation: the Barthel Index, *Maryland State Medical Journal,* **14** (1965) 61-65.
[93] T. Reynolds *et al*, The Camberwell Assessment of need for the Elderly, *British Journal of Psychiatry*; 1999, in press.
[94] A.S. Zigmond and R.P. Snaith, 'The Hospital Anxiety and Depression Scale', *Acta Psychiatrica Scandinavica*, **67** (1983) 361-70.
[95] G. Fillenbaum, Multidimensional functional assessment of older adults: the Duke Older Americans Resources and Services Procedures, Hove: Lawrence Erlbaum Associates, 1988.
[96] F. Ross, Assessment in the community. In I. Philp, I. (ed.), Assessing elderly people in hospital and community care, London: Farrand Press, 1994.
[97] A.J. Tulloch, Preventive care of elderly people: how good is our training? *British Journal of General Practice* (editorial), 1991 354-355.

Author Index

Adam, S.G.M.	135
Albertini, A.	97
Bagnall, A.	27
Baudoin, C.	27
Bień, B.	161
Borgermans, L.	1
Chwalow, J.	27
Döhner, H.	49
Elgrably, F.	27
Figueiro, D.	189
Hässler, R.	237
Hutten, J.B.F.	135
Kofahl, C.	49
Lamura, G.	97
Larizgoitia Jauregi, A.	211
Lothian, K.	255
McKee, K.	255
Melchiorre, M.G.	97
Mengani, M.	97
Mestheneos, E.	75
Nolan, M.	1,255
Philp, I.	1,255
Polityńska, B.	161
Quattrini, S.	97
Sousa, L.	189
Triantifillou, J.	75
Wilmańska, J.	161
Wojszel, B.	161